AF429425

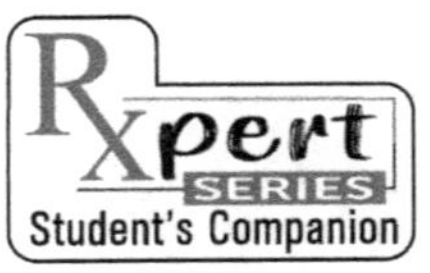

Pharmacognosy and Phytochemistry-I

Theory and Practical

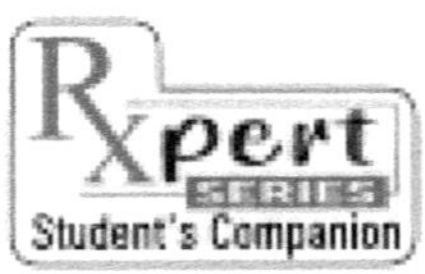

Pharmacognosy and Phytochemistry-I

Theory and Practical

Sharada L. Deore

M.Pharm (Pharmacognosy & Phytochemistry),
Ph.D (Pharmaceutical Sciences), PG Diploma in Patent's law
Associate Professor,
Govt. College of Pharmacy,
Amravati-444604
Maharashtra

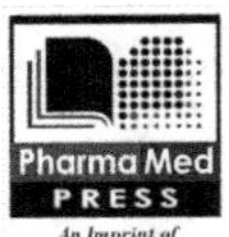

PharmaMed Press

An imprint of BSP Books pvt. Ltd

4-4-309/316, Giriraj Lane,
Sultan Bazar, Hyderabad - 500 095.

Pharmacognosy and Phytochemistry-I, Theory and Practical
by **Sharada L. Deore**

© 2023, *by Publisher*

Published by:

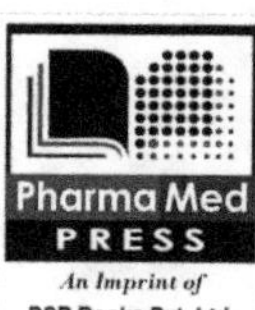

PharmaMed Press

An imprint of BSP Books Pvt. Ltd.
4-4-309/316, Giriraj Lane, Sultan Bazar, Hyderabad - 500 095.
Phone: 040-23445688; Fax: 91+40-23445611
e-mail: info@pharmamedpress.com
www.pharmamedpress.com/pharmamedpress.net

ISBN: 978-93-91910-47-1 (Hardback)

Preface

For centuries the history of pharmacy has been interlinked with the history of pharmacognosy, or the study of materia medica, which is obtained from natural sources—mostly plants. The term "pharmacognosy" was first used in 1811 by Johann Adam Schmidt (1759–1809). It appeared first in the handwritten manuscript Lehrbuch der Materia Medica by Johann Adam Schmidt, though published in 1811.

Rich heritage of traditional medicinal knowledge of different parts of world is becoming global resurgence of interest in these systems especially either for prevention and or improvement in quality of life of chronic disease affected population. Advances in chemistry, analysis and biotechnology expanded the discipline to novel chemical therapeutic agents, quality control standards and plant tissue culture innovations.

Pharmacy Council of India (PCI) has introduced subject ***Pharmacgonosy-I in B.Pharm Fourth Semester*** to make students aware and understand about basics of Pharmacognosy, traditional medicine systems, primary and secondary metabolites, cultivation and conservation of medicinal plants, quality control and plant tissue culture techniques.

Theoretical knowledge of above topics will create well informed academic, clinical, hospital and community pharmacist.

Experimental skills of phytochemical screening of oragnised and unorganised crude drugs, quality control as per Pharmacopeial standards will help student to serve better in herbal industry, community, academics and research establishments.

Present book is strictly designed as per PCI syllabus to cover theory as well as practical syllabus topics to able students to upgrade the desired theoretical plus practical skills.

Subjective as well as specific and related objective (MCQs) questions are added to analyse the topic understanding of students.

I would first and foremost like to acknowledge the authors and publishers of various books, research articles, journals, websites and other sources that have been referred to for putting together to make this book an fine source of reference.

Author is thankful to all her teachers, students, friends and family for motivation of keeping writing as per the need of time and changing scenario in pharma world.

Author would like to acknowledge the excellent efforts of Publisher Anil Shah and Editor Naresh Daver for corrections and suggestions to bring out the theory as well as practical syllabus content in the form of semester book.

- Sharada L. Deore

Contents

Part – I

Pharmacognosy and Phytochemistry-I (Theory)

Part - II

Practical Manual

Part – I
(Theory)

Pharmacognosy and Phytochemistry-I

Unit 1

1.1 Introduction to Pharmacognosy

The term 'pharmacognosy' (combination of two Greek words i.e. pharmakon means drug and gnosis means knowledge) means "acquiring knowledge of drugs" was coined in 1815 by C. A. Seydler, German medical student in his thesis title "AnalyeticaPharmacognostica". Pharmacognosy is defined as "scientific and systematic study of structural, physical, chemical and biological characters of crude drugs along with history, method of cultivation, collection and preparation for the market".

The American Society of Pharmacognosy defines pharmacognosy as "the study of the physical, chemical, biochemical and biological properties of drugs, drug substances or potential drugs or drug substances of natural origin as well as the search for new drugs from natural sources'. It is also called as study of crude drugs.

Thus pharmacognostical studies of plant drugs involves study of synonyms, vernacular names, Biological sources, distribution, morphology, histology, chemistry, qualitative test, various physicochemical tests, pharmacological actions along with commercial varieties, substitutes, adulterants and any other quality control parameters of the drugs.

Scope

- The pharmacognosy has played an important role in the transformation of ***various basic science subjects.*** Pharmacognosy has a vital contribution to the advancement of natural and physical science due to advances in technologies of cultivation, purification, identification, characterization of natural drugs.

- Pharmacognosy has enabled to establish a sound knowledge of the vegetable drugs under ***botany and animal drugs*** under zoology through taxonomy, breeding, pathology and genetics concepts.

- This knowledge used to improve and ***modernise cultivation*** methods of medicinal and aromatic plants to fulfill demand from quality raw material to genetic transformations in plants to get desired characters.

- World Health Organization (WHO) has estimated that 80% of world population depends on herbal medicines for their primary health care. Some of the very ***famous crude drugs*** are senna as a purgative, digitalis as a cardiotonic and rauwolfia as an antihypertensive drug. Pharmacognosy explains thorough knowledge of the history, cultivation, collection, quality control, transport, storage and even economic impact of all these crude drugs.

- Pharmacognosy is ***vital link*** between pharmacology and medicinal chemistry because it enables isolation of purified natural drugs, converts into medicine and evaluates its therapeutic effects.

- Pharmacognosy links basic science, pharmaceuticals, ayurvedic and allopathic system of medicines to each other.

- Pharmacognosy helped to improve plant chemistry (***phytochemistry***) significantly with the knowledge of extraction. Varieties of chemical constituents that are accumulated and synthesized by plants have revolutionized the process of natural drug discovery.

- ***Novel techniques*** like "Bioassay Guided Fractionation" helps in the isolation of phytochemicals based on therapeutic potency. This has led to specific use of medicinal constituents or plant parts and its utilization in disease treatment.

- Recently started studies on natural drug-drug, drug-food ***interactions*** are avoiding the untoward effects of severe interactions and hence helping in obtaining the optimal therapeutic outcomes especially for classes like Blood thinners, Protease inhibitors, Cardiac Glycosides, Imuuno Suppressants.

- In the pharmaceutical ***industry***, various drugs of botanical origin are used in drug manufacturing process. Knowledge of pharmacognosy surely helps as a research tools in the new drug/dosage form development.

- Recent guidelines for quality control of crude drugs are to assure the identity, purity and consistency of drug substances, efficacy to determine the therapeutic responses, indications, ***clinical aspects*** and pharmacological effects, safety to avoid untoward toxic reactions, interactions and contraindications.

- However, this subject is as old as pharmacy and humankind evolution; recently it is evolved as a ***multidisciplinary subject*** focusing many modern disciplines like ethanobotany, ethanopharmcology, phytotherapy, phytochemistry, chemo-taxanomy, biotechnology, clinical trials, herbal drug interaction and even novel drug delivery systems like phytosomes rather only botanical and taxanomical descriptions. Recent advances in extraction methods, analytical hyphe-nated techniques, screening methods continues to hasten major changes in this subject. Modernization of conventional and/or traditional dosage forms is opening doors to "***Industrial Pharmacognosy***".

- Due to most recent technologies and innovative chemical concepts, many new drugs or drug candidates still originated from natural products or derivatives thereof. Even in this era of nanotechnology, natural drugs are important part of primary health care which is giving pharmacognosy professionals new possibilities to exploit the huge diversity designed and generated by nature.

- Due to rapid growth in demand and popularity of natural products, research has been directed towards patentable drug discovery and development in the field of pharmacognosy.

- There is a shortage of established scientists engaged in pharmacognosy research; hence detail knowledge of this subject is till need to be studied by conventional scientists. Thus, actual secret of opportunities in pharmacognosy research is that only the tip of the iceberg seems to have been discovered yet.

History

History of Medicines ranged from folklore, evidence-based medicine to antibiotics, nanotechnology, and gene therapy. Few of most notable historical medicinal texts are as follows:

Region	Medicinal Texts
Egypt	Imhotep, Edwin Smith Papyrus, Ebers Papyrus, Kahun Gynecological Papyrus
Mesopotamia	Diagnostic Handbook, Alkindus, De Gradibus
India	Ayurveda, Sushruta Samhita, Charaka Samhita
China	Yellow Emperor, Huangdi Neijing
Greece	Iliad and Odyssey are the earliest sources of Greek medical practise; Hippocratic medicine
Persia	Rhazes, Avicenna, The Canon of Medicine, The Book of Healing
Spain	Abulcasis, Kitab al-Tasrif
Syria	Ibn al-Nafis, Commentary on Anatomy in Avicenna's Canon, Comprehensive Book on Medicine

Through above literatures, it can be concluded that History of pharmacognosy is as old as mankind. Human being came to know medicines from nature itself. Following table is explaining various historical developments, which together contributed to the progress of Pharmacognosy. Various traditional systems of medicines from different corners of world also played vital role in development of pharmacognosy.

Scientists and their work in the development of Pharmacognosy			
Name	Profession	Work	Period
Ebers Papyrus or Papyrus Ebers	Egyptian medical papyrus	Herbal knowledge	1550 BC
Pedanius Dioscorides	Greek physician	De Materia Medica book is compilation of several plants	78 A.D.
Gaius Plinius Secundus or Pliny the Elder	Roman naturalist	Encyclopedic work entitled Naturalis Historia	25-70 A.D.
Aelius Galenus or Claudius Galenus or Galen	Greek pharmacist	Galenical Pharmacy	131 – 200 A.D.
Hippocrates *Father of Medicine*	Greek scientist	Studied human anatomy and Physiology	460 - 360 B.C
Aristotle *Father of Biology*	Greek Philosopher	Animal kingdom	384-322 B.C.
Theophrastus *Father of Botany*	Greek Philosopher	Plant kingdom	370- 287 B.C.
Carl Linnaeus *Father of Taxonomy*	Swedish botanist	Binomial classification	1753
C A Seydler	German	Coined word Pharmacognosy	1815
Sir Joseph D. Hooker	British botanist	Plant nomenclature	1817 - 1911.
George Bentham	English botanist	Plant nomenclature	1800 - 1884
Charles Darwin	English naturalist	Evolutionary theory	1809 - 1882.
Friedrich Sertürner	German chemist	isolated first alkaloid morphine from opium	1804
Mikhail Tsvet	Russian scientist	Separation of plant pigments by chromatography	1900

1.2   Sources of Crude Drug

Crude Drugs

Crude drugs are the drugs, which are obtained from natural sources like plant, animals or minerals and used as such as they occur in nature without any processing except collection, drying and size reduction. It also defined as the drugs that have not been advanced in value or improved in condition by shredding, grinding, chipping, crushing, distilling, evaporating, extracting, artificial mixing with other substances or any other process beyond that which is essential to its proper packing and to prevention of decay or deterioration during manufacturing. Crude drugs and their constituents are commonly used as therapeutic agents. Source of crude drugs are plant (senna, opium, digitalis and Clove), Animal (Musk, Honey, Shark liver Oil) and Mineral (Shilajit, Talc, Bentonite).

Plant	Plant source is the oldest source of drugs. More than 25% of the drugs prescribed worldwide are obtained from plants and more than 150 active chemical compounds from plants are prescribed. Many synthetic drugs obtained from natural precursors. More than 10 % plant formulations of total are considered as basic and essential by the World Health Organisation (WHO). Plants are very rich source of simple as well as complex and extremely diverse structures. Even many of such chemicals cannot be synthesized in laboratory. ***Examples***: digoxin from Digitalis, quinine and quinidine from Cinchona. vincristine and vinblastine from vinca, atropine from belladonna and morphine and codeine from opium.
Animal	Different animal derived products are always being part of treatment of human ailments or nutritional diet. Example: Honey from honeybee, beeswax from bees, cod liver oil from shark, Bufalin from toad, Insulin from animal pancreas, musk oil from musk, spermaceti wax from sperm whale, woolfat from sheep, carminic acid from colchineal, venoms from snake
Mineral	A mineral is a naturally occurring solid crystalline inorganic substance made up of one element or more elements combined together. Many minerals derived from calcium, sulfur, sodium, iron, zinc, silver, gold, diamond, quartz are practiced as medicine in a highly purified form in traditional Ayurveda, Unanai, Siddha and Chinese systems of medicines . Example: sulfur is a key ingredient in certain bacteriostatic drugs, shilajit is used as tonic, calamine is used as anti-itching agent
Marine	Since thousands of years, marine flora and fauna has provided many compounds which are useful in their natural form or as templates for synthetic modification of bioactives for treatment of many diseases. Marine microorganisms, plants, algae, fungi, invertebrates, and vertebrates are used to isolate more than 10,000 chemical entities. For instance, about more than 1000 patents on bioactive marine natural product have been issued since 1970. Many marine drugs are useful in food, confectionary, textile, pharmaceutical industry as gelling, stabilizing and thickening agents.. Till only 10% of marine flora and fauna have been investigated for therapeutic efficacy. Example: Agar- a jelly like substance from red algae, Carrageenans or carrageenins from red seaweeds, sodium alginate from brown seaweed
Plant tissue culture	Plant tissue culture refers to growing and multiplication of single cell, tissues and organs under aseptic and controlled environment on specific media. This source is very useful for large scale production of plants in limited area, conserve rare and endangered plants, produce genetically varied plants like seedless fruit bearing plants, production of therapeutically important secondary metabolites (example: antihypertensive ajmalicine from callus culture of *Catharanthus roseus*, anti-inflammatory berberine from suspension culture of *Thalictrum minus*, immunomodulatory ginsenoside from callus culture of ginseng)

1.3 Classification of Crude Drug

In Pharmacognosy crude drugs are classified in the following category.

Alphabetical classification: In this classification drugs are classified in alphabetical order using either their Greek name or Latin name. Though pharmaco-poeias, formulary, encyclopedias of various countries follow this classification, but due to lack of scientific value now-a-days this classification is not preferred. **Example:-** Acacia, Bael, Cinchona, Dill, Ergot, Fennel, Ginger, Henbane, Ipecac, Jalap, Kurchi, Licorice, Myrrh, Nux-Vomica, Opium, Podophyllum, Quassia, Rauwolfia, Senna, Tea, Urgenia, Vasaka, Wool Fat, Yam, Zedoary etc. Major Advantage of this method is that it provides quick reference.

Morphological classification: This is most simple classification method where crude drugs are grouped into organized drug (parts of plant like root, rhizome, flower, leaf, fruit, bark, seed, wood etc) and unorganized drug (dried lattices, dried juice, gum, wax, oil etc). But many crude drugs are very similar morphologically and hence difficult to distinguish. Many times crude drug available in powder form that time morphological classification is not so suitable and acceptable.

Difference between organized and unorganized drugs			
Organised crude drugs		**Un-organised crude drugs**	
Parts of plants or animals		Obtained from parts of plants	
Well defined structure		Not well defined structures	
Solid in nature		Semisolid, solid, liquid in nature	
Microscopic studies are useful in quality control		Chemical tests are more useful in quality control	
Examples		*Example*	
Parts	**Example**	**Class**	**Example**
Leaves	Senna, Digitalis, Vasaka, Eucalyptus	Resins	Balsam of tolu, Myrrh, Asafoetida, Benzoin
Barks	Cinchona, Kurchi, Cinnamom, Quaillia	Gums and mucilages	Acacia, Tragacanth, Guar Gum
Woods	Quassia, Sandalwood	Dried latices	Opium
Roots	Rauwolfia, Ipecacuanha, Aconite	Dried juices	Aloes, kino
Rhizomes	Turmeric, Ginger, Valerian, Podophyllum	Volatile oils	Cinnamon oil
Seeds	Nux-vomica, Strophanthus	Fixed Oil	Castor oil and lard
Flowers	Clove, Saffron	Waxes	Beeswax
Fruits	Coriander, Colocynth, Fennel, Bael	Extracts	Catechu
Entire plant	Vinca, Belladonna	Saccharine substances	Honey

Examples of crude drugs based on plant parts	
Plant Part	**Example**
Leaves	Senna, Digitalis, Vasaka, Eucalyptus
Barks	Cinchona, Kurchi, Cinnamom, Quaillia
Woods	Quassia, Sandalwood
Roots	Rauwolfia, Ipecacuanha, Aconite
Rhizomes	Turmeric, Ginger, Valerian, Podophyllum
Seeds	Nux-vomica, Strophanthus
Flowers	Clove, Saffron
Fruits	Coriander, Colocynth, Fennel, Bael
Entire plant	Vinca, Belladonna
Resins	Balsam of tolu, Myrrh, Asafoetida, Benzoin
Gums and Mucilages	Acacia, Tragacanth, Guar Gum
Dried latices	Opium
Dried juices	Aloes, Kino

Taxonomic classification: In this classification crude drugs are arranged according to taxonomic order i.e. phylum, division, class, sub-class, orders, families, genus and species (See chapter 2 for more details).Precise and orderly arrangement of drugs has no ambiguity in this classification. But again this type of classification lacks scientific value and unorganized crude drugs are difficult to classify.

Phylum - Spermatophyta

Division - Angiospermae

Class - Dicotyledons

Sub-class - Sympetalae

Order - Tubiflorae

Family - Solanaceae

Genus - *Atropa*

Species - *belladonna*

Biological or pharmacological classification: In this classification, Crude drugs having similar therapeutic effects or pharmacological activity are grouped together but drugs having more than one therapeutic effect are difficult to classify. It also don't give any idea about chemistry or taxonomy.

Examples of pharmacological classification of crude drugs	
Pharmacological Action	**Drug**
Carminatives	Fennel, Dill, Coriander, Clove.
Purgatives	Cascara, Aloe, Senna, And Rhubarb.
Cardio tonics	Digitalis, Squill, Strophanthus
Anti- cancer	Taxaol, Vinca, Podophyllum
CNS Stimulant	Nuxvomica
Expectorant	Vasaka, Liquorice
Bitter tonic	Gentian, Chirata

Chemical classification: This classification is purely based on chemistry of constituents. Different crude drugs are classified according to the presence of major active constituents. This is most preferred method of classification.

Examples of chemical classification of crude drugs	
Chemical class	**Drugs**
Alkaloid	Cinchona Rauwolfia, Datura.
Volatile oil	Clove, Fennel oil, Coriander
Glycoside	Senna, Digitalis, Licorice.
Resin	Jalap, Ginger, Tolu Balsam
Carbohydrates	Acacia, Honey, Starch, Isapgol
Tannins	Arjuna, Ashoka,
Lipid	Castor oil, Peanut Oil, Mustard,
Proteins Enzymes	Casein, Gelatin
	Papain, Trypsin

Chemotaxonomic classification: Chemo-taxonomy is a technique which establishes relation between chemistry and taxonomy. It is also called as chemosystematics. Morphological characters and chemical constituents are interrelated and have a lot significant for the plant taxonomy. Examples: In case of eucalyptus, feather-veined leaves have high Pinene content in their essential oil, while intermediate veined leaves contain both pinene and Cineole. Chemotaxonomic study starts with exact choice of group, then sound sampling, analysis of chemical content, inter-pretation, comparison and finally classification.

Serotaxonomical classification:

Serology deals with studies of antigen-antibody reaction to provide knowledge of origin and properties of antisera. Serotaxonomic classification involves phytoserology which carries in-vitro immunochemical reaction of plant proteins (antigens or agglutinogens) to detect taxonomic homology based on antibodies (agglutinins) produced in animals. Desipite significant contribution made in the serotaxonomy, it has so far not gained much importance in the plant classification. The most common approach in serotaxonomic classification of plants is "precipitin reaction". Precipitin is antibody which causes precipitation.

Precipitin reaction: After injecting a crude plant protein extract into the blood stream of an experimental animal like rabbit or a rat results in the production of specific antibodies. When animal serum containing antibodies also called antiserum reacts in-vitro with the antigenic proteins as well as proteins from other related taxa, of which the affinities are in question, leads to formation of a precipitate. This is called precipitin reaction. The degree of protein homology is determined by the amount of precipitation and hence it is taken as a phylogenetic marker and taxonomic character. If no precipitation is observed then there is no relation and if high precipitate then close relationship among examined taxas.

Crude protein extracts contain a large number of proteins, which stimulates the production of a vast range of antibodies, which differ in their specificity and reactivity. Some are produced in abundance while others are hardly detectable. But advanced serologic techniques allows to deals with single antigen and antibody. The "antisystematic" reactions have recently been shown to result from variation in the systematic ranges of determinants; and the absorption (presaturation) technique for removing common determinants increases the accuracy of serological placements. Immunodiffusion in Agarose Gels, Rocket Immuno-electrophoresis and Enzyme-Linked Immuno-sorbent Assay (ELISA) are commonly used techniques in serotaxonomy.

Following are Parameters to be analysed in Pharmacognostic study of crude drug

Parameters	Description
Common names	Names in various languages
Biological source	Genus, species and family
Geographical source	Location
History	Discovery of crude drug
Cultivation , collection and preparation for market	Time and method of cultivation, irrigation, climate, fertilizers, collection time, processing etc.
Morphological description	Color, odor, taste, size, shape, extra features
Microscopical description	Cell, tissue type and arrangement, cell inclusions, special characters etc
Chemical constituents	major and minor chemical constituents present
Chemical tests	To Identify crude drug and its chemistry
Uses and pharmacological actions	Various therapeutic applications
Adulterants and Commercial varieties	Useful for quality control
Formulations available in Market	To understand market potential
Quality control and standardization	To establish qualitative and quantitative standards with the help of sophisticated instruments.

1.4 Quality Control of Drugs of Natural Origin

Evaluation of crude drugs involves the process of identification of adulteration and determination of quality of crude drugs. Or Evaluation means *"confirmation of its identity and determination of its quality and purity.* This can be organoleptic or morphological, microscopic, biological, physical and chemical evaluation. Thus to determine impurities is also part of evaluation and one of the major reasons of impurity in crude drugs is **drug adulteration. Adulteration means** sub standardisation of drug with respect to therapeutic and chemical properties by replacing wholly or partially original drug. Types and terminologies related to adulteration are given as follows:

Types of adulteration on the basis of reasons	
Unintentional	
Misidentification	**Due to confusion**: for herb Lakshmana different species are used *Arlia quinquefolia, Ipomea sepiaria* **Due to lack of knowledge of authentic plant**: All plants like *Cressacretica, Selaginella bryopteris, Desmotrichum, fimbriatum, Malaxis acuminata (M. wallichii, Microstyliswallichii), Trichopuszeylanicus*and *Terminalia chebula* are consistently and repeatedly referred as Sanjeevani
Carelessness	Root of *Sida cordifolia* are replaced with the whole plant of *Sida cordifolia*
Geographical Unavaibility	*Plucia lanceolata* is used as Rasna in northern India while *Alpinia galanga* is used as Rasna in southern India.

Table 1.7 *Contd....*

Morphological similarity	*Cassia angustifolia* replaced with *Cassiaacutifolia* and *Euphorbia dracunculoides* Lam. (Euphorbiaceae) with *R. graveolens*
Intentional	
Adulteration with substandard commercial varieties	Rhubarb replaced with Chinese rhubarb or raphnotic rhubarb
Adulteration with superficially similar inferior drugs	Pimpalii *(Piper nigrum)* adulterated by papaya seeds
Adulteration with artificially manufactured substances	Artificial invert sugar are mixed with or replaced with pure Honey
Adulteration of exhausted drugs	Ginger is sold after extraction of its volatile oil
Adulteration with synthetic materials	Addition of synthetic Citral to oil of lime.
Adulteration with harmful substances	Pieces of limestone in asafoetida and of lead in opium.
Intentional	
Adulteration of the species belonging to same family	Mixing or replacement of *Datura metal* with *Datura stramonium*
Adulteration of different species	Mixing of *Tribulus terrestris*(zygophylaceae and *Pedalium murex* (Pedaliaceae)
Adulteration with totally different drugs	Bharangi (*Clerodendron indicum*) is totally replaced with Kantakari (*Solanum xanthocarpam*)
Adulteration with low cost drug	Kumkuma (saffron) being costly herb is substituted by Kusumbha (dried flowers of American saffron -*Carthamustinctorius*)

Terminologies related to adulteration	
Inferiority	Impairment of quality with naturally substandard drug Example: The dried ripe seeds of *Strychnosnuxvomica* contain 1.15% of strychnine. Seeds containing less than 1.15% of strychnine, considered as inferior substandard drug.
Spoilage	Impairment of quality due to addition of Spoiled drug by the action of microorganism and thus renders the crude drug unfit for human consumption.
Deterioration	Impairment of the quality by destruction of any valuable constituent by extraction, moisture attack, heat treatment, microbial attack or by any other means. Example: Coffee that has largely lost its caffeine through over roasting is an example of deterioration.
Admixture	Impairment of the quality by addition of one product to another through accident, ignorance or carelessness. Example: *Senna* containing a few stems
Sophistication	Impairment of the quality by sophistication means the intentional addition of inferior material to any substance. Example: The addition of yellow soil to powdered turmeric powder
Substitution	Impairment of the quality by substitution means entirely different material is used instead of original drug. Example: Cotton seed oil is sold in the place of olive oil

Following are few Examples of Adulterants of various crude drugs	
Crude drug name	**Adulterant**
Aconite	Japanese aconite (*A. unicinatum)* and Indian aconite (*A. chasmanthum*)
Alexandrian senna (Cassia acutifolia)	Dog senna, Palthe senna, Bombay, Mecca or Arabian senna.
Aloes (Aloe barbadensis)	Natal aloes which contain natalion, homonatalion and resin with nataloresinotannol; Mocha aloes, black catechu, pieces of iron and stones.
Arachis oil	Cotton seed oil or sesame oil.
Arjuna	*Terminalia tomentosa* (Etheral extract of arjuna gives pinkish fluorescence, while *T. Tomentisa* gives pale blue)
Artemisia	*Artemisia vulgaris* Linn (Compositae)
Asafoetida	Gum Arabic, rosin, gypsum, red clay, chalk and barley or wheat flour.
Belladonna herb	Leaves of *Phytolacca americana* (Idioblast present), *Solanum nigrum*, and *Ailanthus glandulosa* (needle shaped crystals of calcium oxalate present).
Black pepper	*Piper attenuatum , Piper brachystachyum , Piper longum*
Caraway	Indian dill fruits. *Cuminum cyminum* (contains cuminic aldehyde)
Cardamom	Orange seeds and unroasted coffee grains, *Elettaria cardamom*, Korarima cardamom, Cardamom husk
Chenopodium oil	*Chenopodium ambrosoides, Chenopodium album*
Chirata	*S. Densifolia , S. Ciliate , S. Paniculata.*
Cinchona	Cuprea bark (Remijia pedunculata, a coppery red coloured drug, contain quinine, quinidine and other alkaloid which resemble to those from cinchona bark. The bark contains numerous stone cells. Along with cinchona alkaloids, it also contains cupreine. False cupre bark (*R.purdiena*) contains alkaloids called cusconidine, traces of cinchonine, cinchonamine, but no quinine.
Cinnamon	Jungle cinnamom , Cinnamom chips, Saigolcinnamom, *Cinnamomum loureirii* (Lauraceae), Java cinnamom, *Cinaamomumburmanii* (Lauraceae).
Clove	Mother clove, Blown clove, Clove stalks
Digitalis	Leaves of *Verbascum thapsus* (Schophulariaceae) contain large woolly branched candelabra trichomes. The primrose leaves from *Primula vulgaris* (Primulaceae) contains uniseriate covering trichomes, which are 8 to 9 celled long. Comfrey leaves from *Symphytum officinale* (Boraginaceae) contains multicellular trichomes forming hook at the top.
Dill	*Anethum sowa*
Dioscorea	*Dioscoreaflouribunda* and *D.villosa*Linne
Ephedra	*E. eduisetina* and *E. sinica* (Both Chinese). *E. intermedia, E. major, E. helryetica* and *E. alata,Aconitum napelles* (Ranunculaceae): *Sida cordifolia; and S. rhombifolia*(Malvaceae); *Roemeriarefracta* (Papaveraceae); and *Taxus baccata* (Taxaceae)
Fennel	Exhausted fennel fruits
Ginger	Exhausted ginger
Guggul	Resins of various *commiphora* species like C. abyssinica, *C. roxburghii, C. molmol* and *Boswellia serrata.*
Honey	Artificial invert sugar contains furfural which is detected by Fieh's test and by resorcinol in hydrochloric acid.
Liquorice	Manchurian liquorice from *Glycyrrhiza uralensis*
Male fern	Lady fern Athyrium filix-foemina.
Musk	Beaver (Castor fiber), civet (Viuerrazibetha) and America musk (Fiber zibeythicus), Musk mallow (*Abelmoschus moschantus*)
Myrrh	Arabian myrrh, Yemen myrrh, Indian bdellium (Balsamodendronmukul)

Contd….

Crude drug name	Adulterant
Opium	*Papaver argemone, P. dubium, P.orientate, P. psendoorientale*and *P. bracteatum* which does not contain morphine and hence new source of opiate.
Peppermint oil	Mentha oil
Psyllium seed (Flea seed)	Seeds of *Plantago psyllium*, Seeds of *Plantago lanceolata*
Punarnava	*Trianthemaportulacastrum, Trianthemaobcordata*and *T. decandra*
Rasna	*Apinia galangal* (Java galangal or Greater galangal)
Rauwolfia	*Reserpine containing*: African rauwolfia species(Rauwolfia vomitoria, caffra, R. cumminsfi, R.mombasiana, R. oreogiton, R. obscura, R. rosea and R. volkensii), R.tetraphylla and R. nitida, Alstoniavenenata and A. constricta; *Ajmalicine containing*: Catharanthus roses; *Yohimbine containing*: Pausinystaliayohimba,
Rhubarb (Indian rhubarb)	Rhaphontic rhubarb obtained from rhizome of *R. rhaphonticum*. It lacks rhein , emodin or aloe-emodin butit contains rhaphonticin.
Senega	Indian senega is *Polygala chinesis* Linn which does not contain Spurious Indian senega is *Glinusoppositifolia* family Molluginaceae. It contains a Saponins and starch. It shows several rings of vascular bundles. White senega is root of *Polygala alba* does not show keel
Shankhpushpi	*Canscoradiffusa*
Spermaceti	Mixtures of esters of saturated fatty alcohol and saturated fatty acids
Starch (Maize, Rice, Wheat, Potato)	Tapioca starch or cassava or Brazilian arrowroot obtained from Manihot esculenta (Euphorbiaceae)
Storax	Rosin, olive oil, Red Gum or Sweet Gum or American storax from *Liquidamabarstyraciflia*, Stramonium; *Xanthium strumarium* (Compositae) and *Solanum nigrum* (Solanaceae). Later contain no calcium oxalate crystals.
Crude drug name	**Adulterant**
Thyme	Wild thyme: *Thymus serpyllum* (Labiateae)
Tolu Balsam	Exhausted balsam of tolu, Fictitious tolu Balsam, Colophony
Turmeric	*Curcuma amda*
Turpentine oil	Resin oil, wood turpentine and petroleum jelly
Yellow Bees wax	Colophony, hard paraffin, stearic acid, japan wax, spearmaceti, carnauba wax

Following are WHO parameters for standardization of herbal raw material, extracts and their products	
Preliminary evaluation	Sampling, Foreign matter determination, Determination of total fiber
Morphological evaluation	Qualitative evaluation of color, odor and taste, size, shape, extra features ~~ete~~

Microscopical evaluation:	➢ Qualitative microscopy: histological evaluation of types and arrangements of tissues
	➢ Quantitative microscopy:
	  o *Leaf constant*: assessment of palisade ratio, vein-islet, vein termination, stomatal index, stomatal number
	  o *Lycopodium spore method*
	➢ Powder microscopy

Physical Qualitative evaluation	Solubility, refractive index, optical rotation, melting point, boiling point, density, viscosity, chromatographic and spectroscopic evaluation
Physical quantitative or Physicochemical evaluation	Ash value, extractive value, moisture content, volatile oil determination
Chemical evaluation	➢ *Qualitative chemical evaluation*: to detect different classes of phytochemicals ➢ *Quantitative chemical evaluation*: determination of phytochemicals, assay

Contd....

WHO Specific Parameters	Swelling index Foam index Hemolytic index Bitterness value Total tannin value
Biological evaluation	
Toxicological evaluation	Microbial load determination Aflatoxin detection Pesticide residue determination Radioactive contamination Heavy metal detection
Pharmacological evaluation	In-vivo, ex-vivo evaluation (Animal, animal organ or tissue activities)
Analytical evaluation	Chromatographic (TLC, Paper, HPTLC, HPLC and GC data) and spectroscopic evaluation
Along with above parameters there is need to evaluate herbal formulation for specific pharmaceutical parameters, such as: tablet: weight variation, friability, disintegration, and dissolution.	

Morphological Evaluation

Morphological or organoleptic evaluation is preliminary examination and considered as a first step towards establishment of identity and degree of purity. This is the evaluation by means of organs of senses to evaluate appearance of the drug, its odour and taste, occasionally the sound or snap of its fracture and feel of the drug to the touch. In the case of whole crude drugs, the macroscopic and sensory characters are usually sufficient to enable the drug to be identified. It provides simplest and quickest mean to establish the identity and purity and thereby ensure quality of a particular sample. Judgment may vary from person to person and time to time based on individual's nature. Description of these features are very difficult so that often the characteristic like odour and taste can only described as "characteristic" and reference made to the analyst's memory. The organoleptic characterization is based on the color, odor, shape, size, surface feel, texture of whole crude drug, fracture and appearance of the cut surface.

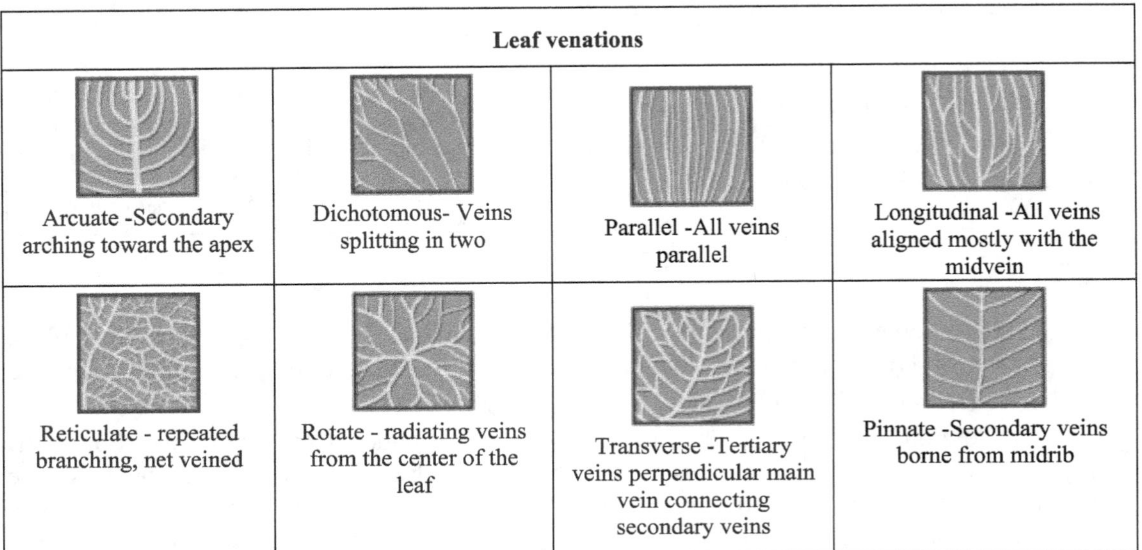

Leaf venations			
Arcuate -Secondary arching toward the apex	Dichotomous- Veins splitting in two	Parallel -All veins parallel	Longitudinal -All veins aligned mostly with the midvein
Reticulate - repeated branching, net veined	Rotate - radiating veins from the center of the leaf	Transverse -Tertiary veins perpendicular main vein connecting secondary veins	Pinnate -Secondary veins borne from midrib

Contd....

Leaf Apex			
Acuminate- Long-tapering point in a concave manner	Acute- Ending in a sharp, but not prolonged point	Cuspidate- With a sharp, elongated, rigid cusp tip	Emarginate- Indented, with a shallow notch at the tip
Mucronate- Abruptly tipped with a small short point	Mucronulate- Mucronate, but with a noticeably diminutive spine	Obcordate- Inversely heart-shaped	Obtuse- Rounded or blunt
Truncate- Ending abruptly with a flat end			
Leaf Margin			
Entire- Even, smooth margin	Ciliate -Hairy	Crenate- Wavy rounded dentate	Dentate -Toothed
Denticulate -Finely toothed	Doubly serrate – Multilayered toothed	Serrate- Saw-toothed	Serrulate- Finely serrate
Sinuate- deep wavy indentations	Lobate- the indentations	Undulate- shallow wavy edge	Spiny - sharp points

Fig. 1.1 Types of leaf venentaions, apex and margin

> **Color:** It is to be examine under an artificial light source and or day light. The color of the sample should be compared with that of a reference material. Example: Senna leaves are fresh green in color while Digitalis leaves are dark green in color.

> **Odour**: Slow and repeated inhalation of the material provides necessary information of its odour. Where no distinct odour is perceptible, crude drug is to be crushed using gentle pressure to verify exact odour. If the material is known to be toxic or dangerous, then determine its odour by other suitable means such as pouring a small quantity of boiling water

on to the crushed sample placed in a beaker. Determine the strength of the odour like weak, distinct, strong, characteristic, and then the sensation like musty, moldy, rancid, fruity, aromatic etc. Example: Essential oil containing crude drugs have aromatic odour while ergot, vinca like crude drugs have disagreeable odour and many of crude drugs are odourless.

➢ **Taste**: Non-toxic crude drugs can be tasted while toxic crude drugs like Nux-vomica, Aconite should not be tasted. Example: Most of alkaloid containing drugs are bitter in taste; senna leaves have mucilaginous taste while digitalis leaves are bitter in taste; Licorice is sweet in taste and cinnamon is in sweet-pungent in taste.

➢ **Size and shape:** The length, width and thickness of the crude materials are of great importance while evaluating a crude drug. Example: Width of Indian senna is smaller than Tinnevelly senna leaves. Length of *Digitalis lanata* leaves is more than *Digitalis purpurea* leaves. Rauwolfia root is wavy (snake like) in shape. Following are shapes of barks:

  ➢ Flat: Arjuna bark

  ➢ Curved: Cassia bark

  ➢ Re-curved: Kurchi bark

  ➢ Channeled: Cinchona bark

  ➢ Quill: Casacara bark

  ➢ Double quill: Cinnamon bark

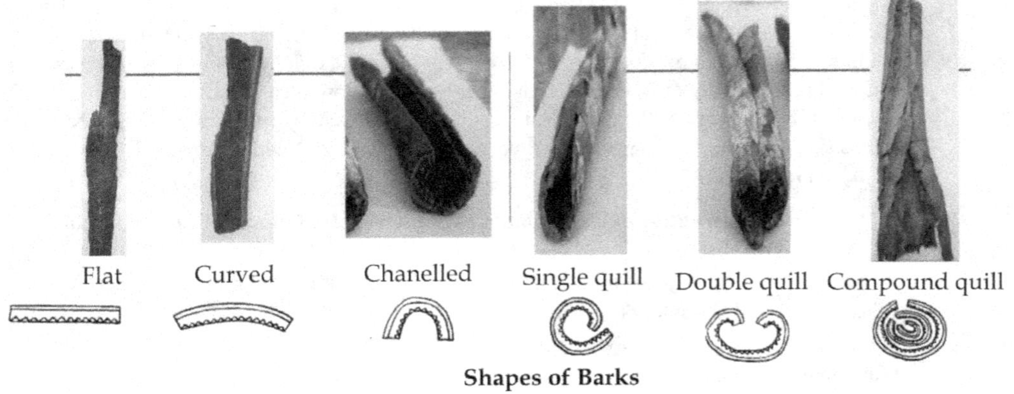

Fig. 1.2 Various shapes of bark

➢ **Extra features:** The texture is best examined by taking a small quantity of material and rubbing it between the thumb and forefinger, it is usually described as 'smooth', 'rough', 'gritty'. Touch of the material describes its softness or hardness. Bend and rupture caused to the sample, provides information of the brittleness.

Following are important morphological characters of bark crude drugs:

  ➢ Lenticle: Pores on stem of woody plant for gaseous exchange

  ➢ Lichens: composite organism from symbiosis association of algae, cyanobacteria and fungi

- ➢ Fissures: Deep cracks
- ➢ Striations: Parallel or longitudinal linings
- ➢ Furrows: Troughs between wrinkles
- ➢ Corrugations: Inner surface wrinkles
- ➢ Fracture: Appearance of broken bark surface

Appearance of the fractured plane as fibrous, smooth, rough, granular, etc. helps in distinguishing bark, stem and root like crude drugs. All these characteristics are valuable in indicating the general type of material and the presence of more than one adulterant components. Example: Nux-vomica seed exhibits smooth silky feel due to presence of trichomes. Outer surface of Rhubarb rhizome shows presence of star spots and cascara bark shows presence of lenticles and lichen.

Microscopical Evaluation

Qualitative microscopical evaluation: It involves histological study of type and arrangement of tissues, presence of characteristic features such as stomata, starch grains, calcium oxalate crystals by using magnification power of microscopes. It utilizes stains to distinguish and identify different microscopical characters. Example: iodine for starch detection, phloroglucinol and HCl for lignin detection, Sudan red –III for oil detection etc.

Starch grains	Starch is composed of amylose and amylopectin, with the level of amylose ranging from 20% to 30% for most cereal starches. Starch grains are typically microscopically identified with either optical or electron microscopy. Starch grains can become clearer if they are stained a darker color with Iodine Stains. Logol's Iodine is one, used for staining starch because iodine reagents easily bind to starch but less easily to other materials. Features that allow identification of starch grains include: presence of hilum (core of the grain), lamellae (or growth layers), birefringence, and extinction cross (a cross shape, visible on grains under revolving polarized light) which are visible with a microscope and shape and size.

Structure and Amylose Content of Some Whole Granular Cereal Starches

Source	Granule Shape	Granule Size (nm)	Amylose Content (%)
Wheat	Lenticular or round	20–25	22
Maize	Round or polyhedral	15	28
Waxy maize	Round	15 (5–15)	1
High-amylose	Round or irregular sausage-shaped	25	52
Barley	Round or elliptical	20–25	22
Rice	Polygonal	3–8	17–19[a] 21–23[b]
Oats	Polyhedral	3–10	23–24

a-Japonica, b-Indica

Adapted from Lineback (1984).

Calcium Crystals		There are two types' of calcium crystals forms due to excess carbonic acid or oxalic acid.
	Calcium carbonate	Rare and generally associated with cell wall They are also called as cystoliths as they appear in the form of grapes in the tissues. Example: *Ficus elastica*

Contd….

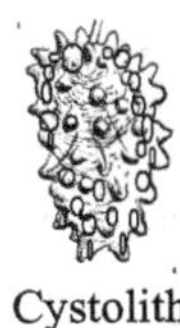

Cystolith

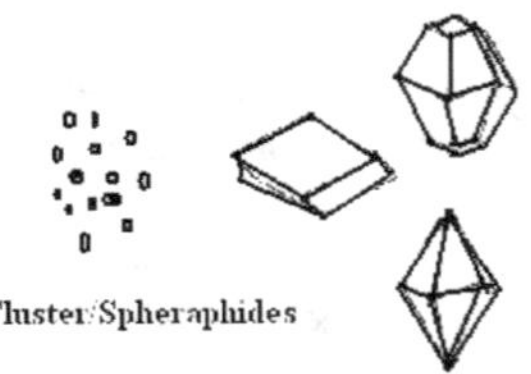

Cluster/Spheraphides

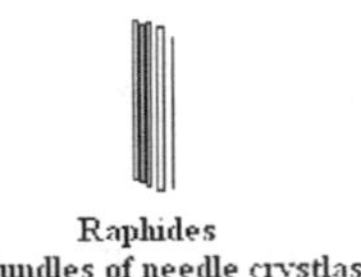

Prism

Raphides
(Bundles of needle crystlas)

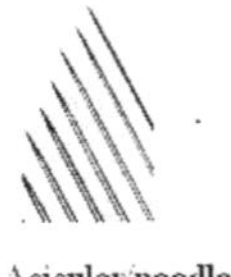

Acicular/needle crystals

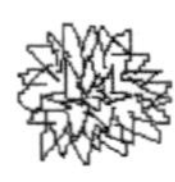

Rossette

Calcium oxalate	Very common and present in almost each part of plant. **Prisms/single crystals**: they are large, single or small groups and well developed. **Cluster crystals/ spheraphides**: they are group of numerous prisms/pyramids. The crystal are projecting, pointed, acute angled, and more or less spherical. **Rosette crystals**: they are large number of crystals in spherical mass (in the centre of which is an organic substance). Components of crystals radiate from the centre to the periphery and form a toothed circumference. **Acicular crystals/ raphids**: they re needle like, slender, long pointed at the ends. They may be single or in bundles. **Microcrystal/ crystal sand / micro sphenoid**: occur like an amorphous mass in cell. They are very minute and are present in large number in a single cell which is usually enlarged than other cells and is called idioblast.

Table 1.1 Common crude drugs and their Calcium crystals

Crude drugs	Type of calcium crystals
Asparagus, Aloe, Centella, Clove Flower Bud, Digitallis, Ephedra, Ginger, Isapgol, Nuxvomica	Absent
Azadircata, Senna, Clove, Rhubarb, Wild cherry bark, Tinosperma	Prism and cluster
Bacopa, Rauwolfia, Vasaka, Liquorice, Clove stalk, Senna, Kurchi, Cocca, Qaussia, Cascara	Prism
Cinchona	Microprism
Caraway	Rosette
Coriander, Dill, Fennel	Microrosette
Cassia, Cinnamon, Gentian	Acicular
Ipecac, Squill	Raphides
Cinnamon	Tubular
Datura	Spherophide crystals
Eucalyptus, Podophyllum	Clusters
Kurchi	Rhomboidal
Vinca	Microtubular, tactoid or needle shaped
Withania, Cinchona, Belladonna	Microsphenoid

Stomata	It is a pore, found in the upper epidermis of leaves, stems, and other organs, that controls the rate of gas exchange. The pore is bordered by a pair of specialized parenchyma cells known as guard cells that are responsible for regulating the size of the stomatal opening.There are different types of stomata and they are mainly classified based on their number and characteristics of the surrounding subsidiary cells. Listed below are the different types of stomata.

Types of stomatas present in Dicots:

➤ *Paracytic(meaning parallel celled) or rubiaceous type:* stomata have one or more subsidiary cells parallel to the opening between the guard cells. These subsidiary cells may reach beyond the guard cells or not. Examples families like Rubiaceae, Convolvulaceae and Fabaceae.

Contd....

> *Diacytic(meaning cross-celled) or caryophyllaceous type*: stomata have guard cells surrounded by two subsidiary cells, that each encircle one end of the opening and contact each other opposite to the middle of the opening. Examples families like Caryophyllaceae and Acanthaceae.

> *Anomocytic(meaning irregular celled) or ranunculaceous type:* stomata have guard cells that are surrounded by cells that have the same size, shape and arrangement as the rest of the epidermis cells. Examples families like Apocynaceae, Boraginaceae, Chenopodiaceae, and Cucurbitaceae.

> *Anisocytic(meaning unequal celled) or cruciferous type:* stomata have guard cells between two larger subsidiary cells and one distinctly smaller one. Examples families like Brassicaceae, Solanaceae, and Crassulaceae.

> *Actinocytic(meaning star-celled)* stomata have guard cells that are surrounded by at least five radiating cells forming a star-like circle. Examples families like Ebenaceae.

> *Hemiparacyticstomata* are bordered by just one subsidiary cell that differs from the surrounding epidermis cells, its length parallel to the stoma opening. Examples families like Molluginaceae and Aizoaceae.

Types of stomatas present in Monocots:

> *Gramineous (meaning grass-like) stomata* have two guard cells surrounded by two lens-shaped subsidiary cells. The guard cells are narrower in the middle and bulbous on each end. This middle section is strongly thickened. The axis of the subsidiary cells are parallel stoma opening. Examples families like Poaceae and Cyperaceae.

> *Hexacytic(meaning six-celled) stomata* have six subsidiary cells around both guard cells, one at either end of the opening of the stoma, one adjoining each guard cell, and one between that last subsidiary cell and the standard epidermis cells.

> *Tetracytic(meaning four-celled) stomata* have four subsidiary cells, one on either end of the opening, and one next to each guard cell. This type occurs in many monocot families, but also can be found in some dicots. Examples families like Tilia and several Asclepiadaceae.

Types of stomatas present in ferns:

> *Hypocyticstomata* have two guard cells in one layer with only ordinary epidermis cells, but with two subsidiary cells on the outer surface of the epidermis, arranged parallel to the guard cells, with a pore between them, overlying the stoma opening.

> *Pericyticstomata* have two guard cells that are entirely encircled by one continuous subsidiary cell (like a donut).

> *Desmocyticstomata* have two guard cells that are entirely encircled by one subsidiary cell that has not merged its ends (like a sausage).

> *Polocyticstomata* have two guard cells that are largely encircled by one subsidiary cell, but also contact ordinary epidermis cells (like a U or horseshoe).

Table 1.2 Common crude drugs and their stomata

Crude drugs	Type of Stomata
Senna, Coca	Paracytic (Rubiaceous)
Centella,Vasaka, mentha, peppermint, spearmint	Diacycytic (Caryophyllaceous)
Belladonna, stramonium, Datura, henbane, Vinca	Anisocytic(Cruciferous or unequal celled)
Digitallis, azadircata, bacopa, eucalyptus	Anomocyctic (Ranunculaceous)

Trichomes   Trichomes on plants are epidermal outgrowths of various kinds.These are fine outgrowths or appendages on plants, algae, lichens, and certain protists.Trichomes can protect the plant from a large range of detriments, such as UV light, insects, transpiration, and freeze intolerance. Glandular trichomes found to store secondary metabolites like volatile oil, flavonoids etc.

Trichome type may assess the number of cells per trichome. A unicellular trichome consists of a single cell and is usually quite small. A multicellular trichome contains two or more cells. Multicellular trichomes can be either uniseriate, having a single vertical row of cells, or multiseriate, having more than one vertical row of cells. The number of cell layers in a trichome can also be diagnostic.

Many trichomes are diagnosed based on their general shape and morphology. Tapering trichomes are those ending in a sharp apex. Malpighian or dolabriform (also termed "two-armed" or "T-shaped") trichomes are those with two arms arising from a common base. (Malpighian is named after the family Malpighiaceae, where this trichome type is common.) Glandular trichomes are secretory or excretory trichomes, usually having an apical glandular cell. Glandular trichomes can be pilate-glandular, with a glandular cell atop an elongate basal stalk, or capitate-glandular, with a glandular cell having a very short or no basal stalk. Branched trichomes include two types: stellate, which are star-shaped trichomes having several arms arising from a common base (either stalked or sessile); and dendritic, which are treelike trichomes with multiple lateral branches. Peltate trichomes are those with a disk-shaped apical portion atop a peltately attached stalk.

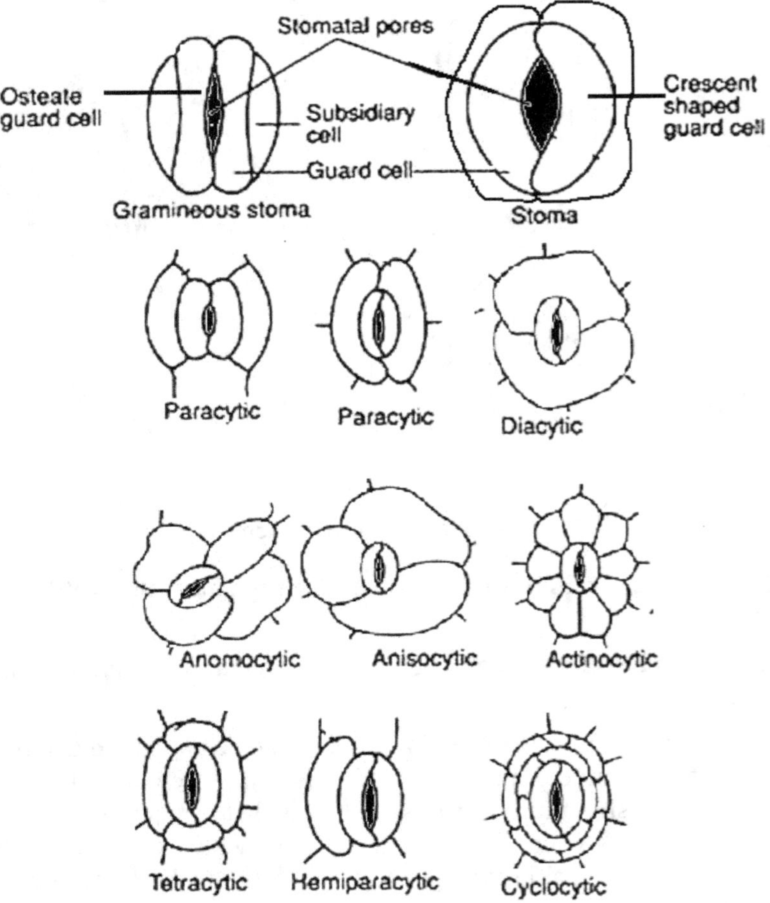

Fig. 1.3 Various types of stomata

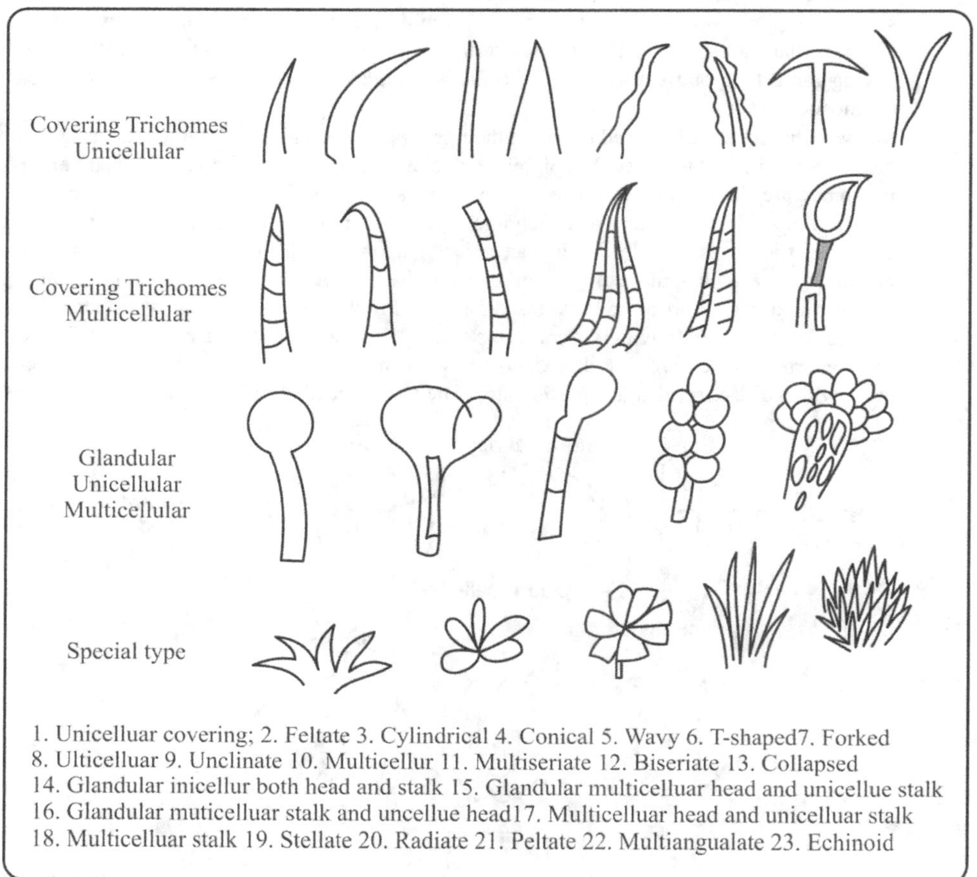

Fig. 1.4 Various types of trichomes

Quantitative microscopical evaluation: It involves determination of quantity of microscopical characters such as

> *Leaf constant*: Palisade ratio, Vein islet number, Vein termination number, Stomatal number, Stomatal index

> *Lycopodium spore method*: Newer technique which can be applied to determine percentage purity of any plant part crude drug unlike leaf constants which are applicable only to leaf crude drugs. Additional significance of this method is that it requires powder form of crude drugs unlike leaf constants which requires fresh or dry whole crude drug. Whole fresh or drug crude drugs cannot available throughout year while powder form of crude drug can be available and stored easily.

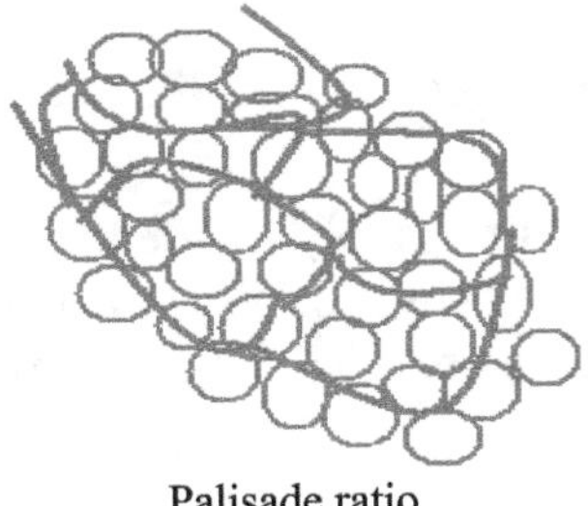

Palisade ratio

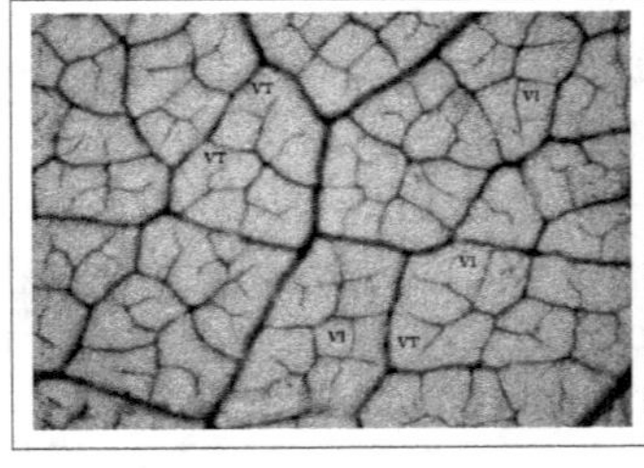
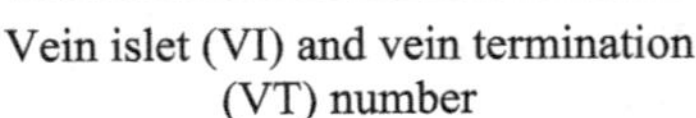

Vein islet (VI) and vein termination
(VT) number

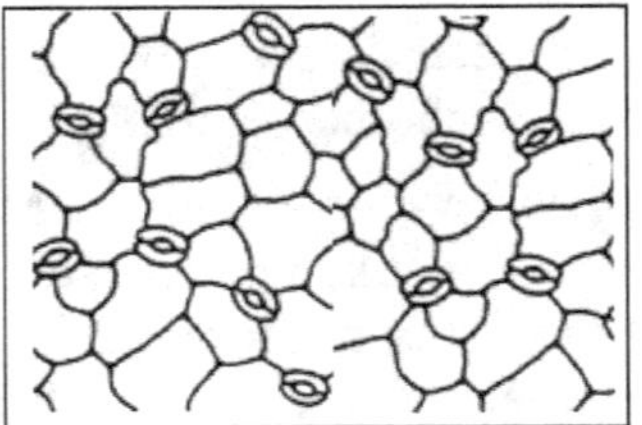

Stomatal number and stomatal index

Fig. 1.5 Leaf constants

Camera Lucida

The name "camera lucida" (Latin for "light chamber") is an optical device used to draw microscopic images. It facilitates accurate sketching of minute objects. Originally the camera lucida performs an optical superimposition of the subject being viewed upon the surface upon which the artist is drawing. The principle is very simple. By looking into the prism from just the right angle, two images will enter the eye; one, of the object to be sketched, the other of the pencil and paper with which you intend to work with. The resulting effect is that your eye perceives illusion of seeing objects in front of the instrument on the drawing surface beneath. This is possible only after proper angle adjustment between mirror or prism and drawing board.

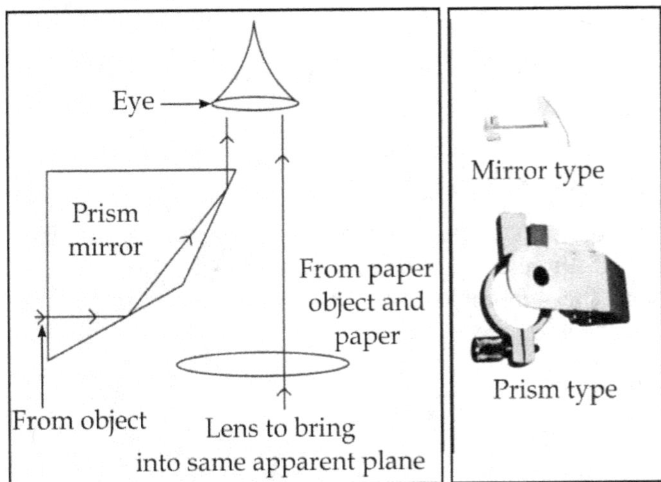

Fig. 1.6 (a) Principle of working camera lucida   **Fig. 1.6 (b)** Types of camera lucida

Two types of camera lucida are available in market as given in figure 1.6 (b). There are three main parts of camera lucida – attachment ring, prism and mirror. Attachment ring attaches camera lucida around the body tube and prism over eyepiece. Prism reflects the image on mirror and then mirror reflect it on paper. Thus it allows passing light from prism to paper and from paper to prism as shown in figure 1.6(a). Thus this is a unique tool to aid perspective drawing and the recording of fine detail.

Micrometer

Micrometer is scale which is used to measure microscopically magnified images like cells, fibers, trichomes, starch grains and calcium oxalate crystals.

Stage micrometers: Stage Micrometer is simply a microscope slide with a finely divided scale of 1 mm marked on the surface. 1 mm is divided into 100 divisions so 1 division is 1/100 i.e. 10 um. This micrometer is just useful to calibrate eyepiece micrometer reticle. Stage Micrometer is removed after calibration and slide of sample is placed.

Eyepiece micrometer: An ocular micrometer is a glass disk with etched scale that fits in place of a eyepiece and this micrometer is actually used to measure the size of magnified objects. In this micrometer scale of 1 mm is also divided into 100 divisions so 1 division is 1/100 i.e. 10 um. But the physical length of the marks on the scale depends on the degree of magnification which varies due to objective/eyepiece combination and mechanical tube length of the microscope. Hence it is very necessary to calibrate eyepiece micrometer divisions by stage micrometer and arbitrary units of the transfer scale (reticle) must be converted to absolute units, such as millimeters or micrometers.

Calibration of eyepiece micrometer: Calibration of the scale is commonly performed by imaging a stage micrometer with the objective to be used for specimen measurements. Put stage and eyepiece micrometer in appropriate place. Superimpose the scale of stage and eyepiece micrometer. Observe any one line of stage micrometer which is coinciding with eyepiece micrometer and then see the next line of stage micrometer which is coinciding with eyepiece micrometer. Count the divisions between these two lines.

Example:

    3 divisions of stage micrometer = 29 divisions of eyepiece micrometer

    But 1 division of stage micrometer = 10 um

    Hence 30 um = 29 divisions of eyepiece micrometer

    So 1 divisions of eyepiece micrometer = 30/29 = 1.03 um

This value is often referred to as the micrometer value, or calibration factor, for that particular objective. Once the value has been determined, the size of any specimen feature may be calculated by multiplying the number of eyepiece reticle divisions spanned by the feature with the calibration factor for the objective in use.

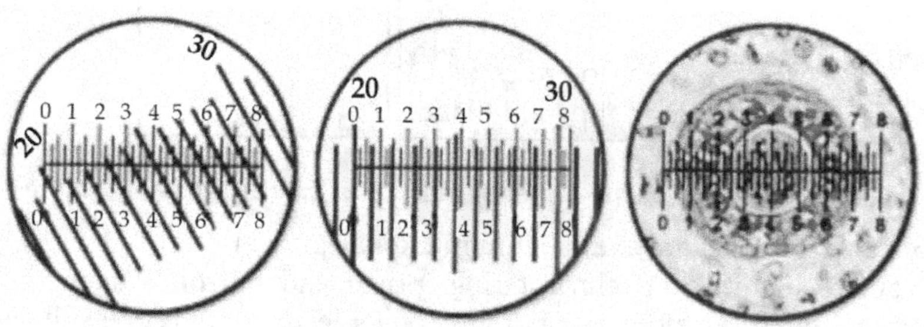

Fig. 1.7 Calibration and measurment by micrometer

Leaf constant determination

Palisade ratio: This is average number of palisade cell beneath each epidermal cell. It can be also determined with powdered drugs.

Procedure: Clear a piece of the leaf by boiling in choral hydrate solution for about thirty minutes. Arrange camera lucida and drawing board for making drawings to scale. Place stage micrometer on the microscope and using 16 mm objectives, draw a line equivalent to 1 mm as seen through the microscope. Construct a square on this line. Move the paper so that the square is seen in the eye piece, in the centre of the field. Place the slide with the cleared leaf (epidermis on the stage). Trace off at least four epidermal cells and draw palisade cells beneath each epidermal cell. Calculate average palisade cell beneath each epidermal cell.

Vein-islet number: This is number of vein-islets per square mm of the leaf surface midway between midrib and margin.

Procedure: Clear a piece of the leaf by boiling in choral hydrate solution for about thirty minutes. Arrange camera lucida and drawing board for making drawings to scale. Place stage micrometer on the microscope and using 16 mm objectives, draw a line equivalent to 1 mm as seen through the microscope. Construct a square on this line. Move the paper so that the square is seen in the eye piece, in the centre of the field. Place the slide with the cleared leaf (epidermis on the stage). Trace off the veins which are included within the square, completing the outlines of those islets which overlap two adjacent sides of the square. Count the number of vein islets in the square millimeter. Where the islets are intersected by the sides of the square, include those on two adjacent sides and exclude those islets on the other sides. (To obtain a critical result for a leaf, 4 sq mm should be used, preferably in one large area of 4 sq mm). Find the average number of vein islets from the four adjoining squares, to get the values for one sq mm.

Examples of Vein-islet numbers of few leaf crude drugs			
Vein-islet numbers	**Species**	**Range of vein-islet numbers**	**Average**
Senna	*Cassia senna*	15–29.5	26
	Cassia angustifolia	19.5–22.5	21
Coca	*Erythroxylum coca*	8–12	11
	Erythroxylum truxillense	15–26	20
Digitalis	*Digitalis purpurea*	2–5.5	3.5
	Digitalis lanata	2–3.5	2.7
		3–8	4.4
	Digitalis lutea	1–1.5	1.2
	Digitalis thapsi	8.5–16	

Vein–termination number: This is number of vein termination per square mm of the leaf surface midway between midrib and margin.

Procedure: Clear a piece of the leaf by boiling in choral hydrate solution for about thirty minutes. Arrange camera lucida and drawing board for making drawings to scale. Place stage micrometer on the microscope and using 16 mm objectives, draw a line equivalent to 1 mm as seen through the microscope. Construct a square on this line. Move the paper so that the square is seen in the eye piece, in the centre of the field. Place the slide with the cleared leaf (epidermis on the stage). Trace off the veins which are included within the square, completing the outlines of those islets which overlap two adjacent sides of the square. Count the number of veinlet terminations present within the square. Find the average number of veinlet termination number from the four adjoining squares, to get the values for one sq. mm.

Contd….

Examples of Vein- termination numbers of few leaf crude drugs	
Veinlet termination numbers	
Atropa acuminata	1.4–3.5
Atropa belladonna	6.3–10.3
Cassia angustifolia	25.9–32.8
Cassia senna	32.7–40.2
Datura stramonium	12.6–20.1
Digitalis purpurea	2.5–4.2
Erythroxylum coca	16.8–21.0
Erythroxylum truxillense	23.1–32.3
Hyoscyamus niger	12.4–19.0

Stomatal number: This is average number of stomata per square mm of epidermis of the leaf.

Procedure: Clear the piece of the leaf (middle part) by boiling with chloral hydrate solution or alternatively with chlorinated soda. Peel out upper and lower epidermis separately by means of forceps. Keep it on slide and mount in glycerin water. Arrange a camera lucida and drawing board for making the drawings to scale. Draw a square of 1 mm by means of stage micrometer. Place the slide with cleared leaf (epidermis) on the stage. Trace the epidermis cell and stomata. Count the number of stomata present in the area of 1 sq. mm. Include the cell if at least half of its area lies within the square. Record the result for each of the ten fields and calculate the average number of stomata per sq mm.

Stomatal index: This is percentage of the number of stomata forms to the total number of epidermal cells each stoma being counted as one cell.

Procedure: Clear the piece of the leaf (middle part) by boiling with chloral hydrate solution or alternatively with chlorinated soda. Peel out upper and lower epidermis separately by means of forceps. Keep it on slide and mount in glycerin water. Arrange a camera lucida and drawing board for making the drawings to scale. Draw a square of 1 mm by means of stage micrometer. Place the slide with cleared leaf (epidermis) on the stage. Trace the epidermis cell and stomata. Count the number of stomata, also the number of epidermal cells in each field. Calculate the stomatal index using the above formula. Determine the values for upper and lower surface (epidermis) separately.

$$\text{Stomatal index} = \frac{\text{Stomatal number}}{\text{Toal number of stomata} + \text{Total number of epidemol cells}} \times 100$$

Examples of stomatal index of few leaf crude drugs		
Stomatal index	**Upper surface**	**Lower surface**
Atropa acuminata	1.7 to 4.8 to 12.2	16.2 to 17.5 to 1.83
Atropa belladonna	2.3 to 3.9 to 10.5	20.2 to 21.7 to 23.0
Cassia senna	11.4 to 12.4 to 13.3	10.8 to 11.8 to 12.6
Cassia angustifolia	17.1 to 19.0 to 20.7	17.0 to 18.3 to 19.3
Datura inermis	18.1 to 18.3 to 18.7	24.5 to 24.9 to 25.3
Datura metel	12.7 to 17.4 to 19.4	21.2 to 22.3 to 23.9
Datura stramonium	16.4 to 18.1 to 20.4	24.1 to 24.9 to 26.3
Datura tatula	15.6 to 20.2 to 22.3	28.3 to 29.8 to 31.0
Digitalis lanata	13.9 to 14.4 to 14.7	14.9 to 16.1 to 17.6
Digitalis lutea	2.5 to 5.5 to 8.4	21.6 to 22.9 to 25.2
Digitalis purpurea	1.6 to 2.7 to 4.0	17.9 to 19.2 to 19.5
Digitalis thapsi	5.9 to 7.0 to 7.8	11.9 to 12.4 to 13.5
Erythroxylum coca	Nil	12.2 to 13.2 to 14.0
Erythroxylum truxillense	Nil	8.9 to 10.1 to 10.7
Phytolacca acinosa	Nil	15.0
Phytolacca americana	2.9 to 4.2 to 5.7	13.0 to 13.2 to 13.4

Lycopodium spore method:

Lycopodium is composed of the spores of *Lycopodium clavatum L.* each spore is tetrahedral in shape, the base is rounded and the three flat sides meet to form three well-marked covering ridges, which join one another at the apex. The whole surface of the spore is covered with minute reticulations and the interior is filled with fixed oil. The spores are exceptionally uniform in size (25 μm), so that one can always know that a definite number of spores represent a particular weight of lycopodium. The whole process can be simplified as 1 mg of spores contains averagely 94000 spores. By this figure one can calculate the weight of any number of spores under any condition under the microscope. If the lycopodium has been fixed with a definite proportion of another substance, one can find immediately how much of the second substance has been added, when examined microsopically. If it is admixed with any fine particles like pollen grains, starch etc. with characteristic countable particles it is possible to calculate the number of such characteristic particles per mg. In this way it is possible to have a standard figure that represents any such material. The number of characteristic particles per unit weight is often constant and is useful in assessing the quality of a sample. To use this method the number of particles in a good quality sample must either be known or first determined.

$$\% \text{ Purity}: \frac{N \times W \times 940000}{S \times M \times P} \times 100$$

where

N = Number of Characteristic particlesof sample in 25 fields

W = Weight of Lycopodium spores taken in mg

S = Number of Lycopodium spores in 25 fields

M = Weight of sample in mg

P = Standard value of number of characteristic samples per mg in taken sample material (Example: 1 mg ginger powder contains 2, 86, 000 starch grains)

Powder Microscopical Evaluation

Powder microscopical evaluation is done using powders of crude drugs unlike to histological studies where whole crude drug is used. Every time it is impossible to obtain fresh or to store whole dried crude drug so powder microscopy is most feasible. All microscopical characters can be observed in disperse form without intact information like exact arrangement of cells, tissues.

Procedure: Clear powder with clearing agents. Spread thin layer of powder on glass slide and observe under microscope. To differentiate cells (lignified and non-lignified, starch grains, oil glands) use staining reagents. Following characters can be observed according to plant parts:

Common Powder characteristics of different plant parts are as follows:

Leaves	Epidermal cells, palisade cells, stomata, trichomes, calcium crystals, starch grains,
Roots/Rhizomes	Cork cell, parenchyma cells, phloem fibers, xylem, calcium crystals, starch grains, stone cells
Bark/wood	Cork cell, parenchyma cells, phloem fibers, xylem, calcium crystals, starch grains, stone cells, pericyclic fibers, sclerides, fibers
Flowers	Epidermal cells, anthers, pollen grains, oil globules, pigments,
Seeds	Endosperm, oil glands, aleurone grains, starch grains, pigment
Fruits	Epidermal cells, pericarp, mesocarp, oil glands (vittae), sclerenchymatous cells

Physical Evaluation

Qualitative Physical Evaluation

This evaluation gives idea about quality of crude drug either pure or impure. This involves determination of following parameters:

➤ *Solubility*: Solubility is the property of a solid, liquid, or gaseous chemical substance called solute to dissolve in a solid, liquid, or gaseous solvent to form a homogeneous solution of the solute in the solvent.

- Fats and oils: soluble in non polar solvents like petroleum, ether, benzene, and hexane
- Carbohydrates, glycosides, tannins, flavonoids: soluble in different types of alcohols or water
- Aglycone part of glycosides, bases of alkaloids: soluble in non-polar solvents

Descriptive Term	Parts of Solvent for 1 part of solute
Very Soluble	Less than 1
Freely Soluble	From 1 to 10
Soluble	From 10 to 30
Sparingly Soluble	From 30 to 100
Slightly Soluble	From 100 to 1000
Very Slightly Soluble	From 1000 to 10,000
Practically Insoluble, or Insoluble	More than 10,000

➤ *Optical rotation* of a liquid is the angle through which the plane of polarization of light is rotated when the polarized light is passed through a sample of the liquid, rotation clockwise or anticlockwise. Clove oil 0 to -1.5 while eucalyptus oil having 0 to +10.

➤ *Melting point*: All solid pure phytochemicals should be evaluated for its melting point. Difference in melting point indicates presence of impurities.

➤ *Boiling point*: This parameter is applicable to all liquid phytochemicals like essential oils or few alkaloids. Shift in boiling point range helps in determining purity of phytochemicals.

➤ *Refractive index (RI)*: The refractive index of a substance is the ratio between the velocity of light in air and the velocity in the substance under test. The refractive index of the material is given by the sine of the angle of incidence divided by the since of the angle of refraction. The RI varies with the temperature; Pharmacopoeial determinations are made at 20°C.

➤ *Viscosity*: Viscous natural drugs like gums, mucilages or pectin like compounds should be evaluated for its viscosity.

➤ *Density, specific gravity determination*: All liquid phytochemicals have to be evaluated for its density and specific gravity. This parameter is very essential for volatile oil standardization.

➤ *Spectroscopic evaluation*: λmax values in UV, wave number values in FTIR, delta values in NMR and m/e values in mass spectroscopy useful to identify impurities and thus to determine purity of samples.

Spectroscopy is the study of the interaction between matter and radiation. It measures radiation intensity as a function of wavelength. Spectroscopic analyses are based on measuring the amount of radiation produced or absorbed by molecular or atomic species of interest. Spectroscopy is a common technique used in analytical chemistry for the identification of substances through the spectrum emitted from or absorbed by them. Spectroscopic methods can be classified according to the region of the electromagnetic spectrum involved in the measurement. The regions that have been used include gamma-ray, X-ray, Ultraviolet (UV), Visible, Infrared (IR), Microwave and Radio frequency (RF). Spectroscopic methods are mostly classified as atomic, molecular or ionic based on whether or not they apply to atoms, molecules or ions. The nature of their interactions can also be used to classify spectroscopic methods. These can be divided in three categories;

➢ Absorption spectroscopy which uses the range of the electromagnetic spectra in which substance absorbs photons. Example: Infrared, ultraviolet, visible and microwave spectroscopy are molecular techniques of absorption spectroscopy.

➢ Emission spectroscopy that uses the range of electromagnetic spectra in which photons are emitted by the substance. Example: Fluorescence spectroscopy, flame photometry

➢ Scattering spectrometry where the amount of light that a substance scatters depends on polarization angles and wavelength. Example: Raman spectroscopy.

➢ *Chromatographic evaluation*: Presence of extra band after development of chromatogram in paper or TLC, HPTLC indicates presence of impuri-ties.

Chromatography is based on the principle where molecules in mixture applied onto the surface or into the solid, and fluid stationary phase (stable phase) is separating from each other while moving with the aid of a mobile phase.

The factors effective on this separation process include molecular characteristics related to adsorption (liquid-solid), partition (liquid-solid), and affinity or differences among their molecular weights. Because of these differences, some components of the mixture stay longer in the stationary phase, and they move slowly in the chromatography system, while others pass rapidly into mobile phase, and leave the system faster.

Based on this approach three components form the basis of the chromatography technique.

➢ Stationary phase: This phase is always composed of a "solid" phase or "a layer of a liquid adsorbed on the surface a solid support".

➢ Mobile phase: This phase is always composed of "liquid" or a "gaseous component."

➢ Separated molecules

The type of interaction between stationary phase, mobile phase, and substances contained in the mixture is the basic component effective on separation of molecules from each other.

Chromatography methods based on partition are very effective on separation, and identification of small molecules as amino acids, carbohydrates, and fatty acids. However,

➢ Affinity chromatographies (ie. ion-exchange chromatography) are more effective in the separation of macromolecules as nucleic acids, and proteins.

➢ Paper chromatography is used in the separation of proteins, and in studies related to protein synthesis;

➢ gas-liquid chromatography is utilized in the separation of alcohol, esther, lipid, and amino groups, and observation of enzymatic interactions,

➤ molecular-sieve chromatography is employed especially for the determination of molecular weights of proteins.

➤ Agarose-gel chromatography is used for the purification of RNA, DNA particles, and viruses.

Types of chromatography

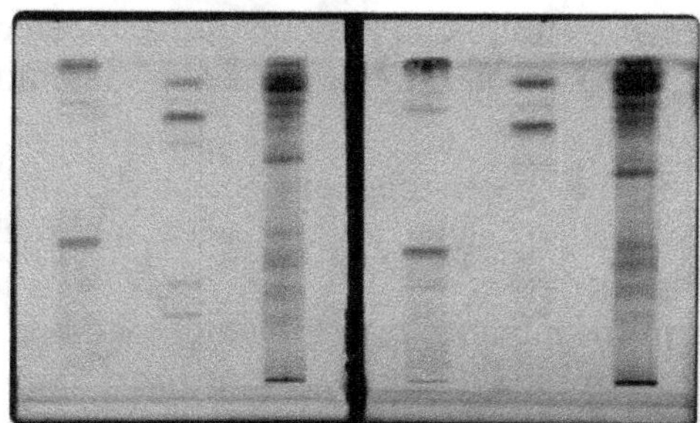

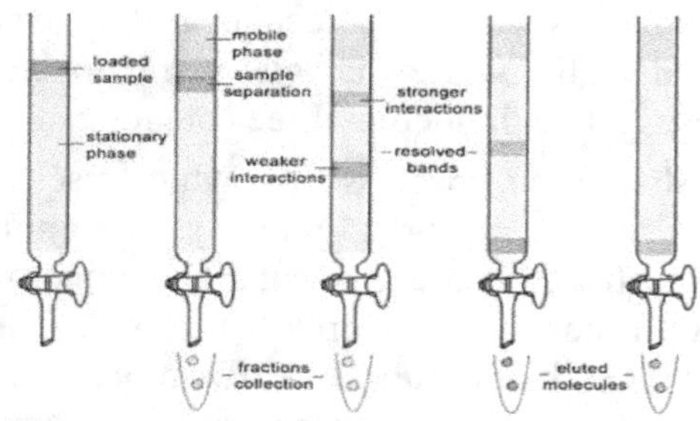

PlanarChromatography

➤ Paper chromatography
➤ Thin-layer chromatography
➤ High Perfomrmace Thin-layer chromatography (HPTLC)

Column Chromatography

➤ Column chromatography
➤ Ion-exchange chromatography
➤ Gel-permeation (molecular sieve) chromatography
➤ Affinity chromatography
➤ Gas chromatography
➤ High-pressure liquid chromatography (HPLC)

Fig. 1.8 Types of chromatography

Quantitative physical Evaluation or Physicochemical evaluation

Ash value determination:

The residue remaining left after incineration of the crude drug is designated as ash. The residue obtained usually represents the inorganic salts naturally occurring in the drug and adhering to it. It varies with in definite limits according to the soils. It may also include inorganic matter deliberately added for the purpose of adulteration. Hence, an ash value determination furnishes the basis for judging the identity and cleanliness of any drug and gives information relative to its adulteration/contamination with inorganic matter, thus ash values are helpful in determining the quality and purity of drug.

Muffle furnace Muffle furnace is an oven type instrument which can reach high temperatures. The furnace achieves the high-temperature on the basis of the insulating material which is fitted inside the chamber. The insulating material which is provided in the chambers acts as a muffle and stops the heat from escaping out of the chamber.

Crucible: There are a number of different types of crucible available for ashingcrude drug samples, including quartz, pyrex, porcelain, steel and platinum. Selection of an appropriate crucible depends on the sample being analyzed and the furnace temperature used. The most widely used crucibles are made from porcelain because it is relatively inexpensive to purchase, can be used up to high temperatures ($< 1200°C$) and are easy to clean. Porcelain crucibles are resistent to acids but can be corroded by alkaline samples, and therefore different types of crucible should be used to analyze this type of sample. In addition, porcelain crucibles are prone to cracking if they experience rapid temperature changes.

Types of ash values

Total ash: The determination of ash is useful for detecting low grade products, exhausted drugs & excess of sandy and earthy material. Total ash is useful to exclude drugs which have been coated with chalk, lime or calcium sulphate to improve their appearance. Example: Ginger and Nutmeg. This test is designed to measure the amount of material remaining after ignition. Physiological ash is derived from the plant tissue. Nonphysiological ash is the residue after ignition of the extraneous matter (Example: sand and soil) adhering to the surface.

Procedure: weigh accurately into previously ignited and tared crucible, usually platinum, silica about 2 to 3 g of the ground material. Spread the material in an even layer in the crucible. Ignite the material by gradually increasing the heat to 450 °C until free from carbon, cool in desiccator and weigh. If carbon-free ash can't be obtained in this manner, cool the crucible and moisten the residue with about 2 ml of water or a saturated solution of ammonium nitrate, dry on a water bath. Then on hot plate and ignite to constant weight without delay. Calculate the content of total ash in mg/g of air-dried material.

Acid-insoluble ash: Acid-insoluble ash is the residue obtained after boiling the ash with dilute Hcl and igniting the washed insoluble matter left on the filter. This determination measures the presence of silica especially sand and siliceous earth. Acid-insoluble ash is useful for detecting the presence of excessive earthy material.

Procedure: To the crucible containing the total ash, add 25 ml of Hcl(70 g/l) TS, cover with a watch-glass and boil gently for 5 mins. Rinse the watch-glass with 5 ml of hot water and add this liquid to the crucible. Collect the insoluble matter on an ash less filter paper and wash with hot water until the filtrate is neutral. Transfer the filter paper containing the insoluble matter to the original crucible, dry on hot plate and ignite to the constant weight. Allow the residue to cool in a suitable desiccator for 10 min and weigh without delay. Calculate the content of acid insoluble ash in mg/g of air dried material.

Water-soluble ash: Water soluble ash is the calculated difference in wt between the total ash and the residue remaining after treatment of total ash with water. Water-soluble ash is useful to detect the presence of material exhausted by water. Example: Tea leaves and Ginger. For the ginger the value of total ash is 2.5-6% and water-soluble ash is 1.9-3.0%.While for the exhausted ginger the value of total ash is 2-4% and water-soluble ash is 0.2-0.5%.

Procedure: To the crucible containing the total ash, add 25 ml of water and boil for 5 min. Collect the insoluble matter in a sintered glass crucible or on an ash less filter paper. Wash with hot water and ignite for 5 min at a temperature not exceeding 450 °C. Subtract the weight of this residue in mg obtained from the weight of total ash. Calculate the content of water soluble ash in mg/g of air dried material.

➢ ***Dry Ashing***: Dry ashing procedures use a high temperature muffle furnace capable of maintaining temperatures of between 500 and 600 °C. Water and other volatile materials are vaporized and organic substances are burned in the presence of the oxygen in air to CO_2, H_2O and N_2. Most minerals are converted to oxides, sulfates, phosphates, chlorides or silicates. Although most minerals have fairly low volatility at these high temperatures, some are volatile and may be partially lost. Example: iron, lead and mercury. If an analysis is being carried out to determine the concentration of one of these substances then it is advisable to use an alternative ashing method that uses lower temperatures. The food sample is weighed before and after ashing to determine the concentration of ash present. The ash content can be expressed on either a dry or wet basis:

$$\% \text{ As(dry basis)} = \frac{M_{ASH}}{M_{DRY}} \times 100$$

$$\% \text{ As(wet basis)} = \frac{M_{ASH}}{M_{DRY}} \times 100$$

where M_{ASH} refers to the mass of the ashed sample, and M_{DRY} and M_{ASH} refer to the original masses of the dried and wet samples.

A number of dry ashing methods have been officially recognized for the determination of the ash content of various foods (AOAC Official Methods of Analysis). Typically, a sample is held at 500-600°C for 24 hours.

Advantages: Safe, few reagents are required, many samples can be analyzed simultaneously, not labor intensive, and ash can be analyzed for specific mineral content.

Disadvantages: Long time required (12-24 hours), muffle furnaces are quite costly to run due to electrical costs, loss of volatile minerals at high temperatures, Example: Cu, Fe, Pb, Hg, Ni, Zn.

Recently, analytical instruments have been developed to dry ash samples based on microwave heating. These devices can be programmed to initially remove most of the moisture (using a relatively low heat) and then convert the sample to ash (using a relatively high heat). Microwave instruments greatly reduce the time required to carry out an ash analysis, with the analysis time often being less than an hour. The major disadvantage is that it is not possible to simultaneously analyze as many samples as in a muffle furnace.

➢ ***Wet Ashing:*** Wet ashing is primarily used in the preparation of samples for subsequent analysis of specific minerals (see later). It breaks down and removes the organic matrix surrounding the minerals so that they are left in an aqueous solution. A dried ground food sample is usually weighed into a flask containing strong acids and oxidizing agents (Example: nitric, perchloric and/or sulfuric acids) and then heated. Heating is continued until the organic matter is completely digested, leaving only the mineral oxides in solution. The temperature and time used depends on the type of acids and oxidizing agents used. Typically, a digestion takes from 10 minutes to a few hours at temperatures of about 350°C. The resulting solution can then be analyzed for specific minerals.

Advantages: Little loss of volatile minerals occurs because of the lower temperatures used, more rapid than dry ashing.

Disadvantages: Labor intensive, requires a special fume-cupboard if perchloric acid is used because of its hazardous nature, low sample throughput.

Ash values of popular crude drugs as per pharmacopoeias			
Ash values	**Name of pharmacopeia**		
	Indian Pharmacopeia Vol-III, [2018]	**Ayurvedic Pharmacopeia Vol-I, [1986]**	**Indian Herbal Pharmacopeia [2002]**
Ashwagandha			
Ash value [NMT %]	7	4	7
Acid insoluble value [NMT %]	2	1	1.2
Turmeric			
Ash value [NMT %]	10	9	9
Acid insoluble value [NMT %]	2	1	1
Sarpagandha (Rauwolfia)			
Ash value [NMT %]	8	8	8
Acid insoluble value [NMT %]	2	1	2
Sunthi (Ginger)			
Ash value [NMT %]	8	6	6
Acid insoluble value [NMT %]	1.5	1.5	1.5

Extractive value determination

Extractive value gives idea about soluble chemical constituents in particular solvents. According to IP, alcohol, Pet. Ether and water soluble extractive values should be determined.

Procedure: Weigh accurately quantity of crude drug and macerate it for 24 hr. With intermittent shaking for first 6 hr and allow to stand for further 18 hr. After 24 hr filter and evaporate filtrate. Residue remains after evaporation is value of extractive value of that particular solvent. While determining water extractive value, add 5% chloroform as a microbial growth inhibitor.

Extractive values of popular crude drugs as per pharmacopoeias			
Extractive values	**Name of pharmacopeia**		
	Indian Pharmacopeia Vol-III, [2018]	**Ayurvedic Pharmacopeia Vol-I, [1986]**	**Indian Herbal Pharmacopeia [2002]**
Ashwagandha			
Ethanol soluble extractive value [NLT %]	10	2	20
Water soluble extractive value [NLT %]	15	8	16
Turmeric			
Ethanol soluble extractive value [NLT %]	6	8	8
Water soluble extractive value [NLT %]	12	12	12
Sarpagandha (Rauwolfia)			
Ethanol soluble extractive value [NLT %]	2	4	9
Water soluble extractive value [NLT %]	5	10	8
Sunthi (Ginger)			
Ethanol soluble extractive value [NLT %]	2	3	2
Water soluble extractive value [NLT %]	10	10	10

Determination of moisture content:

An excess of water in medicinal plant material will lead to deterioration through microbial growth or enzyme mediated hydrolysis in glycoside containing plants. Therefore limits for the amount of water should be set for every plant material. Methods of determination of moisture content include:

Loss on Drying: (Gravimetric method):	This test determines loss of both water and volatile matter by drying thermostabel substance at 100-105 °C in oven or thermo labile substances in a desiccators over phosphorus Pentoxide R under atmospheric or reduced pressure and temperature for a specified period of time. In an LOD test, the sample is weighed, dried, and weighed again. The difference in the two weights (Loss on Drying) is then compared with either the original weight (Wet-base test) or final weight (Dry-base test) and the moisture content calculated. Tests can be manually conducted (weigh, oven dry, weigh) or automated (integrated weight and heating unit) with systems called Moisture Determination Balances. Depending on the balance and heating mechanism, a wide array of precision and accuracy is available. Today there are even micromoistureanalyzers, using microbalances that can provide moisture measurement to the PPM level, consistent with the limits of KF testing.LOD Moisture Measurement can be done by: • Forced air ovens. • Convection ovens. • Vacuum ovens. • Infrared moisture balances. • Microwave (drying) ovens. *Procedure:* Take accurately weighed quantity of (about 2-5 g) of the material to be tested in silica crucible and dry the sample by one of the following techniques until constant weight is obtained. Calculate the loss of weight in mg/gof air dried material. ➢ Dry in an oven at 100-105 °C for 4 hr ➢ Dry in desiccator over phos-phorouspentaoxide R under
Azeotropic Method (Toluene distillation method): 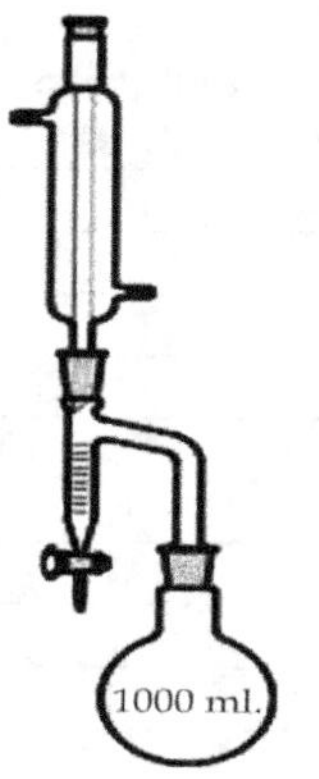 **Fig. 1.9** Water content determination apparatus (Dean Stark apparatus)	This method gives a direct measurement of the water present in the material being examined. When the sample is distilled together with an immiscible solvent, such as toluene R or xylene R. The water present in the sample is absorbed by the solvent, they are distilled together and separated in the receiving tube on cooling. *Procedure:* Take accurately weighed quantity of the material expected to give about 2-3 ml of water into the flask. Heat the flask gently. When boiling begins, distill at a rate of 2 drops/sec until most of the water has distilled over, and then increase the rate of distillation to about 4 drops/sec. After complete distillation, rinse the inside of condenser tube with toluene R. Continue the distillation for 5 more min and again wash any droplets of water adhere to the walls of the receiving tube with toluene. Allow the water and toluene layers to separate and measure volume of the water. Calculate the content of water in % using the formula: % of Water = 100 (n'- n) / w where w = the weight in g of the material being examined. n = the number of ml of water obtained in the first distillation n'= the total number of ml of water obtained in both distillations.

Contd....

Karl Fischer Method	In this methodcolored solution of Karl Fischer reagent (pyridine, sulfur dioxide, iodine, and anhydrous methanol) reacts quantitatively with water to form a colorless solution. This is coulometric or electrochemical titration method to determine water only unlike other methods of moisture content determination where volatile components are also estimated. *Principle:* The working electrode is an iodine electrode, while the reference electrode is a platinum electrode. The reaction involves converting solid iodine into hydrogen iodide in the presence of sulfur dioxide and water. <u>Pyridine</u>, which is a base, is often used to counteract the formation of sulfuric acid. All reagents must be <u>anhydrous</u> for the analysis to be quantitative. Procedure: The main compartment of the titration cell contains the anode solution plus the analyte. The anode solution consists of an alcohol (methanol or diethylene glycol monoethyl ether), a base Pyridine, Sulfur dioxide (SO_2) and iodine (I_2). The titration cell also consists of a smaller compartment with a cathode immersed in the anode solution of this main compartment. A dehydrating solvent suitable for the sample is placed in this flask. The sample is then added. Titration is carried out using a titrant. According to Faraday's laws, the iodine is produced in proportion to the quantity of electricity. This means that the water content can be determined immediately from the coulombs required for electrolytic oxidation. $$\text{1 mg of water = 10.71 Coulombs}$$ Water reaction with Karl-Fischer reagent: $$H_2O + I_2 + SO_2 + 3\ C_5H_5N \rightarrow 2(C_5H_5N{+}H)\ I + C_5H_5N \cdot SO_3$$ $$C_5H_5N \cdot SO_3 + CH_3OH \rightarrow (C_5H_5N{+}H)\ O\text{-}O_2 \cdot OCH_3$$ 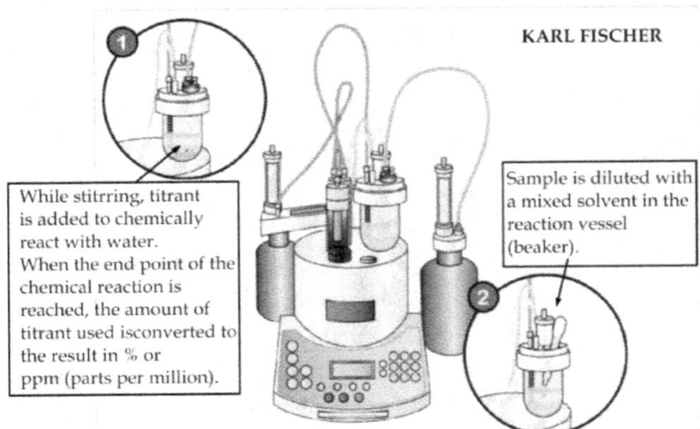 **Fig. 1.20** Karl Fischer apparatus
Modern Methods of moisture content determination	Electrical Methods, Microwave, Nuclear and Near-Infrared methods

> ## Determination of volatile oils

This determination is important standardization parameter for volatile oils containing plant materials. Initially in round bottom flask, add sufficient quantity of xylene R or the solvent given for the material, attach condenser and graduated collector tube. Heat the liquid in the flask until it begins to boil and adjust the distillation rate to 2-3 ml/min. Stop the heating after 30 min, turn off the heater and at least 10 min later, record the volume of solvent xylene collected in the graduated tube. Take the accurately weighed crude plant material and introduce into the flask and continue the distillation. After further 10 min, record the volume of the oil collected in the graduated tube and subtract the volume of the solvent (xylene) previously noted. The difference represents the volume of the volatile oil in the weight of plant material taken. Calculate the content in ml of oil per 100 g of plant material.

Chemical Evaluation

Qualitative Chemical Evaluation: This involves various chemical tests to identify different phytochemicals. For example, Alkaloids can be detected by Mayer's reagent, Dragendroff's reagent, Wagner's reagent; cardiac glycosides by killer killani tests etc.Specific chemical tests can also be helpful in chemical evaluation. For example, Thalleoquin test for quinine.

Quantitative Chemical Evaluation:Quantitative Chemical Assay procedure (Radio immuno assay, Enzyme-linked immunosorbent assay), values (Acid value, iodine value, saponification value for fats and oils whileester value, acetyl value, aldehyde content for volatile oil) and quantitative estimation of individual phytochemicals by using chromatography, spectroscopy etc. are parameters of quantitative chemical evaluation.

Biological Evaluation

When potency of crude drug or its preparations is measured by its effect on microorganisms, organs or tissues of animal then it is known as biological evaluation and if on whole animals like rat, mice, monkey, guinea pig then it is known as pharmacological evaluation. When strength of drug in its preparation is to be evaluated then it is named as bioassays. This is preferred method when chemical or physical evaluation is not satisfactory for material.

In vivo methods	In vivo means "within the living. In this method drug effects are tested on whole, living organisms or cells, usually animals, including humans and plants. Animal testing and clinical trials are major elements of in vivo research. **Anti- inflammatory activity determination** Method/Model : Carrageenan rat paw edema model Animal : Rats Standard drug : Diclofenac Disease inducing agent : Carrageenan Duration : 3 hr Method of evaluation : Measurement of paw edema by using Plethysmometeror vernier caliper Calculations : Percentage of inhibition of
In vitro methods	In vitro studies are performed with microorganisms, cells, or biological molecules outside their normal biological context in labware such as test tubes, flasks, Petri dishes, and microtiter plates **In vitro anticancer activity on determination using animal cells or tissues:** In metabolic assays in which, the cellular reduction of a colorless tetrazolium salt (MTT or XTT) yields a colored formazan in proportion to viable cell number. The formazans could be measured con-veniently in an automated colorimeter.

Contd....

	Procedure: Take cancer cells of 3 x 105 cells/well concentration in a 96 well plate except at least three wells without cells to serve as a control for the minimum absorbance. Incubate plate overnight at 37°C in a humidified incubator, 5% CO2 for the cancer cells to grow and adhere to the surface. Add Test compounds in to the plate. Include replicates for a range of concentrations. Include negative controls (including vehicle control) and a positive control. The final volume will be 100µl per well. Incubate plate for overnight (or for some other appropriate time) at 37°C in a humidified incubator, 5% CO2. Then add 3-(4,5-dimethylthiazol-2-yl)-2,5-diphenyltetrazolium bromide (MTT) reagent (20µl/100µl per well of the 96 well plate). Incubate at 37°C for 3 hours then add 2.0 ml of 10% Trichloroacetic acid to stop further reaction and shake plate at room temperature for a minimum of 1 hour. After the 1 hour incubation, ensure the formazan precipitate is dissolved by pippeting each well up and down until no precipitate is visible. Read the plate on a plate reader using wavelength at 572 nm. Tabulate results and calculate the % viability.
	Antimicrobial activity Three methods can be useful to determine antimicrobial activity i.e. agar well method, turbidometric method and bioautographic method. In agar well method, select media specific to microorganisms and prepare plates of solid media Add microbial strains of optimum dilutions and then prepare well in plate by bore, add sample and standard solution in wells, incubate it for 24 hr for bacteria and 72 hr for Fungi. Measure zone of inhibition in mm by scale and compare with standard. In turbidometric method, prepare tubes of liquid media; add strains and sample solutions, incubate it 24 hr for bacteria and 72 hr for Fungi. Measure turbidity of liquid solutions by spectrophotometer and compare with standard. Bioautographic method involves use of TLC plates where media and microbial strain is applied over pre developed plates and allowed to incubate for 24 to 72 hr depending upon microorganism. Sepa-rated fractions on TLC having antimicro-bial activity would show zone of inhibition in visible light or after spraying with reagents like MTT which are able to differentiate between live or dead cells. 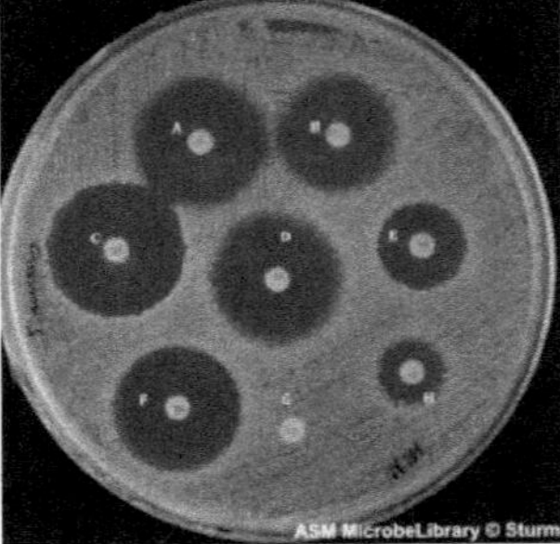 **Fig. 1.21** Zone of inhibition area indicates antimicrobial potency
Ex vivo methods	Ex vivo refers to experimentation or measurements done in or on tissue from an organism in an external environment with minimal alteration of natural conditions. Ex vivo conditions allow experimentation on an organism's cells or tissues under more controlled conditions than is possible in in vivo experiments (in the intact organism), at the expense of altering the "natural" environment. Tissues may be removed in many ways, including in part, as whole organs, or as larger organ systems.
In silico methods	Experiments are performed on computer or via computer simulation. Virtual screening (VS) is a computational technique used in drug discovery to search libraries of small molecules in order to identify those structures which are most likely to bind to a drug target, typically a protein receptor or enzyme. There methods can be ligand-based, structure-based or hybrid techniques.

Subjective Questions

1. Define Pharmacognosy. Write in brief about scope and developments of Pharmacognosy.
2. What are different sources of crude drugs?
3. How to classify crude drugs? Explain with suitable examples.
4. What is difference between chemotaxonmy and serotaxonomy?
5. Define adulteration and explain how crude drugs are adulterated?
6. What is oraganoleptic evaluation? Explain with suitable examples.
7. What is stomata? What are different types of stomata. Explain with examples.
8. What is trichome? What are different types of trichomes. Explain with examples.
9. What is cystoliths?
10. What is quantitative microscopy? Explain with suitable examples.
11. Write note on leaf constants.
12. What is formula for stomatal index determination?
13. What is formula for determination of percentage purity by Lycopodium spore method?
14. What is difference between vein islets and vein termination?
15. Write a note on Lycopodium spore method.
16. Why spores of Lycopodium are useful for quantitative microscopy.
17. What is camera lucida and how it is useful in Pharmacognosy?
18. What is micrometer? How it is useful in pharmacognosy?.

Multiple Choice Questions (MCQs)

1. .... is one of the oldest as well as famous surviving document belonging to 1600 B. C
   a. Papyrus Ebers
   b. Materia medica
   c. Samhita
   d. Analecta pharmacognostica

2. ....is the oldest chinese herbal doccument written by emperor Shen Nungarround 3000 B. C
   a. Huang Di Nei Jing
   b. Pen-t' sao
   c. Internal medicine
   d. None of the above

3. *Charak Samhita* and *Sushrutha Samhita* are well known treaties in
    a. Homeopathy
    b. Sidha
    c. Unani
    d. Ayurveda

4. Which one of the following is known as "father of Medicine"?
    a. Hippocrates
    b. Aristotle
    c. Galen
    d. None of the above

5. Which one of the following is known as first pharmacist to introduce opium as a pain relieving material in his apothecary?
    a. Hippocrates
    b. Galen
    c. Aristotle
    d. Dioscorides

6. Paracelsus (1493 - 1541) is doccumented in history for
    a. Development of mineral salts as drug
    b. Development of sea salts as drugs
    c. Development of rock salts as drugs
    d. Both a and b

7. The importance of extraction method and alcohol as an extractant was reported by…………..
    a. William Withering
    b. Serturner
    c. Le'mery
    d. None of the above

8. Who isolated narcotine from opium in 1803?
    a. Serturner
    b. Derosne
    c. both a and b
    d. None of the above

9. In 1806, morphine was isolated from opium by………………..
    a. Derosne
    b. Serturner
    c. Pelletier
    d. None of the above

10. In 1852 extraction process for alkaloids was first introduced by.........................
    a. Stass and Otto
    b. Posslet and Reimann
    c. Gerrard and Hardy
    d. Neumann

11. Nicotine was first time isolated in 1828 by............................
    a. Stass and Otto
    b. Posslet and Reimann
    c. Gerrard and Hardy
    d. Neumann

12. The term "Pharmacognosy" was first coined by German scientist................
    a. Seydler in 1815
    b. Seydler in 1820
    c. Pelletier in 1815
    d. Pelletier in 1820

13. Coccaine was first discovered by.......................
    a. Reimann
    b. Neumann
    c. Neuton
    d. Neimann

14. Pharmacognosy deals with
    a. Crude drugs from natural origin
    b. Crude drugs from synthetic origin
    c. Both a and b
    d. None of the above

15. Pharmacognosy is important link between.................
    a. Pharmacology
    b. Medicinal chemistry
    c. Both a and b
    d. None of the above

16. Crude drug materials which represent a part of the plant are classified as,
    a. Organized crude drugs
    b. Unorganized crude drugs
    c. Both a and b
    d. None of the above

17. Crude drugs representing a diverse group of solid and liquid materials which do not consists of parts of plants and obtained from natural sources are classified as,

    a.   Organized crude drugs
    b.   Unorganized crude drugs
    c.   Both a and b
    d.   None of the above

18. Dried latex, gums, mucillages comes under category of

    a.   Organized crude drugs
    b.   Unorganized crude drugs
    c.   Both a and b
    d.   None of the above

19. Quinine was first isolated in

    a.   1818
    b.   1819
    c.   1820
    d.   1821

20. Ephedrine was first discovered by ....

    a.   Neumann
    b.   Nagai
    c.   Kuersten
    d.   Gerrard

21. In pharmacopoeias, crude drugs are arranged in alphabetical order of their .... and .... names

    a.   Latin and English.
    b.   German and English.
    c.   French and English
    d.   Italian and English

22. Which one of the classification is based on phylogeny among plants or animals?

    a.   Alphabetical
    b.   Taxonomic
    c.   Chemotaxonomic
    d.   Therapeutic

23. In the drug name, *Glycerrhiza glabra, Glycerrhiza* represents

    a.   Species.
    b.   Genus.
    c.   Family
    d.   Class

24. Which one of the following drug belongs to solanaceae family?
    a. *Hyoscyamus Niger.*
    b. *Atropa belladonna.*
    c. *Glycyrhhiza glabra*
    d. Both a and b

25. *Myroxylonbalsamum* belongs to family
    a. Solanaceae.
    b. Apocynsceae.
    c. Scrophulariaceae
    d. Leguminosae

26. The drug isabgol according to morphology, classified as
    a. Seeds.
    b. Husk.
    c. Leaves
    d. Bark

27. Cinnamon drug represents ……….. part of plant
    a. Wood.
    b. Roots.
    c. Rhizomes
    d. Bark

28. Gelatin comes under the category of
    a. Dried juices.
    b. Dried latices.
    c. Dried extracts
    d. None of the above

29. Choose correct pair from following
    a. Glycosides   1. Eucalyptus
    b. Alkaloids.   2. Vinca
    c. Tannins.   3. Cinchona
    d. Lipids   4. Ashoka
    a. A-2
    b. C-4
    c. B-1
    d. C-3

30. Papain chemically classified as
    a.   Vitamins and hormones.
    b.   Proteins and enzymes.
    c.   Resins
    d.   Glycosides
31. Which drugs acts as purgative?
    a.   Cascara.
    b.   Colocynth.
    c.   Senna
    d.   All of the above
32. Which one of the following drug classified as both anti-malarial as well as bitter tonic?
    a.   Cascara
    b.   Kurchi.
    c.   Cinnamon
    d.   Cinchona
33. Choose the correct pair from following
    A.   Emetic.   A. Ipecacunha
    B.   Expectorant.   B. Morphine
    C.   Antitussive.   C. Pilocarpus
    D.   Cholinergic.   D. Liquorice
    a.   AA
    b.   BB.
    c.   CC.
    d.   DD
34. Which one of the following acts as skeletal muscle relaxant?
    a.   Opium.
    b.   Coffee
    c.   Datura.
    d.   Curare
35. Which one of the following acts as smooth muscle relaxant?
    a.   Coffee.
    b.   Curare.
    c.   Opium
    d.   Ipecacunha

36. Coca is therapeutically characterized as
    a. Antidepressant.
    b. Analgesic.
    c. Local anaesthetic
    d. CNS stimulant

37. .... is therapeutically classified as anti-expectorant
    a. Vasaka.
    b. Ipecacunha.
    c. Liquorice
    d. Stramonium leaves

38. Which one of the following is therapeutically catagorized as analeptic?
    a. Camphor.
    b. Lobelia.
    c. Both a and b
    d. None of the above

39. Chemotaxonomic classification mainly deals with
    a. Understanding of biological evolution of plant and their chemistry
    b. Understanding of therapeutic activities
    c. Understanding of morphology
    d. None of the above

40. DNA hybridisation and taxonomy are involved in
    a. Pharmacology.
    b. Serotaxonomy.
    c. Chemotaxonomy
    d. None of the above

41. Adulteration is
    a. Debasement of natural drug
    b. Substitution of original crude drug partially or wholly with spurious substances
    c. Performed deliberately for commercial benefits
    d. All of the above

42. Impairment in quality of drug is known as
    a. Admixture.
    b. Sophistication.
    c. Substitution
    d. Deterioration

43. Admixture is the practice in which one article is added to another due to

    a.   Carelessness.

    b.   Ignorance.

    c.   Accidental

    d.   All of the above

44. The term used for deliberate or intentional adulteration is called

    a.   Substitution

    b.   Sophistication

    c.   Both a and b

    d.   None of the above

45. ....occurs when some totally different substance is added in place of original drug

    a.   Substitution.

    b.   Sophistication.

    c.   Deterioration

    d.   d. Both b and c

46. Spoilage is due to

    a.   Microorganisms.

    b.   Minerals.

    c.   Heat

    d.   Cold

47. In terms of adulteration, inferiority means

    a.   High standard drug

    b.   Low standard drug

    c.   Substandard drug

    d.   Both a and b

48. Strychnusnux-vomica is commercially adulterated with

    a.   Strychnusnuxblanda

    b.   Strychnuspotatorum

    c.   Both a and b

    d.   None of the above

49. Alianthus leaves are inferior quality substitution for

    a.   Catharanthus rosus.

    b.   Atropa belladonna.

    c.   Azadirecta indica

    d.   CentellaAsiatics

50. Saffron is usually adulterated with inferior quality
    a.   Carthamus victorious.
    b.   Carthamus tinctorius.
    c.   Carthamus tinctona
    d.   Carthamus roseus

51. Evaluation of crude drug is necessary because
    a.   Biochemical variation of a drug
    b.   Deterioration due to treatment and storage
    c.   Substitution and adulteration
    d.   All of the above

52. Morphological or organoleptic evaluation is technique of
    a.   Qualitative investigation
    b.   Quantitative investigation
    c.   Both
    d.   None

53. Microscopy is
    a.   Study of form of crude drug
    b.   Description of form of crude drug
    c.   Both
    d.   None

54. Morphology is
    a.   Study of form of crude drug
    b.   Description of form of drug
    c.   Both
    d.   None

55. Chemo-microscopy involves
    a.   Application action of chemicals to micro constituents of drug before study under microscope
    b.   Application of chemicals to micro constituents of drug after study under microscope
    c.   Application of chemicals to microscope
    d.   None of the above

56. A drop of phlroglucinol and concentrated hydrochloric acid gives ....stain in the presence of lignin
    a.   Yellow.
    b.   Green.
    c.   Violet
    d.   Red

57. In powdered microscopic of aloe, different varieties of aloe can be identified based on
    a.   Number of stomata
    b.   Number of calcium oxalate crystals
    c.   Presence or absence of raphide crystals
    d.   Presence or absence of chloroplast pigments

58. The diameter of starch grains in *Cinnamomum cassia* is
    a.   9 micron.
    b.   11 micron.
    c.   10 microns
    d.   12 microns

59. Palisade ratio of leaf drug *Digitalis purpura*
    a.   3.1 – 4.2.
    b.   3.2 – 4.2.
    c.   3.7 – 4.2
    d.   3.8 – 4.2

60. In microscopic evaluation, which one of the following represents quantitative analysis?
    a.   Lycopodium Assay
    b.   Vein islet number
    c.   Stomatal index.
    d.   All of the above

61. Which types of stomata are present in coca and senna leaves?
    a.   Paracyclic
    b.   Rubiaceous.
    c.   Both a and b
    d.   Anisocytic

62. Which type of trichome is present in *Calendula officinalis*?
    a.   Unbranched triseriate.
    b.   Unbranched biserriate.
    c.   Unbranched uniserriate
    d.   d. None of the above

63. Diameter of Lycopodium spores is
    a.   20 micrometer.
    b.   22 micrometer.
    c.   23 micrometer
    d.   25 micrometer

64. 1 milligram of powdered Lycopodium contains on an average
    a.   95000 spores.
    b.   94000 spores.
    c.   10000 spores
    d.   99000 spores

65. Which one of the following technique is used for separation of components of volatile oils?
    a.   Extraction.
    b.   Distillation.
    c.   Sublimation
    d.   Fractional crystallization

66. Which one of the following method is used for purification of alkaloids from extracts?
    a.   Sublimation.
    b.   Steam distillation.
    c.   Fractional crystallization
    d.   d. Fractional liberation

67. Foam test is specifically used for identification of
    a.   Tannins.
    b.   Saponins.
    c.   Alkaloids
    d.   Glycosides

68. Melting point range of cocoa butter
    a.   30 – 33.
    b.   25 – 30.
    c.   35 - 40
    d.   40 – 45

69. Camera Lucida is specifically used for determination of leaf constants like
    a.   Stomatal number.
    b.   Vein islet number.
    c.   Palisade ratio
    d.   All of the above

70. Volatile oil content in clove is....................
    a.   Not less than 15.0 (%w/w).
    b.   More than 15% w/w.
    c.   Not less than 10% w/w
    d.   More than 10% w/w

Answer Key

1.a	2. b	3. d	4. a	5. b	6. a	7. c	8. b	9. b	10. a
11.c	12. a	13. b	14. a	15. c	16. a	17. b	18.b	19. c	20. b
21.a	22.b	23. c	24. d	25. d	26. a	27. d	28. c	29. b	30. b
31. d	32. d	33.a	34. d	35. c	36. c	37. d	38. c	39. a	40. b
41. d	42. d	43. d	44. b	45. a	46. a	47. b	48. c	49. b	50. b
51. d	52. a	53. b	54. a	55. a	56. d	57. c	58. a	59. c	60. d
61. c	62. b	63. d	64. b	65. b	66. d	67. b	68. a	69. d	70. a

Unit 2

2.1 Cultivation and Collection of Medicinal Plants

Due to popularity of medicinal plants for primary health care and prevention of diseases, natural resources of these plants are destroyed by human being. But sound knowledge of Cultivation technology has resulted in gradual depletion of raw material from wild sources. Cultivation of medicinal plants requires knowledge, skills, and technologies used to grow intensively produced plants for human food and non-food uses and for personal or social needs. Actual work involves plant propagation and cultivation with the aim of improving plant growth, yields, quality, nutritional value, and resistance to insects, diseases, and environmental stresses. Wild medicinal plant collection damages natural environment due to extinction of a species and many times it is difficult to collect correct plant from remote areas like mountains, forests etc. So cultivation of medicinal plants allows preservation of endangered medicinal plants and thus natural resources improves quality and quantity as well as yield of drugs and builds up national economy.

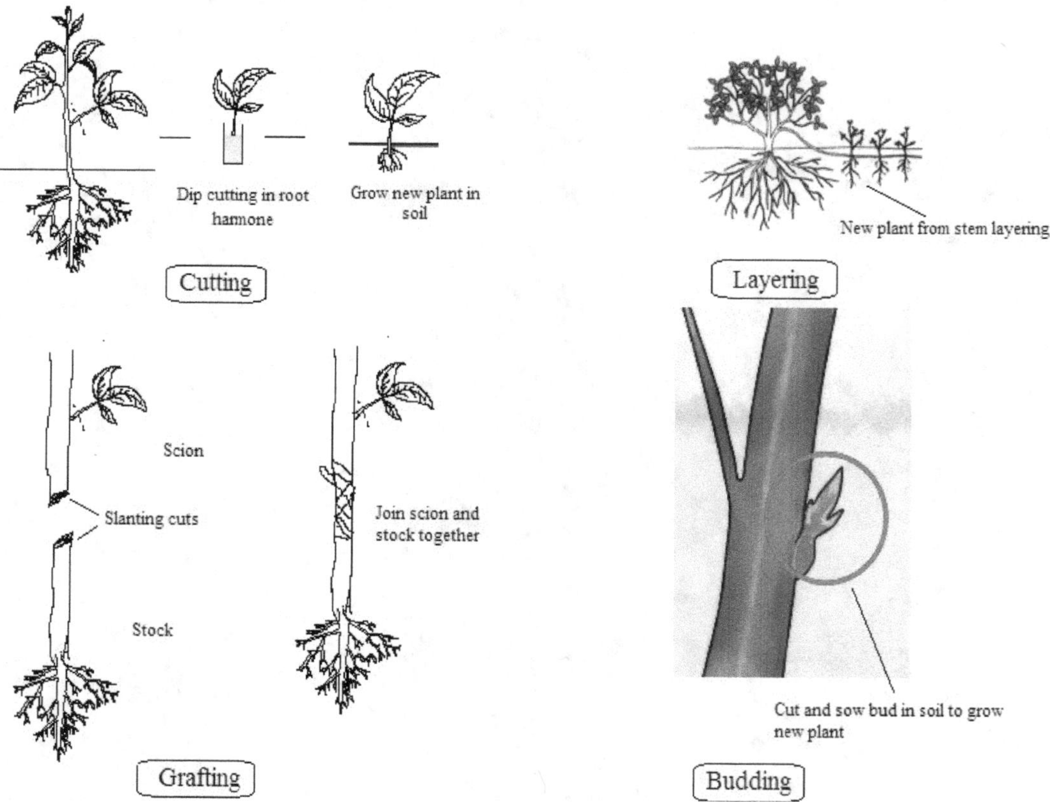

Fig. 2.1 Different Asexual (vegetative) propagation methods

Following are Methods of propagation				
Method	**Sexual (seed) propagation**	**Asexual (vegetative) propagation**		
Material of propagation	Seeds are sowed by broadcasting (scattering of extremely small seeds) or dibbling (sowing of large size seeds into holes) method	**Natural**: Bulbs (garlic), tubers (aconite), offsets (aloe), corms (saffron), rhizomes (ginger), roots, suckers (banana), stolons (licorice)	**Artificial**: Cuttings (rose, brahmi), layering (lemon), grafting (mango), budding (hibiscus)	**Tissue culture**: Laboratory developed cultures of plants (Example: Banana)
Advantages	Cheap method of raising Seedlings which are long-lived, sturdy and suitable for plants which cannot be propagated by asexual method	Uniformity in yield and other characters, fast in growth, seedless, nutrients improved or disease resistant varieties can be obtained		
Disadvantages	Time consuming and costly as to grow seed-lings first and then actual plant, poor uniformity in yield of seedlings,	Poor adaptability to climatic changes and hence short lived		

Collection

Collection of drugs from cultivated plants always ensures a true natural source and reliable products. This may or may not be this case when drugs are cultivated from wild plants.

Following are factors to be considered at the time of collection	
Labour	Drugs may be collected from wild or cultivated plants and the task may be undertaken by casual, unskilled native labour. Example- Ipecacuanha
	Drug may be collected by skill worker in a highly scientific manner. Example- Digitalis, Cinchona, Belladona
Season	The season at which each drug is collected is also important, since the amount and sometimes the nature of the active constituents is not constructed through the year. Example- Podophyllum, Ephedra, Rhubarb, Aconite
	Rhubarb contains no anthraquinone derivatives in winter but contain anthranols which on the arrival of warmer weather are converted by oxidation into anthraquinone.
Age	The age of plant is also considerable important and governs not only the total quntity of active constitute produced but also the components of the active mixure. Clove (volatile oil): Cloves contain about 11-21% oil while mother blown cloves contain very little oil. Datura (alkaloids): The hyoscine/hyoscyamine ratio falls from about 80% in young seedlings to about 30% in mature frutings plants.
Geographical location	Geographical location also affects the cultivation in a certain extent. Location helps in development of the desired type and amount of constitutes. Example- *Ammi vianaga* growing wild in the mediteranean area contains variety of a coumarins and chromones in its seeds, however same plant cultivated in Arizona, found to produce plenty seeds practilly devoid of the desired constituents

Harvesting

Harvesting is the process of collection of the highest quality crude drug from its original source in the appropriate season and time of the day.

Leaves are collected from plants during the flowering season when the plant is very active.

➤ Bark is collected in spring or early summer.

➤ Flowers are collected about the time of pollination in dry weather in the forenoon when the dew has disappeared and dried in shade.

➤ Roots and tubers are collected in autumn when the plant is inactive and the vegetative process has ceased and contain the maximum active constituents.

Drying is essential for maintaining the quality of crude drugs after collection to avoid decomposition, microbial growth, enzyme activation and other possible chemical changes. Herbal raw drugs are dried prior to extraction to avoid detoriation on storage and transport as well as to facilitate grinding. In the preparation of crude drugs, drying is usually designed to yield a stable, homogenous product which is easy to manupulate in subsequent operation of storage and packaging.

Drying is defined as the removal of a liquid or moisture contents from a material (herbal drugs) by the application of heat and is accomplished by the transfer of a liquid or moisture content from a surface into an unsaturated vapour phase.

Proper and successful drying depends on control of temperature and regulation of air flow. Drying process is to be done depending upon source of herbal crude drug and its chemical nature.

• If enzymatic action is to be encouraged, slow drying is necessary at moderate temperature. Example- Orris rhizome, Vanilla pods, Cocoa seed, Gentian root.

• If enzymatic action is not desired, drying should take place as soon as possible after collection. Drugs containing volatile oil are liable to lose their aroma if not dried or if the oil is not distilled from them immediately.

Two types of drying are classified as follows:

1. Natural drying (sun drying)

(a) ***Direct sun drying (outdoor drying)***: The crude drugs can be dried directly in sunshine if the contents of crude drugs are quite stable to the temperature and sunlight. Example: Gum acacia, seeds, fruit are dried by direct sun drying method.

(b) ***Shed drying:***Shed drying is prepared when the natural colors of the drug (digitalis leaves, clove, senna leaves) and volatile principles of the drug (Example- Peppermint) are to be retained. Drying in the shed at the air temperature is frequently adopted especially for leaves containing oil.

2. Artificial drying

(a) ***Tray dryer: (truck dryer):*** This is most commonly used method in the pharmaceutical plant operatation. Tray dryers are used for drying heat stable plant material. Example-roots, barks. In this process, hot air of desired temperature is circulated through the dryers and this facilitates the removal of water content of the drugs. This is simplest and inexpensive method. Disadvantage of tray dryers is deterioration of material due to high residence time at high temperature.

(b) *Vaccum dryer:* In this method, vaccum facilitates drying of plant material at low temperature. It can handle stiky, free flowing, hygroscopic, heat sensitive plant meterials. Examples- Tannic acid, Digitalis leaves.

(c) *Spray dryer:* This is used for non-hygroscopic products. This is continous, thermally efficient dryer where filtered atmospheric hot air comes in contact with atomized fine mist of the feed and instantly evaporates the water in the feed droplets. The fluidized mixture of air and powder get separted in cyclone separator. This method of drying retains all the original properties of plant material such as color, aroma, efficacy, density etc.

Pulverisation

Pulverisation or comminution is a process of fragmenting a substance into small particles by mechanical forces. It is one of the important process operation and inevitable in very first step of herbal extraction. Comminution of different parts of the herbal drugs can be explained as followed.

Crude Drug	Details and type of mills useful
Leaf drugs	Leaf drugs are predominant in herbal industry. • Shredding mills - medicinal leaves and herbs with high content of stem and stalk • Hammer mills- for resinous and friable leaf drugs • Pin mills – leaf drugs with high fat content or ethereal oil.
Roots and barks	Roots and barks are moderately hard or woody but sometimes brittle and friable also. Example- Cinnamon, Quercus, Ipecacuanha • Shredder mills- cutting and shredding • Hammer mills- grinding
Seeds and fruits	The comminution of seeds and fruits offer proves to be particularly difficult because of their content of fats and ethereal oils. Example- coffee and cocoa beans. • Shredder mills – comminution
Other drug plant materials	These include flowers, part of flowers and products such as alginates, agar, and gelatins • Shredder mills – comminution

Garbling

The next step in preparation of crude drug for market after drying is garbling which is the final step of the preparation of crude drug. The process is desired when sand, dirt and foreign parts of the same plant, not constituents are required to be removed. If extraneous matter to be removed permitted in crude drugs, the quality of crude drugs suffers and at times it doesn't pass pharmacopoeial limits. Example: 1. excessive stem in case of lobelia and stramonium need to be removed. 2. Stalks, in case of cloves are to be detected. 3. Drugs constituting rhizomes need to be separated carefully from roots and rootlets and also stem bases. 4. Pieces of iron must be removed with the magnet in case of caster seeds before crushing 5. Shifting in case of vinca and senna leaves. 6. Pieces of bark should be removed by peelings as in gum acacia.

Packing

The morphological and chemical nature of the drug, its ultimate use and effect of climatic conditions during transportation and storage should be taken into consideration while packing of drugs.

- Colophony and balsam packed in kerosene tins.
- Asafoetida is stored in well-closed container to prevent loss of volatile oil.
- Cod liver oil is sensitive to sunlight so it should be stored in such containers, which will not affect the sunlight.
- Leaf drug like senna, vinca are pressed and baled.
- Drug (like digitalis, ergot, squills) which very sensitive to moisture and costly at the same time need special attention.
- Colophony needs to be packed in big masses to control auto oxidation.
- Crude drugs like roots, seeds and other part packed in gummy bags.
- Weight of certain drug in lots also kept constant e.g. Indian opium.

Packing material and specific storage of Raw Herbs

1. Woody in nature like stem, heartwood, bark etc. : Gunny bags and woven sacks
2. Soft in nature like creepers, leaves etc. : High gauge HMHD bags, woven sacks with LD liner, High gauge polyethylene bags
3. Fleshy in nature like fruits, rhizomes etc.: High gauge HMHD bags, woven sacks with LD liner, wooden boxes.
4. Flowers, anthers, stigma, petals, seeds etc. : Corrugated box with polypropylene woven sacks, HDPE containers, Fiber board's drums
5. Volatile contents: Air tight HDPE containers, Air tight HDPE carboys, Card board box with polyethylene liners
6. Herbal extracts and compounds: Air tight HDPE containers, corrugated box with polyethylene woven sacks and fiber board's drums with polyethylene bags. HDHM (High molecular weight high density polyethylene), LD liner (Low density liner bags), HDPE (High density polyethylene)

Storage of Herbal Raw Drug

1. Proper storage and preservative are important factors in maintaining a high degree of quality of the drug.
2. Warehouse should preferably be of fire proof, steel, concrete or brick construction, and unheated and rodent proof.

3. Hard packed bales usually reabsorb little moisture. This is also true of barks and resinous drug but leaf, herbs, and roots drugs that are not well packed tend to absorb moisture up to 10%, 15%, or 30% of weight of drug.

4. Excessive moisture not only increases the weight of the drug. Thus reducing the % of active constituents but also favours enzymatic activity and facilitates fungal growth. Eg. Digitalis glycoside is deteriorate when moisture in the drug reaches 8% or higher.

5. Liquid adversely affects drugs, which are higher colored, rendering them unattractive and possibly causing undesirable changes in constituents. It has been shown that polarized light changes more rapidly the ordinary light.

6. The oxygen of the air increase oxidation of the constituent so of the drugs, especially when oxidases (oxidizing enzymes) are present.

7. Insects also attack on crude herbal drugs so to prevention of their attacks a number of methods have been employed. The simple method of all being to expose the drug to a temperature of 65°C. They also prevent form determination.

8. The fumigation of large lots of crude drugs such as stored in warehoused and manufacturing plants, the use of methyl bromide.

9. Small lots of drugs may readily be stored in air-light, moisture proof and lightproof containers.

10. If drugs in small quantities are stored in air-tight containers, insect attack can be controlled by the addition of a few drops of chloroform or CCl_4.

11. Certain drugs such as biologics must be stored at a temperature between 2° and 10°C

2.2 Processing of Herbal Raw Materials

Before using a crude drug for production of herbal formulations, it should be properly processed so that, the active constituents and the appearance of the drug do not deteriorate before being used. The information on the raw material(s) and the solvents/reagents or vehicles used for the Herbal Stock(s) and final dilution preparation should be evaluated. For raw materials of botanical origin, the scientific name -genus, species, variety, chemo type, part employed and other names should be provided. For raw materials of biological origin, the scientific name (e.g., animal), -genus, species- tissue(s), fluid(s), parts of organ(s) or organ(s) used and other names should be evaluated. For minerals or chemicals, the international non-proprietary name (I.N.N), chemical and other names should be evaluated. For raw materials of botanical origin, the state (e.g. fresh, dried) of the material used and, where applicable, information on pharmacological active, toxic constituents or marker compound(s), if applicable, should be analyzed. Additionally a macroscopic and microscopic description of the raw material should be evaluated. For raw materials of biological origin, information on the physical and/or anatomical and histological state (where applicable) should be evaluated. For minerals or chemicals, physical form, structural formula, molecular formula and relative molecular mass, where applicable, should be evaluated. The preparation of a crude drug for the market depends on the following major processes.

2.3 Factors Affecting Cultivation

These factors include the environmental and ecological factors. These factors not only influence the production but also activity of the crude drugs.

Exogenous / Extrinsic Factors	Endogenous/ Intrinsic Factors
1. Climate: Temperature, Light radiation, Humidity, Day length 2. Soil And Soil Fertility 3. Altitude and latitude 4. Fertilizers 5. Age of plant/ stage of development 6. Pests and pest control 7. Allelopathy	These are the factors related to the genetics of plants, which affects the cultivation process. Members of given species are rarely homogenous. The difference in the genetic makeup can cause not only morphological variation but also bio-chemical diversity, i.e., they can bring about difference in the amount and type of chemical constituents present. Main intrinsic factors involved: ➢ Selection ➢ Mutation ➢ Polyploidy ➢ Hybridization ➢ Chemodemes ➢ Plant growth regulators

Following are details of Exogenous / Extrinsic Factors	
Climate	Climate e.g. temperature, rainfall, length of day and altitude, plays an important role in the growth of plants. Plants should be cultivated in conditions which are similar to the plant's natural habitat. **Weather** -Different crops require different climatic pattern. The growth of plant and flower and fruiting condition depends upon the climate and light. Example: In cloudy weather the amount of carbohydrates in leaves is decreased, since photosynthesis is light-dependent. **Temperature**- Temperature is an important factor controlling the development and metabolism of plants by affecting various biochemical reactions. Excessive as well as very low temperature also affects quality of medicinal plants adversely. Examples: Camphor and coffee can't withstand frost whereas saffron needs only cold climate. Fixed oil produced at lower temperature contains fatty acid with a higher content of double bonds than those formed at higher temperature. **Irrigation or Rainfall**- Medicinal plants require great care in managing proper irrigation or sufficient rainfall distribution for desire growth as it affects humidity as well as water holding capacity of soil. Examples: cinchona and cinnamon need high rainfall. High rainfall causes loss of volatile oil from leaves. Continuous rainfall is responsible for loss/leaching of water-soluble substances like glycosides, tannins and flavonoids and some volatile oils through leaves and roots. **Moisture or Humidity**- The moisture present in the drug depends upon the relative moisture present in the atmosphere, which is expressed in terms of humidity. Humidity condition for storage in underground cellars will depend upon the nature of soil. Examples: In high humidity conditions materials like starch, squill, gentian, gelatin, etc. will absorb deleterious amount of moisture. In digitalis moisture content of more than 5% will activate various enzymes undergoing a rapid change. **Light**- Light is also essential for rooting, cutting, germination of seeds, Shooting multiplication of plants, flowering, ripening of fruits etc. Sunny location increases the alkaloidal contents of belladona plant. Peppermint gives less menthol but more menthone when cultivated in the shady location than in open field. The color of light is also helpful in many plant processes. The daily variation in the proportion of secondary metabolites is probably light controlled. Example: Red light enhances seed germination, blue light enhance *in-vitro* bud regeneration of potato. In full

Contd...

	sunshine gives a higher content of alkaloids than in shade. In short day light, peppermint contains menthofuran in more amount, but in long day lightmenthol, menthone, and traces of menthofuran.
Soil and Soil Fertility	Soil is the top cover of earth and it is most important resource as it supports growth of all plants. Soil contains minerals, organic matter, water, etc. The commonly known soil is the shallow upper layer and is the friable material in which plant finds foot-hold and nutrition. Soil contains the macro and micro nutrients and help in the growth of the plant. Plant growth depends upon following factors of soil: - Physical arrangement - Nature of soil particles - Organic matter content - Types of organisms present in the soil Soil affects the plant in the following ways: - It provides surface for the growing plants - It provides water to the plants - It provides nutrition - it provides the mechanical strength to the plant

Types of soil based on particle size	
Types of soil	**Particle size**
Fine clay	Less than 0.002 mm
Coarse clay or slit	0.002-0.02 mm
Fine sand	0.02-0.2 mm
Coarse sand	0.2-2 mm

Types of soil based on their percentage covered	
Soil type	**Percentage covered**
Clay	More than 50% of clay
Loamy	39-50% of clay
Slit loam	20-30% of clay
Sandy loam	10-20% of clay
Sandy soil	More than 70% of sandy soil
Calcareous soil	More than 20% of lime

Minerals: Minerals present in the soil are mostly $CaCO_3$, mixture of oxides of aluminium, iron with small amount of magnesium oxide and titanium oxide. And on the basis of various minerals present, the soil is classified as-Calcareous soil<20% of $CaCO_3$ **and** Peatic soil-80-90% of humus darker in color etc.

Organic Matter: It consists of legworm, fungi, bacteria, and insects. The residue from the decay is called humus and provides: nutrition, holds water. Soil contains the water in moisture form. And the capillary water is good for the plants. Examples of plants which grow in various types of soil:

- Clay- rauwolfia
- Clay loamy- rauwolfia
- Loamy sand- isabgol
- Loamy soil- dill, nutmeg, ginger, peppermint, squill, licorice, cinnamon, digitalis, vinca, etc.

Contd…

	Fertility of Soil: It is the capacity of soil to provide nutrients to the plant in adequate amount and in balance proportions. Soil fertility can be maintained by addition of animal manures, nitrogen fixing bacteria or by application of chemical fertilizers e.g. manuring of belladona with nitrate and farmyard manure raises the alkaloid content. A soil good for plant growth should have half of the pore spaces filled with water and rest with air, since good aeration is essential for root development. A soil can be said fertile, if it is having: - God variety of minerals and organic matter - High percentage of capillary water content - Good aeration - High nutrient handling capacity - Permeability, calorific value, capillary of soil ***pH of Soil:*** pH is the measure of hydrogen ion concentration and it can affect the germination of seeds, rooting of plants and micro-propagation of explants. pH also determines the presence of various types of nutrients and organisms in the soil. The maximum availability of plant nutrients is in between the pH range of 6.5-7.5. Due to heavy rainfall, the upper soil is having high % of acids and it can be removed by application of gypsum or by removing the upper surface of soil. pH of soil can be raised by injecting dolomite limestone into the soil and it can be lowered by injecting H_2SO_4 and phosphoric acid. Depending upon pH soil can be divided into: - Neutral soil: Peppermint and opium requires the neutral soil with pH 6-9. - Acidic soil: *Datura stramonium* requires pH 6-8. *Majorana hortensis* requires pH 5.6-8.2. - Alkaline soil: Dill requires the slightly acidic soil with pH 8-10.
Altitude and Latitude	Altitude and Latitude are very important factors in cultivation of medicinal plants. It can't be produced artificially. ❖ Senna can be cultivated at sea level while Digitalis and Pyrethrum grows at higher altitude. Cinnamon, clove and cardamom are grown at a height of 500-1000m. Tea, cinchona, Camphor and eucalyptus are cultivated favorably at an altitude of 1000-2000 m. ❖ The bitter constituents of *Gentiana lutea* are increased with altitude. The alkaloids of *Aconitum napellus* and *Lobelliainflata* and the oil content of Thyme and Peppermint decrease with altitude. Tropical region contains largely saturated fatty acids (palm oil, cocoa butter) and Subtropical plants contain large proportion of unsaturated fatty acids (oleic acid is predominat in almond oil, clove oil).
Age of Plant	Age of plant plays an important role in yield of the medicinally active plant material obtained. Also the age of plant plays an important role if its short cutting is used for the vegetative propagation. Example- Camphor tree accumulates more and more camphor from year to year, for this reason this is not used for camphor production until it has reached the age of about 40 years, in order to give reasonable yield. Medicinal rhubarb contains more anthrax-quinone in spring and during flowering than winter season. Rhizomes are generally collected when they get aged. The alkaloid content is highest in young plant, Example-strychnos seed, but generally the alkaloid content increases with age in perennial plants.
Fertilizers	These are added to soil to provide proper nourishment to the plant in order to utilize their genetic potential fully. It supplies nutrients to the plant for their nutritional demand. For the vegetative growth, plants need CO_2, sunlight, water and mineral matter. Plants are also in need of 16 nutrients for synthesizing various compounds. Oxygen, carbon and chlorides are provided to plants from water and rest of them can be provided by fertilizers and compound manure. These are primary and secondary nutrients: - Primary nutrients: Nitrogen, Phosphorus, Potassium - Secondary nutrients: Manganese (Mn), Calcium, Sulphur - Trace elements: copper (Cu), Iron (Fe), Boron, Magnesium

Contd...

	Types of fertilizers: - Nitrogen fertilizers - Ammonium fertilizers - Multinutrient fertilizers - Foliar spray - Potash fertilizers - Phosphate fertilizers

Pest and Pest Control	Large quantity of crude drug is wasted and destroyed by pest. Also loss in quality occurs when these pest are allowed to grow on products. The control of pests thus, assumes primary importance in the context of cultivation of medicinal and aromatic plants.
	
	Types of pests
	➢ Fungi and viruses
	   o *Cercosporaatropa:* leaf spot
	   o *Ascochyta atropae:* leaf necrosis
	   o *Phytophthora nicotianae:* falling of leaves
	   o *Verticilumalbotarum:* wilt
	   o *Puccinia manthae:* rust
	➢ Insects: Agrotis species, flea beetles, e.g.: *Laphygmaexigua* on mentha species, *Plautiaveridicolis* on Rauwolfia. Others are cutworms, termites, spiders, ticks, and mites etc.
	➢ Weeds: Weeds are undesired plants. Because of weeds there is loss of nutrients, water, light, and space, increase of cost of labour and equipment, low product quality.
	➢ Non-insect pests: These are of two types: Vertebrates like rats, monkey, birds, rabbits, etc. and invertebrates like nematodes, crabs, snails, mites, etc.
	
	Methods of Pest Control:
	➢ Mechanical method
	➢ Agricultural method
	➢ Biological method
	➢ Chemical method

Allelopathy	Living organisms constantly exert an influence upon each other. Such interactions are called allelopathy. These interactions may be beneficial or it may be detrimental. Allelopathy is the direct or indirect effects of chemicals produced by plants or microorganisms on the growth, development, and distribution of other plants and microorganisms in natural and agricultural ecosystems. When different plants are grown side by side the effect may be upon: ➢ Germination of seeds ➢ Growth promotion or growth sup-pression. ➢ Leaf development ➢ Leaf shedding ➢ Maturation of fruits. *Symbiosis*: Some organisms depend upon each other to such an extent that they can exist only when living together. Such an allelopathic interaction is termed as symbiosis. *Antibiosis*: When allelopathic interaction causes distribution of other animals. It is termed as antibiosis. **Examples:** ➢ Growth of belladonna is suppressed when grown together with mustard plant, but with *Artemisia absinthium*, the constituents and total production is increased.

Contd...

	➢ Allopathic effect among plants is transmitted by means of exhalation from leaves or secretion from roots. ➢ Pure culture of stramonium growing gave 34% of total alkaloids in leaves. When grown with peppermint this was greatly reduced to 0.15% and with lupin it increased to 0.37%. ➢ Symbiotical existence: nitrogen fixing bacteria living symbiotically with leguminous plants.

Following are details of Endogenous/ Intrinsic Factors

Selection	The process of choosing and cultivating plants with desirable characters (advanced nutritional value, high yield of secondary plant metabolites, disease resistant etc) is called as selection. Desirable characters may exist already in the plant or may be introduced in the plant. Selection procedure must be done very carefully. Continued collection and breeding of most desirable individual characters may result in a population, which will show a greater response towards improvements in the particular quality chosen. *Examples of selection:* ➢ By selection work on *Cinchona ledgeriana* (~5% alkaloids) yield increased upto 15% alkaloids. ➢ By selection work on *Mentha arvensis* caused development of draught resistant and rust resistant type.
Mutation	Sudden change in genotype which is inheritable is called mutation. Change in phenotype is not inheritable called *adaptation* or *modification*. Mutation causes the qualitative and quantitative alteration of genetic material. Characters of mutation are sudden Irreversible, Inheritable, beneficial or harmful changes Mutation is of two types. Chromosomal mutation is change in position or amount of genetic material takes place. Point mutation is change within the gene or cistron of DNA molecule takes place. Spontaneous mutation occurs naturally because of some unknown reasons. Artificial mutation is induced by artificial means. For example: By some reagents or electromagnetic radiations. Hence, such agents are called mutagens. *Types of mutagens* 1. Chemical: Some mutagens like nitrogen mustard, formaldehyde, HNO_2, and ethyl ethane sulphonates alter chemical constitution of DNA bases and cause transitional substitution in DNA. Some mutagens like 2-aminopurine, 5-bromouracil, urethane, coffins, triazine, and phenol act as a base analog and bring out copy error mutation in DNA. 2. E.M.R i.e. electromagnetic radiations like U.V. rays, X-Rays and Y-Rays also causes mutations <table><tr><td colspan="3" align="center">Mutation mediated changes in medicinal plants</td></tr><tr><td>Solanum khasianum</td><td>Chemical mutagen</td><td>increase solasod in content</td></tr><tr><td>Dioscorea bulbifera</td><td>Radiation</td><td>increased diosgenin content</td></tr><tr><td>Mentha piperita</td><td>Irradiation</td><td>wilt disease resistant</td></tr></table> **Applications:** Mutation leads to improved varieties that are directly used for commercial cultivation and new genetic stocks with improved traits like increased yield, enhanced nutritional quality, resistance to pest and disease, early maturity, drought and salt tolerance, etc.

Contd...

Polyploidy	The condition in which the nuclei of the cell contain more than two chromosomes sets is known as polyploidy such as 2n (diploidy), 3n (triploidy), 4n (tetraploidy), etc. Usually each living cell contains in its nucleus two sets of chromosomes. Since chromosomes in nuclei are present in duplicate, the normal cell is referred to as diploid cell. Euploidy is a type of polyploidy in which genome contain whole set of chromosome. Aneuploidy is any deviation from the exact multiplication of the haploid number of chromosomes whether fewer or more. Mainly two types of polyploidy: ➢ Autoploidy: → multiplication of chromosomes is of single species, i.e. self pollination or cross pollination between cliff members of same species. ➢ Alloploidy: → multiplication of chromosomes following hybridization between two species. Example: when *Primula verticila* (infertile) croosed with *Primula floribunda* (infertile) produced *Primula kewensis* (fertile). *Spartina strica* [2n=56] when crossed with *Spartina alternifolia* [2n=70] gave *Spartina townscndii* (2n=126). Techniques of polyploidy: (A) Natural polyploidy: This occurs naturally and randomly due to change in the environment and climate. (B) Artificial polyploidy: Done artificially by: ➢ EMR (X-Rays) ➢ Physical methods like tem-perature (by extreme change in temperature) ➢ Chemical methods: Chemical agents cause disturbance to mitotic spindle of diploid cells and causes non-regulation of already duplicated chromo-somes and thus converts diploid cells into tetraloid cells. It uses colchicines, veratrine, sulphani-lamide, $HgCl_2$, chloral hydrate, hexachlorocyclohexane etc. **Applications** • *To overcome the sterility*: The induction of polyploidy is a common technique to overcome the sterility of a hybrid species during plant breeding. For example, triticale is the hybrid of wheat (*Triticum turgidum*) and rye (*Secale cereale*). • *Seedless fruits:* The seedless trait of triploids has been desirable especially in fruits. • *Bridge crossing:* Another breeding strategy that utilizes the reproductive superiority of polyploids is bridge crossing. • *Ornamental and forage breeding*: One of the immediate and obvious consequences of polyploidy in plants is an increase in cell size which in turn leads to enlarged plant organs, a phenomenon termed gigas effect • *Production of apomictic crops:* Apomixis provides another avenue for use of polyploids in breeding. Apomixis provides an avenue for the production of seeds asexually through parthenogenesis. Most apomictic plants are polyploid but most polyploid plants are not apomictic. • *Disease resistance through aneuploidy:* Aneuploidy has been applied in breeding to develop disease resistant plants through the addition of an extra chromosome into the progeny genome. An example is the transfer of leaf rust resistance to Tricumaestivum from Aegilops umbellulata through backcrossing. The enhanced production of secondary metabolites such as alkaloids and terpenes in polyploids may concurrently offer resistance to pests and pathogens. • *Chemical constituent production*: In vitro secondary metabolite production systems that exploit polyploidism have also been developed. Following are few examples.

Contd...

Examples of Polyploidy and plant secondary metabolite enahncemnet				
Plant	**Constituents**	**2n plant**	**4n plant**	**Others**
Atropa belladonna	Tropane alkaloids		Increase of about 68% over 2n	
Datura stramonium	Tropane alkaloids		Increase of about 60-150% over 2n	
Cinchona succirubra	Quinine	0.53	1.12	
Opium poppy	Morphine			Increase upto 100% in 3n plants
Cannabis sativa	Marihuana	1.4	2.6	
Artemisia annua	ntimalarial sesquiterpene artemisinin	1.2		Increase upto 6 times in 3n plants
Digitalis lanata	Glycosides		Lower or same as in 2n	
Mintha spicata	Volatile oil content	0.48	0.05	

Hybridization	Hybridization is the process through which hybrids are produced. Hybrids are an organism, which result from crossing of two species or two varieties which differ from each other, at least in one set of characters. Example: when Plant A having high yield is crossed with disease resistant Plant B, it gives Plant C showing high yield, disease resistance.
	Hybridization can be categorized into two; sexual and somatic. Sexual hybridization, also referred to as wide or distant hybridization involves combining two genomes from different parental taxa through pollination, either naturally or by induction. Somatic hybridization involves the fusion of somatic cells instead of gametes, which highly depends on the ability to obtain viable protoplasts and eventually differentiate them to whole plants in vitro.
	Inbreeding means cross between two different plants of same species. By inbreeding we can get pure plants. Sometimes pure lines can't be obtained by hybridization. Monohybrids are hybrids with one pair of different characters. Dihybrids are hybrids with two pairs of different characters. Poly hybrids are hybrids with more than two pairs of different characters.
	Hence hybridization helps in inducing the desirable characters in a single variety of plant or species and sometime producing new and favourable characters which are not present in both the parents. The recent development in hybridization is through the medium of tissue culture. In this the protoplast cultures are employed, such protoplast cultures can be fused together which is called protoplast fusion or asexual hybridization.
	The impacts of hybrids can either be positive or negative. Among the positive attributes of hybrids that have been exploited is heterosis, which results either from dominance, over-dominance or epistasis. Negative ones include sterility, arrested growth of the pollen tube and embryo abortion. To overcome these problems, chromosome doubling, the use of hormones such as 2, 4-Dichlorophenoxyacetic acid (2, 4-D) and embryo rescue have been employed to overcome sterility, arrested growth of pollen tubes and embryo abortion respectively. After the development of hybrids, different hybrid identification techniques have been used to test them such as the use of molecular and morphological markers, cytogenetic analysis and fluorescent in situ hybridization. The use of hybridization techniques in plant improvement remains a vital tool to cross

Contd...

<table>
<tr>
<td></td>
<td>

species barriers and utilization of important attributes in unrelated crop plants which could not have been achieved through conventional techniques of plant breeding.

Types of Hybridization

➢ Intergenic: hybridization of two plants from different genus

➢ Interspecific: hybridization of two plants from different species

➢ Intraspecific: hybridization of two plants from same species

Examples: *Cinchona succirubrs* 3.4% and *Cinchona Ledgeriana* 5.1% producedHybrid with quinine 11.2%

Applications:

Applications of hybridization involves inclusion of the desirable characters, development of disease free plant, making new species of plant and increase in content of secondary plant metabolites. Hybrid plants are derived either from hybrid seed (e.g., maize) or from vegetative cuttings (e.g., apples). Many fruit and vegetable plants are vegetatively propagated hybrids, that is, vegetative clones of a hybrid plant, with particularly desirable traits, derived from a sexual cross of two parental plants (e.g., apples, strawberries, holly, and cassava); propagation may be by cuttings, or bulbs. Some vegetable and field crop plants are hybrid plants, derived from F1 hybrid seed, and valued because of enhanced yield of seed (e.g., corn), vegetation (e.g., kale, carrot, and onion), or fruit (e.g., tomatoes).

</td>
</tr>
<tr>
<td>

Chemical Races/Chemo Demes

</td>
<td>

Chemo demes are defined as chemically distinct population within a species and have similar phenotype but different genotype and are identical in external appearance but differ in their chemical constituents. Existence of Chemo demes can be confirmed only by growing different plants of a species in identical condition preferably from the seeds and for many generations. Chemo demes can be made by simple mutation (naturally) or induces (artificially) in laboratory or can be produced by polyploidy. This can offer considerable scope for the improvement of the therapeutic value and also the increase in the overall yield.

Examples:

➢ Linoleic acid enriched oil producing sunflower varieties found convenient for harvesting because of having large single flower head and no side shoots.

➢ Few *Prunus communis* varieties showing different morphological features and without presence of amygdalin or few varieties showing similar characters but differ in presence or absence of glycosides.

➢ Selection of 0.7% morphine containing capsules and collection of its seeds for further cultivation raised average morphine content to 0.765% from previously reported average morphine content of poppy capsule is 0.385%.

➢ Different species of digitalis shows different proportions of cardiac glycosides.

➢ Few of Eucalyptus species shows piperitone as chief constituent of volatile oil while other shows phellendrene or cineole and even few species produce oil consisting other intermediate as chief constituents.

</td>
</tr>
</table>

Plant Growth Regulators

Naturally occurring organic compounds responsible for growth and development of plants are known as plant growth regulators or Plant hormones or phytohormones. Growth hormones allow synchronization of plant development. These are physiological intercellular messengers that are needed to control the complete plant life cycle including germination, rooting, growth, flowering, fruit ripening and death. In addition plant hormones are secreted in response to environment factors such as abundance of nutrients, drought conditions, light, and temperature, chemical or physical stress and thus level of hormones will change over the lifespan of a plant and depend upon season and environment.

Characteristics

➢ These are specific in their action

➢ Active in very low concentration

➢ Regulate cells enlargement, cell division, cell differentiation, organogenesis, senescence, and dormancy.

➢ The main role of hormones has on production of secondary metabolites and tissue culture

Classification

❖ **Traditional plant growth regulators:**

   ❖ Auxins

   ❖ Gibberellins

   ❖ Cytokinins

   ❖ Ethylene

   ❖ Abscisic acid

❖ **Nontraditional plant growth regu-lators:**

   ➢ Jasmonates

   ➢ Brassinosteroids

   ➢ Oligosaccharides

   ➢ Salicylate

   ➢ Nitric oxide

   ➢ Polyamines : Putrescine, Spermine, Spermidine

| 1. *Auxins:* | *Nature:* It is also known as cell elongators. Large amount of auxins had been found in shoot apical meristems, young leaves and fruits. Typical concentration of auxins varies between 0.01 to 10 mg/L.
History: It was first studied by Dutch workers in 1931 who isolated two growth regulating acids namely auxin-a and auxin-b from human urine and cereal products respectively. These had similar properties to Indole-3-acetic acid (IAA) and found particularly in actively growing tissues.
Structure:
Biosynthesis: An essential amino acid tryptophan is the precursors for the biosynthesis of auxins i.e. IAA. There are mainly three routes of biosynthesis in plants that are from Indole-3-pyruvic acid, from Indole-3-acetonitrile and from tryptamine. In some bacteria or transformed plants IAA is synthesized by tryptophan independent pathway.

Classification:
Natural auxins
  ➢ Indole-3-acetic acid
  ➢ Indole-3-acetonitrile
  ➢ Phenyl acetic acid
  ➢ 4-chloro Indole-3-acetic acid |

Contd...

Synthetic auxins:

- Indole-3-butyric acid
- 1-Napthalene acetic acid
- 2,4-D
- 2,4,5-T
- 2-NOA
- 1-NAD

Mode of action: Indole acetic acid has been involved in interaction with auxin binding protein 1(ABP 1) which is responsible for plant growth and morphogenesis.

Indoleacetic   acid (IAA)

2,4 – Dichlorophenoxyacetic acid (2 , 4 – D)

Naphthaleneacetic acid (NAA)

Biological effects of auxins:

- *Cell expansion*: Auxin and GA promote cell elongation through Acid growth" hypothesis where Auxin stimulates proton pump in the cell membrane. Proton pump secrets H^+ into cell wall, acidifies the cell wall, which activates pH dependent enzymes and break bond between Cellulose microfibrils. This wall loosens and pressure expands the cell.

- *Tropisms*: Tropisms are defined as directional response of a plant organ to a stimulus in the environment. Tropic movements allow the plant to adjust itself or orient in responds to surrounding environment for optimal uptake of energy, nutrients, and water. Auxin has a major role in tropic stimuli. It is of two types Phototropism: When plants are illuminated by light from one-direction phenomena of positive photo-tropism is exhibited.

  Gravitropism: It is the plant growth response towards gravity. Plant shoots display negative gravitropism and roots display positive gravitropism, so they grow down.

- *Apical dominance:* The phenomenon in which growth of shoot apex inhibits the development of lateral buds on the stem beneath is called apical dominance. Auxins produced at the apex repress the outgrowth of lateral buds. The decapitation (removal of auxin source) increases the cytokinin content of xylem exudates. The effect of auxin on cytokinin concentration in xylem exudates suggest that auxin can influence apical dominance by inhibiting cytokinin synthesis or export from roots.

Contd…

	➢ Auxin can inhibit or promote (via ethylene production) leaf/fruit abscission. It stimulates root initiation on stem cutting. It stimulates the production of ethylene at high concentration. ➢ Auxin plays important role in producing plants through tissue culture. It produces lateral root development in tissue culture. The process of embryogenesis is initiated in media containing high level of auxin but embryo does not develop until auxin concentration is reduced. Synthetic auxin namely 2, 4-D used to initiate callus culture. Chlorophyll formation Auxins are inhibitory to chlorophyll formation in callus culture. ***Commercial Application of Auxin:*** *Propagation:* In low concentration to accelerate the rooting of woody and herbaceous cuttings. IBA is most commonly used for this because it is stable, insensitive to auxin degrading enzymes. E.g. IBA was successfully used in cinchona cuttings, saving two or three years compared with growth from seed. *Fruit Set:* In California, early spring crop of tomato is treated with 4-CPA at 20-25 ppm to stimulate fruit set at a time of the year when cool night temperature that inhibit fruit set in tomato are likely. This treatment results in an increase in yield and earlier harvest. *Chemical thinning:* Removal of excessive number of young fruits is common orchard management practice for apple and pear. NAA is used for chemical thinning of apple and pear. *Prevention of fruit drop:*2, 4, 5 –TP is mainly used for preventing fruit drop for a longer period in apple, pear, lemon and grape fruit. *Herbicidal action:* Auxin in higher concentration to act as a selective herbicides or weed–killers so used in horticulture and agriculture. E.g. 2, 4-D is particularly toxic to dicotyle-donous plants while, in suitable concentrations having little effect on monocotyledonous. So, 2, 4- D is used to destroy dicotyledonous weeds as dandelion and plantain form grass lawns. (Certain carbamate and ureas derivatives have an opposite effect and can be used to destroy grass without serious injury to dicotyle-donous crops.)
2. ***Gibberellins***	*Nature*: Gibberellins are diterpenoids derived from four isoprenoids unit forming a system of four rings. Gibberellins are little change in chemical but much varied in their biological activities. The 20th carbon atom is not a part of the four rings but belong to the side chain. Gibberellins are found in leaves, immature seeds and fruits of some plants. *Classification:* **Unlike classification of auxins, which are classified on basis of function, gibberellins are classified on basis of structure and function as well. It is named as GA_1 to GAn in order of discovery. Right now 136 gibberellins have been discovered among them GA_3 is well- known a namely Gibberellinic acid (GA). All GAs are found in plants, fungus and bacterias.** 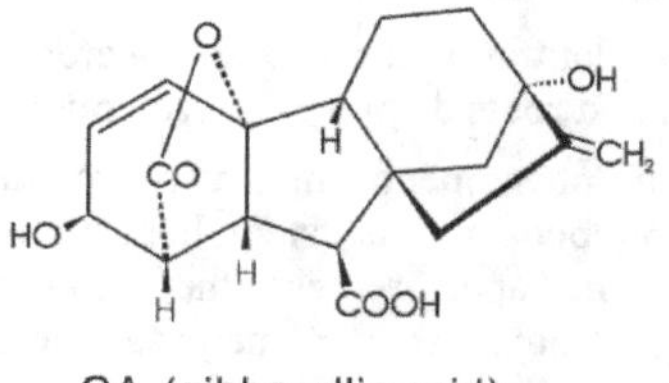 GA_3(gibberellic acid) 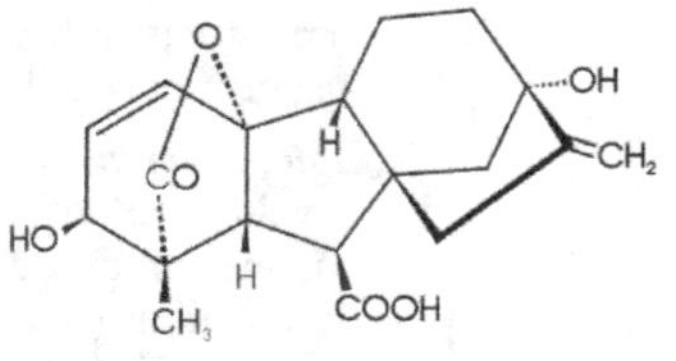 GA_1

Contd...

History: Origin for search of Gibberella was started by Japanese plant physiologist, Kurosawa who investigating cause of "Bakane" (foolish seedlings) disease, which seriously lowered the yields of rice crops in Japan, Taiwan and Asian countries and also isolated responsible known as Gibberellin.

Structure

Biosynthesis and metabolism: Gibberellins are synthesized from acetyl coA by mevalonic Acid pathway.

Mechanism of action: Gibberellins have effects on enzymes involved in gluco-neogenesis during early stages of germination which leads to conversion of lipid to sucrose and thus helps in growth and development. It also includes the synthesis of alpha-amylase and other hydrolytic enzymes, involved in mobilizing seed storage reserve during germination and seedling emergence.

Biological effects of GAs:

➤ Cell elongation

➤ Flower induction and development: Flower formation is controlled by number of external factors like light or low temperature after addition of GA3 flowering can occur even without necessary external signals.

➤ Fruit development: Developing seeds contain highest concentration of GAs, which have a promotive effect on cell division, expansion, and development of ovaries.

➤ Seed development and germination

➤ Break seed dormancy in some plants, which require light to induce germination.

➤ Development of parthanocarpic fruit

➤ Delay senescence in leaves and citrus fruits

➤ It has also effect on secondary metabolites production. Treatments of gibberellins lower the alkaloid content in *H. niger, R. serpentina, C. roseus, T. sinensis*, while increase in Belladonna leaves.

➤ The GA treatment of *Chenopodium ambrosioides*, afforded a 33% increase in the volatile oil content.

3. Cytokinins	*Nature:* Cytokinins are compounds very similar to adenine and promote cell division. These are called as Cytokinins because the compound has ability to promote cytokinesis (cell division). Today more than 200 natural and synthetic cytokinins are evaluated. *History:* In 1950, Miller isolated crystalline substance from autoclaved herring sperm DNA, capable of inducing cell division in tobacco culture and named as a kinetin, which is a 6-furfural amino derivatives. Further, some adenine derivatives were also found having similar biological activity and were also found, collectively known as 'kinins' among them zeatin are the natural cytokinin. ***Structure*** Biosynthesis: • Biochemical modification of adenine leads to conversion of many of cytokinins. • It has been synthesized from mevalonic acid pathway. • Isopentenyl pyrophosphate (IPP) is the main precursor involved in synthesis of various cytokinins. • IPP is isomerizes, this isomer react with AMP with an enzyme isopentenyl AMP synthase leads to synthesis of isopentenyl AMP. • Removal of phosphate by phos-phatase leads to conversion of Isopentenyl adenosine from that removal of ribose group results into Isopentenyl adenine which finally converts into 3 major forms of natural occurring cytokinins

Contd...

Metabolism: Degradation of cytokinin occurs largely due to enzyme cytokinin oxidase. This enzyme removes the side chain and release adenine. Derivatives also be made but the pathways are more complex and poorly understand.

Mode of action: *Cytokinins have a main role in cell division of plants and typical concentration is 0.1 to 10 mg/L. It activates RNA synthesis and stimulates protein synthesis and enzyme activity too.*

Classification: *It is of mainly two types*
Naturally occurring cytokinins: They are N6- substituted adenine deriva-tives like Zeatin Dihydrozeatin
Synthetic cytokinins: Synthetic cytokinins have been prepared because the natural cytokinins cannot be employed due to their high cost.

➢ Substituted purines.: E.g. BAP (6-Benzyl amino purine) or benzyl adenine

➢ Phenyl urea derivatives: E.g. 1,3 – diphenyl urea

Native
Synthetic
NH₂
Adenine
Kinetin
Zeatin
Benzyladenine (BA)
Diphenylurea
2 iPA

Biological effects of cytokinins:

➢ Cell division and development: Auxin and cytokinin together stimulates cell division and control morphogenesis.

➢ Cytokinins and increased levels of auxin: the exogenous application of cytokinin results in more auxin.

➢ Anti-ageing effects: cytokinins have remarkable anti-ageing effects

➢ Cell cycle control

➢ Stimulates morphogenesis (shoot initiation/bud formation) in tissue culture.

➢ Stimulate the growth of lateral buds: release of apical dominance.

➢ Stimulate leaf expansion from cell enlargement.

➢ May enhance stomatal opening in some species.

➢ It also has effects on secondary metabolites production. Cytokinin stimulates auxin synthesis in tissue culture of tobacco. Leaves of coffee plant on treatment with kinetin shows 10% increase in caffeine content.

4. Ethylene	*Nature:* Ethylene, unlike the most of plant hormone compound is a gaseous hormone. It is the only member of its class having simplest structure. It is produced in all higher plants but usually associated with fruit ripening. ***History:* In 1864, Russian scientist Dimitry was identified gas leaked from streetlight was found to have effect on plant growth and abnormal thickening of stems.**

	Structure:
	Biosynthesis: Ethylene has been synthesized from sulphur containing amino acid L-methionine.
	Metabolism: *Ethylene can be metabolized by plant tissue to ethylene oxide and ethylene glycol.*
	Biological effects of ethylene ➢ Stimulate fruit ripening ➢ Stimulates flower and leaf sene-scence. ➢ Stimulate leaf and fruit abscission. ➢ Stimulates flower opening ➢ Promoting role in adventitious root formation ➢ Stimulates the release of dormancy. ➢ Ethylene protects plants from pathogenic attack.
	Application of ethylene ➢ Ethephon increases latex flow in rubber by 50-100% ➢ Ethephon stimulates fruit ripening e.g. tomatoes, mango ➢ Ethephon promotes abscission. After treatment with Ethephon quality of nuts Cherry and walnuts is also increased because they do not remain more time on tree after maturation and also avoid decomposition due to heat and disease
5. *Abscisic Acid (ABA)*	*Nature:* ABA is a single compound unlike auxins, gibberellins, and cytokinins. It was called "abscisin II" (effect on abscission of fruits) and "dormin" (effect on bud dormancy). Abscisic acid is mainly found in leaves, stem and green fruits. Both cis and trans isomer of ABA may be extracted from plant tissues.
	Structure *Biosynthesis* ➢ ABA is a naturally occurring sesquiterpens produced via mevalonic acid pathway in chloroplasts and plastids because it is synthesized partially in chloroplasts.
	Functions of ABA: ➢ Stimulates the closure of stomata as water stress increases ABA synthesis. ➢ Inhibit shoot growth but no effect on roots or may even promote growth of roots. ➢ Inhibits the effects of gibberellins on stimulating de novo synthesis amylase. ➢ Effect on induction and mainte-nance of dormancy ➢ Induce gene transcription especially for proteinase inhibitor in response to wounding which may explain an apparent role in pathogen defense. ➢ Anti-transpirant properties on crops such as burley and coffee ➢ Certain ABA analogs have been found to delay flowering in peach.

Plant Disease

A disease affects normal growth, development and quality of wild as well as cultivated plants by interrupting or modifying its vital functions.

A plant disease is a natural ecological factor that keeps balance between living plants and animals.

Different plants are susceptible to different and characteristic diseases. Occurrence and prevalence of disease depends on type of plant, environment and presence of pathogen.

Plant pathology is a branch which studies plants diseases as follows:

➤ Infectious diseases caused by pathogens/ Organisms (like fungi, oomycetes, bacteria, viruses, viroids, virus-like organisms, phytoplasmas, protozoa, nematodes and parasitic plants).

➤ Physiological factors mediated diseases caused by environmental conditions like temperature, relative humidity, soil moisture, soil pH, soil type and soil fertility

Genetics of plant determines its resistance or susceptibility to a particular disease. Specific pathogens vary in their ability to infect different plant species. **Example:** Late blight: Solanaceous plants like tomato, potato are susceptible to this fungus however cucumber, beans and other types of plants are not found susceptible.

2.4 Conservation of Medicinal Plants

Plants hold medicinal, ecological, commercial and aesthetic recreational value. Endangered species must be protected and saved so that future generations can experience their presence and value. In fact about 40 % of all prescriptions written today are composed from the natural compounds of different species. Plant and animal species are the foundation of healthy ecosystem. The growing herbal market and its commercial benefit might pose a threat to biodiversity through over harvesting of the raw materials for herbal medicines. If not controlled these practices may lead to the extinction of endangered species and the destruction of natural habitats and resources. India has a rich resource base of medicinal plants, with about 8,000 different species due varied climatic conditions and topography. Hence it has been considered as "Botanical garden' or "Herbarium "of the world. Today, according to the World Health Organization (WHO), as many as 80% of the world's people depends on traditional medicine for their primary health care needs by Ayurveda, Sidha, Unani and Tibetan systems. But increased demand is creating extensive destruction of plant-rich habitats and bad news is that these Indian herbs are now going to extinct. Unfortunately very fewer efforts are taken to face threat related to biodiversity. Plant species become endangered or extinct mainly because of following factors:

➤ Forest depletion due to over exploitation of natural resources due to population growth, urbanization and unrestricted collection, Illegal trade

➤ Environmental factors like desert encroachment, Pollution and drastic climatic changes including flood, wide spread use of pesticides.

➤ Agricultural intensification

➤ Destructive harvesting methods and Unsuitable collection practices

➤ Increase in demand and collection due to increase in popularity.

➤ Scant information about the information of these endangered medicinal plants

The in situ conservation of medicinal plants relates to the conservation of wild population of medicinal plant populations in their natural habitats. Question arises that what is need of conservation of medicinal plants and answer is that plants hold medicinal, ecological, commercial and aesthetic recreational value. IUCN has classified endangered species as:

- ➢ ***Rare species:*** Species with small population restricted geographically with localized habitats. They aren't in immediate danger of extinction. e.g. Saraca indica. It is also consider rare if, a few individuals only represent it over a large area.
- ➢ ***Vulnerable species***: Species are under threat of or actually decline in number. e.g. Garcinia indica
- ➢ ***Endangered [threatened] species***: Species with low population number that are in considerable danger of becoming extinct .e. g. Dioscoreadeltoidea
- ➢ ***Critically endangered species:*** When specie is facing an extremely high risk of extinction in wild in the immediate future.e.g. Cosciniumfenestratum
- ➢ ***Extinc species: Species*** which can't be found in areas where they recently been inhabited. e.g. Drosera indica

Following are examples of Endangered Medicinal Plants			
Plant	**Use**	**Threat status**	**Parts used**
Ephedra gerardiana [Ephedraceae]	Asthma, hay fever	Vulnerable	Aerial shoots
Garcinia indica [Guttiferae]	Nutritive, demulcent	Vulnerable	Fruit pulps seeds
Cosciniumfenestratum	Dyspepsia, eye disease	Endangered	Root, stem
Aegle marmelos [Rutaceae]	Antidiabetic, asthma	Vulnerable	Fruits
Decalepishamitonii [Periplocaceae]	Flatulence removal	Endangered	Roots
Frillariaroyelihook [Lilliceae]	Antipyretic, epectorant	Endangered	Bulb
Ampelocissus araneosa	Astringent, cooling	Vulnerable	Fruit pulps
Artemisabrevifolia [Compositae]	Anthelmintic	Threatened	Flowers
Swertia chirata [Gentianaceae]	Bitter tonic, febrifuge	Threatened	Entire herbs

Following are examples of Threatened Medicinal Plants		
Threatned / Endangered Medicinal Plants of India	**Some species which are on verge of extinction**	**Some species, which will become extinct due to over harvesting**
Podophyllum [*Podophyllumhexandrum*] Rhubarb [*Rheum emodi*] Belladona [*Atropa acuminate*] Rauwolfia [*Rauwolfia serpentine]* Dioscorea [*Dioscoreadeltoidea*]	Aconite [*Aconitumheterophyllum*] Salabmisri [*Orchis muscula*] Kutki [*Picrrhizakurroa*] Katphala [*Myrica nagi*] Ashoka [*Saraca indica*]	Senna [*Cassia angustifolia*] Isaphgula [*Plantago ovata*] Kumari [*Aloe barbadensis*] Shatavari [*Asparagus racemosus*] Ashwagandha [*Withaniasomnifera*]

Conservation methods:

- ➢ Medicinal plants are globally valuable sources of herbal products, and they are disappearing at a high speed. A highly conservative estimate states that the current loss of plant species is between 100 and 1000 times higher than the expected natural extinction rate and that the Earth is losing at least one potential major drug every 2 years. According to the International Union for Conservation of Nature and the World Wildlife Fund, there are between 50,000 and 80,000 flowering plant species used for medicinal purposes worldwide. Among these, about 15,000 species are threatened with extinction from overharvesting and habitat destruction and 20 % of their wild resources have already been nearly exhausted with the increasing human population and plant consumption. Although this threat has been known for decades, the accelerated loss of species and habitat destruction worldwide has increased the risk of extinction of medicinal plants, especially in China, India, Kenya, Nepal, Tanzania and Uganda.

➤ Both conservation strategies (e.g. *in situ* and *ex situ* conservation and cultivation practices) and resource management (e.g. good agricultural practices and sustainable use solutions) should be adequately taken into account for the sustainable use of medicinal plant resources. Biotechnical approaches (e.g. tissue culture, micropropagation, synthetic seed technology, and molecular marker-based approaches) should be applied to improve yield and modify the potency of medicinal plants.

Following are Medicinal Plants Conservation strategies	
In situ (conservation in Natural Habitat)	Protected Areas Wildlife sanctuary National Parks Biosphere reserves(marine and Terrestrial)
	Forest and lakes
Ex situ Conservation (conservation away from Natural Habitat)	Seed bank
	Gene bank
	In vitro (Tissue culture callus) storage
	Pollen storage
	Arboretum
	Cryopreservation

1. Bio technological methods:

➤ Micro propagation is a field dealing with the ability to regenerate plants directly from explants. Nodal segments, epicotyls, rhizome roots and leaf and other different explants are used for conservation of species through micro–propagation.

➤ Genetic modification can alter the genetic nature of plants by various techniques like protoplast fusion, tissue culture etc for development of Disease resistant plant, Pest resistant plants and Plants resistant to environmental changes and stress.

➤ Seeds of species can be stored for years. Seeds of species remain dormant for thousands of years if stored at low temperature [-200C] and low humidity [5-10 %].

➤ Cryopreservation involves storage of cells from embryos, shoot tips in liquid nitrogen at relatively low temperature so as to stop the metabolism.

2. Project Works/Workshops/Organizations/Conservation Agencies:

➤ Researchers can collect the scientific and local names of the plants, together with their descriptions, illustrations and places of the occurrence and determined the ailments for which they are used, the parts of the plants that are used, the form in which they are used [fresh, dried, processed etc], how they are preserved and the reasons why the plants are rare or endangered. Some efforts can be made to educate herbalists and the general public on the dangers of exhausting medicinal [plant resources. Seminars and workshops can be held in each project area to train traditional healers in non–destructive methods of harvesting and better methods of preserving. Pamphlets and posters on the conservation and propagation of medicinal plants can be distributed to schools, local communities and policy makers and messages were put out over the mass media. The nurseries and gardens can become training centers for communities; motivating residents start their own backyard cultivation of several medicinal plant species.

➢ Workshop can be arranged to educate participants upon various issues regarding endangered medicinal plants and their conservation.

➢ The World Health Organization on 10 Feb. 2004 released guidelines for good agricultural and collection practices for medicinal plants. These WHO guidelines for medicinal plants are an important initial step to ensure good quality, safe herbal medicines and ecologically sound cultivation practices for future generations.

➢ There are many individuals, groups and organization concerned with conservation of plants in private as well as in Government sectors. Govt. has framed so many agencies and project works in conserving the plants. Some of the international agencies working for conservation of endangered species are:

➢ Royal Society for Nature Conservation [RSNC]

➢ Joint Nature Conservation Commit-tee [JNCC]

➢ Nature Conservancy Council [NCC]

➢ International Union for the Conservation of Nature and Natural Resources [IUCN]

3. Government Steps:

➢ For preservation of endangered plants, Govt. of India has approved 1000 crore for medicinal plants in order to implement the scheme of "Sustainable Conservation" of medicinal plants which involves:

➢ Providing support, aid to farmers to maintain traditional agricultural practices in environmentally sensitive areas.

➢ Conserving some places under the name of special areas for conservation 'SAC' and taking special efforts to conserve the area.

➢ Protecting, restoring habitats, forests and establishing national parks, natural reserves and botanical gardens for protecting plants

➢ Reducing the use of pesticides

➢ Restricting trades of endangered species

➢ Maintaining, protecting the earth ecosystem and biodiversity and avoiding environmental degradation

➢ Educating herb sellers, cultivators regarding importance of conservation of plants and creating awareness among the public

➢ Legal approach to the problems through Government

Subjective Questions

1. How to cultivate and collect crude drugs?

2. How to process crude drugs? Explain with suitable examples.

3. How to store crude drugs? Explain with suitable examples

4. What is polyploidy? Explain with suitable examples

5. What is hybridization? Explain with suitable examples.

6. How mutation relates with polyploidy?

7. How to conserve medicinal plants? Explain with suitable examples.

8. What is difference between ex situ and in situ conservation?

9. What are different factors influence cultivation of medicinal plants? Explain with suitable examples.

10. Give suitable examples of crude drugs affected by factors like age, season and temperature.

11. What are different mills used to pulverize crude drugs? Give example based on type of crude drugs?

12. Give suitable examples of different storage containers used for crude drugs.

Multiple Choice Questions (MCQs)

1. Cinchona plants were first cultivated in the Nilgiri Hills in..................................
   a. 1857
   b. 1957
   c. 1860
   d. 1960

2. Which states in India own Cinchona plantations and factories?
   a. Maharashtra and Gujarat
   b. Kerala and Tamil Nadu
   c. West Bengal and Tamil Nadu
   d. West Bengal and Andhra Pradesh

3. Which one of the following tuberous medicinal plant is grown at altitudes of 1000-3000 meters in throughout Himalayas?
   a. *Withaniasomnifera*
   b. *Dioscoreadeltoidea*
   c. *Curcuma zedoria*
   d. None of the above

4. In which state of India, *Cassia anguistifolia* is commercially cultivated?

   a. Andhra Pradesh

   b. Kerala

   c. Maharashtra

   d. Tamil Nadu

5. Which state in India provides one of the important export drug Papain, which covers approximately 70% of world requirement?

   a. Gujarat

   b. Aasam

   c. Himachal Pradesh

   d. Maharashtra

6. Which one of the medicinal plant oil is known as, 'Liquid gold of Karnataka'?

   a. *Jasminum officinale*

   b. *Coriandrum sativum*

   c. *Santalum album*

   d. *Eucalyptus citriodora*

7. Cultivation ensures……………………………

   a. Quality of medicinal plants

   b. Purity of medicinal plants

   c. Both a & b

   d. None of the above

8. The method of agricultural production which avoids use of synthetic products like fertilizers, pesticides, growth regulators and livestock feed additives is known as ………………..

   a. Organic farming

   b. Inorganic farming

   c. Modern farming

   d. None of the above

9. Seedlings are the result of

   a. Sexual method of propagation

   b. Asexual method of propagation

   c. Both a and b

   d. None of the above

10. The germination capacity of seeds is tested by.................................
   a.   Rolled towel test
   b.   Excised embryo test
   c.   Only a
   d.   Both a and b

11. Colchicum and saffron are propagated by sowing............................
   a.   Bulbs
   b.   Tubers
   c.   Stolons
   d.   Corms

12. Which one of the altitude height is suitable for cultivation of Eucalyptus?
   a.   1000 – 2000 m
   b.   2000 – 3000 m
   c.   3000-4000 m
   d.   4000 – 5000 m

13. Cardamom requires optimum temperature
   a.   60 – 75 F°
   b.   50 – 100 F°
   c.   55 -70 F°
   d.   70 – 90 F°

14. Which one of the following is highly weathered portion of soil consisting of finest particles?
   a.   Clay
   b.   Sand
   c.   Rock
   d.   None of the above

15. Particle size (diameter) of fine clay......................
   a.   More than 0.002 mm
   b.   0.002 mm
   c.   Less than 0.002 mm
   d.   0.003 mm

16. Any type of soil containing organic matter less than 0.5% is considered as
   a.   Poor quality
   b.   Moderate quality
   c.   high quality
   d.   None of the above

17. Which one of the following plant growth hormone promotes elongation of coleoptile tissue?
    a. Auxin
    b. Gibberellins
    c. cytokinins
    d. Both a and b

18. Gibberellin was first time isolated from ………………..
    a. Algae
    b. Fungi
    c. Plant
    d. Both a and b

19. Which one of the following is natural cytokinin?
    a. Kinetin
    b. Zeatin
    c. Both a and b
    d. None of the above

20. Which one of the following is natural growth inhibitor?
    a. Ethylene
    b. Indole acetic acid
    c. Abscisic acid
    d. Phenyl acetic acid

21. When the organism contains more than two genome, it is called as …………………..
    a. Euploidy
    b. Monoploidy
    c. Diploidy
    d. Polyploidy

22. Which one of the following is the causative agent of polyploidy?
    a. Colchicine
    b. Veratrine
    c. Sulphanilamide
    d. All of the above

23. A group of plants of a species which have identical morphological characters, but differ in their chemical nature are known as………………………
    a. Chemodemes
    b. Chemosomes
    c. Chemozomes
    d. Chromozomes

24. The higher solasodine content in *Solanum khasianum* is achieved by applying..............
    a.   Radiation mutation
    b.   Chemical mutation
    c.   Both a and b
    d.   None

25. Recombinant DNA technology involves
    a.   Gene splitting to change characters of plants
    b.   Implantation of genes from other organisms or species
    c.   Crossing of two species
    d.   Both a and b

Answer Key

1.c	2.c	3. b	4. d	5. d	6. c	7. c	8. a	9. a	10. d
11. c	12. a	13. b	14. a	15. c	16. a	17. d	18. b	19. c	20. c
21. d	22. d	23. a	24. a	25. d					

Unit 3

3.1   Introduction

Plant tissue culture broadly refers to "*in vitro* technique of growing plant cells or tissues into plant parts or whole plant in a sterile environment on an appropriate nutrient medium."

Need of plant tissue culture is due to:

- Agriculture demand for fast commercial propagation of crops, enhanced *nutritional value plants, pest resistant plants, virus free plants etc.*

- *Pharmaceuticals* demand for enhanced secondary metabolite production, need of cloning of rare and endangered plants.

One of the most important events in life cycle of organism is fertilization which involves the fusion of two gametes of opposite sex resulting in formation of a zygote. This forms multicellular and multiorgan body. But all structures are morphologically and functionally diverse. The process involved in the manifestation of these variations is called **differentiation.** Unlike animals, where differentiation is generally irreversible, in plants even highly mature cell retain the ability to regress meristematic state as long as they have an intact membrane and viable nucleus. The phenomenon of a mature cell reverting to the meristematic state forming undifferentiated callus tissue is called as **dedifferentiation.** The ability of this callus to form whole plant or plant organ is called as **redifferentiation.**

3.1.1   Basics of Plant Tissue Culture

Totipotency: Cell's inherent ability to develop into whole plant or plant organs in *in-vitro* condition is known as totipotecy. Not all plant cells are totipotent, however, there are a sufficient number of totipotent cells in the plant (e.g. in the pith). The cell theory (Schwann 1839) gave birth to the concept of totipotency. Single cell give rise to whole plant or organism. Manifestation of variation from single cell to morphologically and functionally different organs is known as **differentiation**. The process of mature cell reverting to the merista-matic state and forming undifferentiated callus tissue is termed as **dedifferentiation**. Then ability of these dedifferentiated cells to be cultured indefinitely on fully defined medium and their capacity to regenerate in to whole plant is known as **redifferentiation**. Reason of redifferentiation is presence of sufficient number of inactive genes that are able to express only under adequate culture condition.

Cellular Totipotency = Dediffentiation + Redifferention

Thus cellular totipotency is an important attribute of plant cells. It is of interest in basic as well as applied areas of plant science.

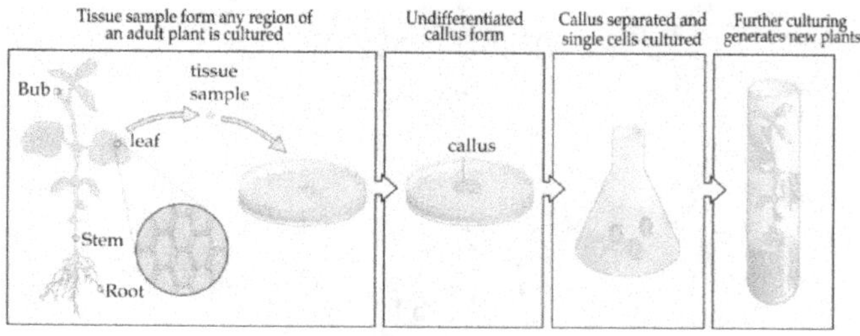

Fig. 3.1 Concept of Totipotency

❖ ***Explant***: Detached portion of cell or tissue from plant organ to start *in vitro* cultures is known as explant. Age and type of explants plays vital role in formation of callus. Choice of explant is always based on desired research Explant can be obtained from bud, roots, nodal segments, apical meristem, seed, embryo, anthers, pollens and or protoplast cells.

❖ ***Callus***: It is mass of actively dividing undifferentiated cells produced by plant tissue explants. Callus can be re-suspended in liquid media to create a suspension culture of single totipotent cells or differentiated into plant with the appropriate manipulations of culture conditions.

❖ ***Plant Regeneration:*** In broad terms, two methods of plant regeneration are widely used in plant transformation studies, i.e. somatic embryogenesis and organogenesis.

Somatic embryogenesis: In somatic (asexual) embryogenesis, embryo-like structures, which can develop into whole plants in a way analogous to zygotic embryos, are formed from somatic tissues with provision of high concentration of 2,4-D during initial stages of embryo formation. These somatic embryos can be produced either directly or indirectly. In direct somatic embryo-genesis, the embryo is formed directly from a cell or small group of cells without the production of an intervening callus. (usually reproductive tissues such as the nucellus, styles or pollen). In indirect somatic embryogenesis, callus is first produced from the explant. Somatic embryo-genesis from carrot is the classical example of indirect somatic embryo-genesis.

Organogenesis: Organogenesis relies on the production of organs, either directly from an explant or from a callus culture. Plant regeneration via organo-genesis depends on adventitious organs (develops from abnormal positions/ embryos from any cell other than the zygote) arising either from a callus culture or directly from an explants. Organogenesis relies on the inherent plasticity of plant tissues, and is regulated by altering the components of the medium.

3.2   Historical Development

1892	Klercker	first attempt to isolate protoplasts mechanically
1902	Haberlandt	first cultivation experiments with isolated plant cells. Gottlieb Habelandt is known as Father of plant tissue culture.
1904	Hanning	establishment of embryo culture for the first time
1909	Kuster	first observation of fusng cells
1922	Kotte and Robins	*in vitro* cultivation of root tips
1925	Laibach	demonstrate the practical application of zygotic embryo culture in the field of plant breeding
1934	White	first permanent root culture. It as a breakthrough in plant tissue culture history
1942	Gautheret	first permanent callus culture of *Dacus* using B-vitamins and auxin
1942	Gautheret	observation of secondary metabolites in plant callus culture
1946	Ball	Micropropagation
1954	Muir	first suspention culture of single cell or cell aggregates of *Tagetes, Daucus*)
1955	Moths and Kala	first report of secondary metabolite production in liquid media
1958	Wickson and Thimann	establishment of axillary branching somatic embryogenesis in tissue culture of *Daucus*

Contd…..

1959	Tulecke and Nickel	first report of large scale culture of plant cells by of *Ginkgo, Lolium, Rosa*
1960	Bergmann	cell clones obtained from single cultures cells plated in an agar medium of *Nicotiana phaseolus*
1960	Jones	hanging drop culture in conditioned medium of *Nicotiana*
1960	Cocking	method for obtaining large numbers of protoplasts from plant tissue of *Lycopersicon*
1962	Murashige and Skoog	Developed MS media
1965	Morel	clonal multiplicaton of horticulture plants through tissue culture of *Cymbidium*
1965	Vasil and Hilderbrandt	regeneration of a plant from one single cell of *Nicotiana* cultivated in a hanging droplet
1966	Kohlenbach	first cell division and culture of differentiated mesophyll cells
1967	Kaul and Staba	reports of the yields of certain products in cell culture equal to those in the intact plants
1967	Bourgin and Nitsch	*in vitro* production of haploid plants of *Nicotiana, Datura* from immature pollen within cultured anthers
1970	Carlson	isolation of auxotrophic mutants from cultured cells (Nicotiana)
1971	Nagata and Takebe	regeneration of plants from cultured protoplasts of *Nicotiana*
1972	Carlson	first inter-specific somatic hybrid plant from fused protoplasts of *Nicotiana*
1978	Melchers	first inter-genetic somatic hybrid plant from fused protoplasts
1978	Zenk	manifold increase in product yield by selection over parent plant documented for a variety of plant metabolites
1979	Brodlius	alginate beads used to immobilize plant cells for biotransformation and secondary metabolite production
1981	Shuler	use of hollow fiber reactor for secondary metabolite production
1983	Mitsui petrochemical	first industrial production of secondary plant products by suspension culture
1994	Calgene	Production of novel transformed plants
1995	Phyton Newsletter	taxol produced from PTC

3.3   Plant Tissue Culture Establishment and Nutritional Requirement

3.3.1 Plant Tissue Culture Lab

Following are Rooms required in tissue culture laboratory

Media preparation and storage	Preparation and storage in same room. Like kitchen with no. of shelves and counter space for storage of chemicals and stocks. pH meter, autoclave, media dispersing equipment, washing area, adequate ventilation
Transfer room (Heart of lab)	Isolation and establishment of plant tissue, Initiation and subsequent culturing performed in aseptic cabinet or laminar flow bench.. It must be provided with AC
Culture room (Largest area of lab)	Cultured explants stored in incubators with provision of desired light and temperature along with adjustment of day night
Cold storage (2-4°C)	To provide chilling requirements for crops such as apples

Necessary equipments as well as sterilization facility details are as follows:

➤ Incubator: Suitable size provided with temperature control, air circulation

➤ Autoclave: Sterilization of water, solution etc

➤ Refrigerator: For storage of reagent, culture stock solutions

➤ Microscope: To study morphology to find out deterioration

➤ Washing up equipments: To wash glasswares

➤ Oven: For sterilization of glasswares

➤ Water purification:

➤ Centrifuge: To obtain concentrated cell mass for suspension culture

➤ Shakers: rotary or reciprocal shaker necessary for suspension culture

➤ Shelves: To place culture vessels

➤ Laminar air flow bench: To perform inoculation in sterile conditions

➤ Culture cabinet: To provide optimal conditions of temperature, p^H, humidity

➤ pH meter: To obtain optimum pH 5.6-6.0 (Affects uptake of nutrients)

3.3.2 Nutritional Media

Plants in nature can synthesize their own food material. In contrast, plants growing *in vitro* are heterotrophic i.e. they cannot synthesize their own food material. Growth and morphogenesis of plant tissues *in vitro* are largely governed by the composition of the culture media. Although the basic requirements of cultured plant tissues are similar to those of whole plants, in practice nutritional components promoting optimal growth of a tissue under laboratory conditions may vary with respect to the particular species. Role of various media components is as follows:

❖ *Mineral (17 essential elements)*: This is essential part of PTC media due to following importance of few macromolecules:

  N: enhances embryogenesis and organo-genesis, part of amino acids, vitamins, nucleic acids; Ca for Organization of middle lamella of call wall; Mg for constitution of chlorophyll molecule; P for essential element of nucleic acid, DNA, RNA, cell membrane; Fe for chlorophyll synthesis and oxidation, reduction; Other elements as catalytic agents.

❖ *Organic compounds*: These are energy and carbon skeleton source. Sucrose is most preferred cheap source of carbon. Glucose, maltose, galactose, and sorbitol are also preferred in some cases.

❖ *Vitamins*: These are not mandatory but growth found to be enhanced in presence of vitamins like thiamine, pyridoxine, nicotinic acid, biotin, citric acid, ascorbic acid, inositol etc.

❖ *Growth regulators*: Auxins is important forroot differentiation and cytokinins are for shoot differentiation. Gibberellins are useful for seed or embryo culture.

❖ *Water* of usually pH 5.0-5.7

❖ *Complex extracts* are supplementary growth substances which promotes tissue growth. Example: coconut milk, tomato juice, yeast extract,

❖ *Solid support*: For callus culture agar is most preferred solidifying agent. Now a day's gelatin, alginate, silica gel are also used.

❖ *Activated charcoal* is used to adsorb toxic tissue residues

Following are Composition of commonly used tissue culture media (mg/1)								
Components	Murashige and Skoog, 1962	Gamborg et al., 1968	White, 1963	Lloyd and McCown, 1981	Vacin and Went, 1949	Modi-fiedKnud-son, 1946	Mitra et al., 1976	Nitsch and Nitsch, 1969
Macronutrients								
$Ca(PO_4)2$					200			
NH_4NO_3	1650			400				720
KNO_3	1900	2500	80		525	180	180	950
$CaCl_22H_2O$	440	150		96				166
$MgSO_47H_2O$	370	250	720	370	250	250	250	185
KH_2PO_4	170			170	250	150	150	68
$(NH_4)_2SO_4$		134			500	100	100	
$NaH_2PO_4H_2O$		150	16.50					
$Ca(NO_3)_24H_2O$			300	556		200	200	
Na_2SO_4			200					
KCl			65					
K_2SO_4				990				
Micronutrients								
KI	0.83	0.75	0.75			80	0.03	
H_3BO_3	6.2	3	1.5	6.2		6.2	0.6	10
$MnSO_44H_2O$	223		7		0.75	0.075		25
$MnSO_4H_2O$		10		29.43				
$ZnSO_47H_2O$	8.6	2	2.6	8.6			0.05	10
$Na_2MoO_42H_2O$	0.25	0.25		0.25		0.25	0.05	0.25
$CuSO_45H_2O$	0.025	0.025		0.25		0.025		0.25
$Co(NO_3)_26H_2O$							0.05	
Na_2EDTA	37.3	37.3		37.3		74.6	37.3	37.3
$FeSO_47H_2O$	27.8	27.8		27.8		25	27.8	27.8
$MnCl_2$						3.9	0.4	
$FeCC_4H_4O_5)_32 H_2O$					28			
Vitamins and other Supplements								
Inositol	100	100		100				100
Glycine	2	2	3	2				2
Thiamine HCl	0.1	10	0.1	1		0.3	0.3	0.5
Pyridoxine HCl	0.5		0.1	0.5		0.3	0.3	0.5
Nicotinic acid	0.5		0.5	0.5			1.25	5
Ca-panthothenate			1					
Cysteine HCl			1					
Riboflavin						0.3	0.05	
Biotin							0.05	0.05
Folic acid							0.3	0.5

3.3.2.1   Media Preparation

Preparation of stock solutions: Basic medium without organic solutions or phyto hormones. Components should be in molar units rather than weight to get accurate concentration

Media preparation:
1. Macronutrients are dissolved in 200ml of distilled water
2. Micronutrients are dissolved in 200ml of distilled water
3. Vitamins are dissolved in 100ml of distilled water in a separate flask and stored at refrigerated conditions
4. Growth hormones are dissolved in separately in 100 ml of distilled water and stored in a cool place
5. To prepare 1 lit of the media the above solutions are mixed together
6. Sucrose and amino acids are added to the medium
7. The volume of the media up to 950ml by the addition of distilled water
8. The pH of this solution is adjusted to 5.6 with 0.1 M sodium hydroxide solution or hydrochloric acid solution. Bcoz at low pH agar fail to gel.
9. Finally the volume of this media is made up to 1 liter with distilled water
10. Transfer media into conical flask and plugged with cotton.
11. If solid media is required add 2% agar.
12. The above conical flasks are autoclaved [microfiltration (0.22mm) for thermo labile components] and used for tissue culture.

3.3.3   Explant Selection and Surface Sterilization

Cell, tissue or organ of a plant that is used to start in vitro cultures is called as explant. Age of explants plays vital role in formation of callus. Choice of explants is based on desired research. Explants can be obtained from buds, roots, nodal segments, apical meristem, seed, embryo, anthers, pollens and or protoplast. As explants are always contaminated with microorganisms so it becomes necessary to carry out surface sterilization. Commonly used sterilizing agents are: Sodium hypochlorite 1-2%; Bromine water: 1-2%; Hydrogen peroxide: 10-12%; Mercuric chloride: 0.1-1%; Silver nitrate: 1% The aerial portion of plants such as bud, leaf, stem sections are sterilizes by submerging 2-3 min in 70% ethanol followed by 2-3 rinses with sterilized distilled water.

Callus Culture/Solid Medium culture: Surface sterilized explant is transferred onto solidified nutrient medium in flasks and then incubated at 26-28^{0}C. About 3-4 weeks callus forms about 3-4 cm. Divide callus into small pieces i.e. about 5-10mm and transfer into fresh medium. This is called sub culturing which should be done at regular intervals of 4 weeks. *Conditions*: Suitable media with IAA, NAA, Kinetin and vitamins, appropriate balance between auxin and kinetin and Suitable intensity light for 12 hr or continuous.

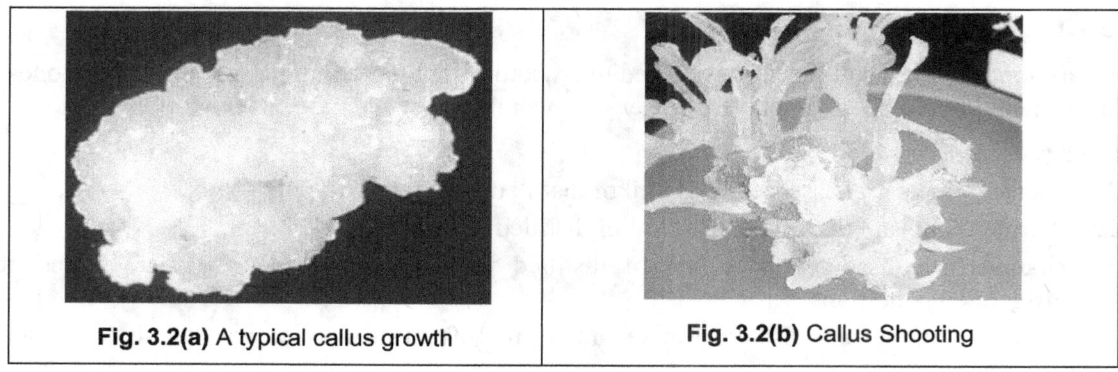

Fig. 3.2(a) A typical callus growth

Fig. 3.2(b) Callus Shooting

3.3.4 Suspension Culture/Liquid Medium Culture

Explant which is previously homogenized to give single cell or Cell cluster is dispersed in a liquid medium. Cell suspension culture actively grows under agitation preferably by shaker and aeration. This culture can be subculture by pippeting out and adding to fresh medium. Advantage: Growth rate is higher than agar culture as cells are surrounded by nutrient media and hence material formed is more uniform. The suspension cultures are broadly grouped as:

1. Batch cultures,

2. Continuous cultures, and

3. Immobilized cell cultures

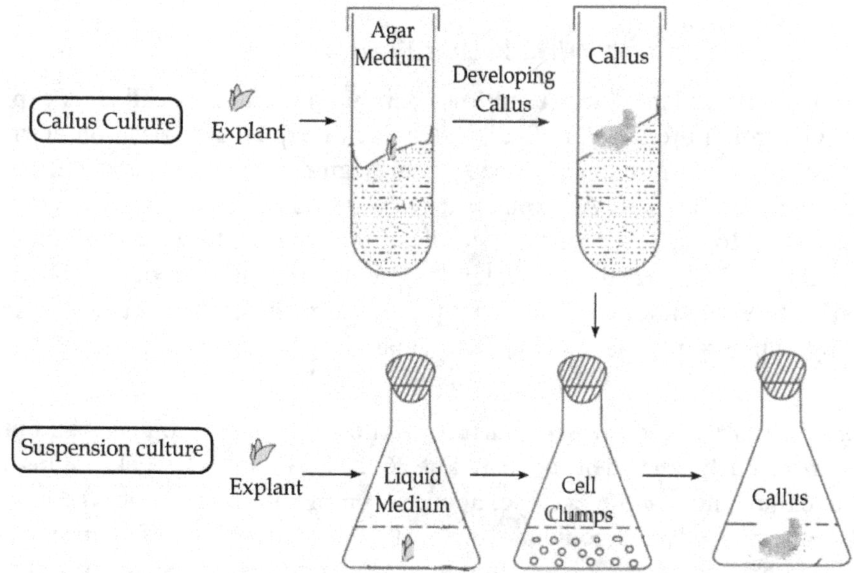

Fig. 3.3 Callus and suspension culturing

3.4   Tissue Culture Growth Measurement

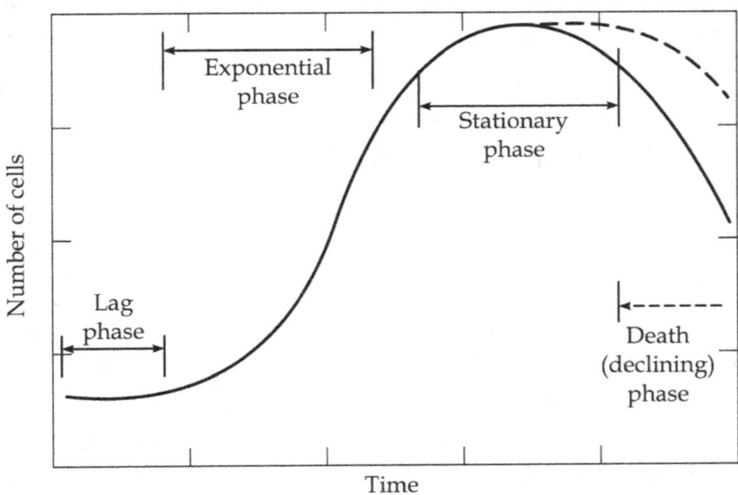

Fig. 3.4 Growth Profile for PTC

The cell number or biomass of a batch culture exhibits a typical sigmoidal curve having *Lag phase* during which the cell number remains unchanged, *Logarithmic* (log) *phase* when there is a rapid increase in cell number and finally ending in a stationary phase during which cell number does not change. The lag phase duration depends mainly on inoculum size and growth phase of the culture from which inoculum is taken.   The log phase lasts about 3-4 cell generations (time taken for doubling of cell number), and the duration of a cell generation may vary from 22-48 hr mainly depending on the plant species.   The stationary phase is forced on the culture by depletion of the nutrients and possibly due to an accumulation of cellular wastes. If the culture is kept in stationary phase for a prolonged period the cells may die.

1. ***Fresh and dry weight measurement***: Fresh and dry weights are the most commonly used measures of growth of both suspension and callus cultures. In case of callus cultures, the cell mass is placed on a pre weighed dry filter paper or nylon filter and weighed to determine fresh weight. Cells from suspension cultures are filtered onto a filter paper or nylon filter, washed with distilled water, excess water removed under vacuum and weighed along with the filter; the filter is pre weighed in wet condition. For dry weight determination the cells and the filter are dried in an oven at 60°C for 12 hr and weighed; the filter is pre-weighed in dry condition. Fresh and dry weights may either be expressed as per ml (suspension culture) or per culture.

2. ***Cell counts***: Callus mass is dissociated into individual cells by gentle treatment with mixture of 10% chromic acid and 10% nitric acid for 5-10 min at 60 Oc. After cooling vigorously shaken and pectinase added to break cluster mass. This cell suspension is then diluted, stained and counted by using heamo-cytometer.

3. ***Packed cell volume***: PCV is a percentage of volume of the pellet to the entire culture volume. The entire content is centrifuged at 200 rpm for 5-10 min or until supernatant is free from cells. Volume after centrifugation is measured and expressed in percentage.

4. ***Cell Viability Test***: Cell viability can be determined by Phase contrast microscopy, and staining with any one or combinations of following staining reagents:
   1. 2. 2, 3, 5-triphenyltetrazolium chlo-ride (TTC),
   3. Fluorescein diacetate (FDA) and
   4. Evan's blue.

   Live cells show cytoplasmic streaming and a well defined healthy nucleus which are easily observable with a phase contrast microscope or even a light microscope. Cell masses can be stained with 1-2% solution of TTC, which is reduced by living cells to formazan that yields red colour.

   Formazan can be extracted and measured with a spectrophotometer to give a quantitative estimate of viability, but it is not suitable for single or few cells. Cells are treated with 0.01 % solution of FDA. Live cells cleave FDA by esterase activity and produce fluorescein, which can not cross plasma membrane. With UV exposure, fluorescein gives green fluorescence so that live cells appear green, while dead cells do not fluoresce. Evan's blue (0.025%) is not taken up by live cells, while it freely enters into damaged dead cells. Therefore all cells that take up stain are dead. Evan's blue is usually used in conjunction with FDA.

5. ***Protein content:*** collect cells and washed with boiling 70% ethanol and dry this material with acetone. Transfer it to 1M NaOH solution, boil for one and half hour to hydrolyze proteins which is then further estimated by routine methods such as Biuret method.

6. ***Mitotic index:*** Fresh cell suspension is transferred to micro slide. To it add aceto-orcein and heat for 5 min. Then observe this slide under oil immersion to observe stages of cell division for about 1000 cells. Percentage showing mitotic stage is called mitotic index.

7. ***Plating of cell suspension:*** To establish the clones of single cell origin. For this 2 ml of aliquot of cell suspension is inoculated in 8 ml of sterile medium containing 0.6 % agar. It is then mixed and transferred to 9cm petriplates and allowed to incubate for 3 weeks. Cellular units are then counted by using stereo binocular microscope and the plating efficiency is then calculated by following formula.

$$PE = \frac{No. \, of \, colonies \, / \, plate}{No. \, of \, cellular \, units \, / \, plate} \times 100$$

3.5   Types of Culture

Type	Explant	Uses
Meristem culture	Shoot apex with few primordial leaves	Clonal propagation. Production of virus free germplasm. Mass production of desirable genotypes. Cryopreservation (cold storage) or *in vitro* conservation of germplasm.
Root cultures	Explants of the root tip of either primary or lateral roots	Clonal propagation. Production of virus free germplasm.
Shoot tip culture	Shoot apex	Somaclonal variation and transformation of plants in disease free plants
Anther or pollen culture	Anthers or isolated pollen grains, flower buds with small anthers	Production of haploids.
Ovary Culture	Un-fertilised ovaries	Production of haploid plants, studies on fruit development. Preferred explant for the initiation of somatic embryogenic cultures.
Seed culture	Seeds	Production of clean seedlings for explants or meristem culture
Embryo culture	Egg, zygote, proembryo, mature embryo,	Overcoming seed dormancy and self-sterility of seeds. Due to embryo rescue, interspecific or intergeneric hybridisation is possible. Shortening of breeding cycle. Production of haploid plants.
Protoplasts culture	Plant cells without cell wall.	To produce somatic hybrids, asymmetric hybrids or cybrids. Production of organelle recombinants. Transfer of cytoplasmic male sterility.
Hairy root culture plant disease caused by *Agrobacterium rhizogenes*Conn., a Gram-negative soil bacterium.	Hypocotyl, leaf, stem, stalk, petiole, shoot tip, cotyledon, protoplast, storage root.	Genetic Transformation studies. Transgenic plant production.

Protoplasts culture: Protoplasts are plant cells without cell wall. Protoplasts are most commonly isolated from either leaf mesophyll cells or cell suspensions, although other sources can be used to advantage. Protoplasts are fragile and easily damaged, and therefore must be cultured carefully. Liquid medium is not agitated and a high osmotic potential is maintained, at least in the initial stages. The liquid medium must be shallow enough to allow aeration in the absence of agitation. Protoplasts can be plated out on to solid medium and callus produced. Whole plants can be regenerated by organogenesis or somatic embryogenesis from this callus. Proto-plasts are ideal targets for transformation by a variety of means.	
Protoplast isolation	Two general approaches to removing the cell wall (a difficult task without damaging the protoplast) can be taken— • *Mechanical* isolation, although possible, often results in low yields, poor quality and poor performance in culture due to substances released from damaged cells.

	Enzymatic isolation is usually carried out in a simple salt solution with a high osmoticum, plus the cell wall degrading enzymes. It is usual to use a mix of both cellulase and pectinase enzymes, which must be of high quality and purity.
Protoplast Fusion	A number of strategies have been used to induce fusion between protoplasts of different strains/species; of these the following have been relatively more successful. 1. *Spontaneous*: Fuses automatically during isolation 2. *Mechanical*: This type of fusion can be achieved by following way: *Intimate physical contact* Micromanipulator and perfusion micropipette like mechanical devices are useful to bring forced close contact under microscope *Electro fusion*: A more selective and less drastic approach is the electro fusion technique, which utilizes low voltage (65-80 V cm-I) electric current pulses to align the protoplasts in a single row like a pearl-chain. The high voltage creates transient disturbances in the organization of plasma lemma, which leads to the fusion of neighboring protoplasts. The entire operation is carried out manually in specially designed equipment, called electroporator. 3. **Chemical**: *High pH¬ high Ca2+ treatment:* Protoplasts of desired strains/species are mixed in almost equal proportion; generally they are mixed while still suspended in the enzyme mixture. The protoplast mixture is then subjected to a high pH (10.5) and high Ca2+ concentration (50 m mol I-I) at 37°C for about 30 min (high pH¬ high Ca2+ treatment). This technique is quite suitable for some species, while for some others it may be toxic. *Polyethylene glycol (PEG) induced protoplast fusion*: It is the most commonly used as it induces reproducible high frequency fusion accompanied with low toxicity to most cell types. The protoplast mixture is treated with 28-50% PEG (MW 1,500-6,000) for 15-30 min, followed by gradual washing of the protoplasts to remove PEG; protoplast fusion occurs during the washing. During the washing process, PEG molecules may pull out the plasma lemma components bound to them. This would disturb plasma lemma organization and may lead to the fusion of protoplasts located close to each other.

The above fusion techniques are nonselective in that they induce fusion between any two or more protoplasts except electro fusion as later induced selective fusion.

Uses: Combining genomes to produce somatic hybrids, asymmetric hybrids or cybrids (hybrids of mitochondrion genome with nuclear genome), production of organelle recombinants, transfer of cytoplasmic male sterility.

Hairy root culture: Hairy root is a plant disease caused by *Agrobacterium rhizogenes*Conn., a Gram-negative soil bacterium and is capable of infecting a wide range of plant species, causing hairy root disease. It has natural transformation abilities.

When *A. rhizogenus* infects a plant cell, it transfers a copy of its T-DNA, which is a small section of DNA carried on its (Tumour inducing) plasmid. This T-DNA is flanked by two (imperfect) 25 base pair repeats. Any DNA contained within these borders will be transferred to the host cell when used as transformation vector. Most plant materials, such as hypocotyl, leaf, stem, stalk, petiole, shoot tip, cotyledon, protoplast, storage root or tuber can be used to induce hairy roots. However, for different species, the proper explant material may vary and the age of the material is most critical, with juvenile material being

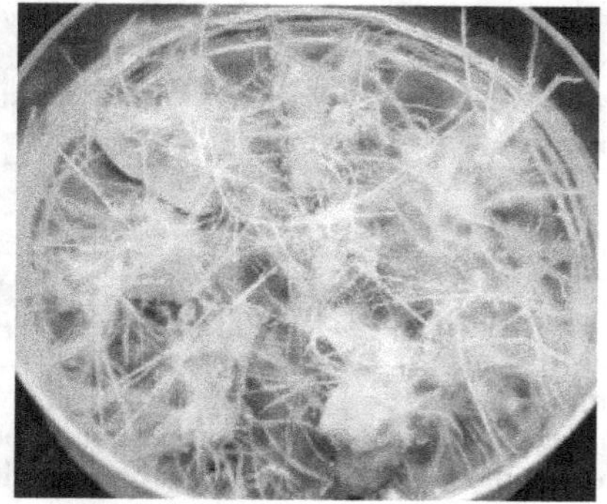

Fig. 3.5 Hairy root growth

optimal. To induce hairy root, explants are separately wounded and co-cultivated or inoculated with *A. rhizogenes*. **e.g.** *Atropa belladonna* produces atropine and scopolamine at significantly higher levels than conventional plant roots.

Wounded site produces phenolic (e.g. acetosyringone, 3', 5'-dimethoxy-4'-hydroxy acetophenone) which attracts *A. rhizogenes* by chemo-taxis. Other phenolics include hydroxyl acetosyringone, coniferyl alcohol, and sinapinic acid. All these stimulate efficient *vir* gene expression. It causes roots to proliferate rapidly at the infection site causing hairy root disease.

This typical disease syndrome is characterized by numerous fast growing, highly branched adventitious roots at the site of infection, which continue to grow in-vitro in a hormone free culture medium. This typical phenotypic response results from the insertion into the plant genome of T-DNA (transfer DNA), carried on the bacterial *Ri* plasmid (root inducing plasmid), coding for auxin synthesis and other rhizogenic functions.

The transformed segment T-DNA contains genes for opine biosynthesis and sensitivity. Products of virulence (vir) genes located on non transferred segment of the Ri plasmid, are responsible for the excision of the T-DNA for transfer into the plant cell, and possibly for chromosomal integration in the nucleus for the recipient cell. Transferred genes often act as dominant. The roots can be removed from the parent tissue and cultured indefinitely in simple defined medium free of plant growth hormones.

Establishment of hairy root cultures: To succeed in establishing a hairy root culture system for a certain plant species, several essential conditions should be taken into consideration. These conditions include the bacterial strain of *A. rhizogenes*, an appropriate explant, a proper antibiotic to eliminate redundant bacteria after cocultivation, and a suitable culture medium. Based on the types of opines produced, the strains of A. rhizogenes can be separated into five lines: octopine, agropine, nopaline, mannopine, and cucumopine. Agropine strains are the most often used strains owing to their strongest induction ability. Most plant materials, such as hypocotyl, leaf, stem, stalk, petiole, shoot tip, cotyledon, protoplast, storage root, or tuber, can be used to induce hairy roots. However, for different species, the proper explant material may vary and the age of the material is most critical, with juvenile material being optimal. To induce hairy root, explants are separately wounded and co-cultivated or inoculated with *A. rhizogenes*. Usually two or three days later, the explant can be transferred into solid media with antibiotics such as cefotaxime sodium, carbencilin disodium, vancomycin, ampicillin sodium, claforan, streptomycin sulphate, or tetracycline, ranging in concentration from 100 to 500 µg/mL, to kill or eliminate redundant bacteria. The hairy roots will be induced within a short period of time, which varies from one week to over a month depending on different plant species. The decontaminated hairy roots can be subcultured on phytohormone-free medium. Optimizing the composition of nutrients for hairy root cultures is critical to gain a high production of secondary metabolites. Factors such as the carbon source and its concentration, the ionic concentration of the medium, the pH of the medium, light, phytohormones, temperature, and inoculum are known to influence growth and secondary metabolism. Heavy metal ions and the concentrations of phosphate, nitrate, and ammonia have also been well studied. The addition of auxin and elicitors often increases the levels of secondary metabolites. Because of these factors and the fact that individual hairy roots may have different requirements for nutrient conditions, the culture conditions should be optimized separately for each species and for individual clones.

3.6 Applications of Plant Tissue Culture in Pharmacognosy

1. *To study respiration and metabolism:* Studies of respiration of growing callus provides means of separating between normal and disease growth. Enzyme levels provide idea regarding composition of media and growth parameters of developing callus. Changes in the composition of the medium alter different phases of metabolism that control cell enlargement. For example: changes in media cause increase or decrease in respiration and ascorbic acid oxidase activity in cultured tobacco pith parenchyma.

2. *To study proliferation and organ function:* Tissue culture allows to study different types of proliferation such as Sections may proliferated as an layer over cut surface; Proliferation may be from preexisting cambia; Many times sections develop roots or bud meristems; Parenchymatous cultures may develop vascular bund; Out-standing efforts have been made to clarify cell growth, cell division, callus formation and organ differentiation in terms of growth substances and balance s of common metabolites.

3. *Single cell culture of higher plant cells:* Due to tissue culture technique it is possible to isolate and grow single cell of higher plant. But question remains whether all cells in callus are similar or not? This single cell method enables to evaluate additional chemical, morphological, genetical and pathological similarities and differences. Even clarification and location of virus infection can be studied by single cell. E.g.: Tobacco plant

4. *Genetic transformation:* The transfer and expression of foreign genes into plant cells. Many different explants can be used, depending on the plant species and its favored method of regeneration as well as the method of transformation. Introduction of foreign DNA to generate novel (and typically desirable) genetic combinations which is also used to study the function of genes. **e.g.** chimeric gene containing DNA of the coat protein protect the plant against cucumo virus (CMV), alfalfa mosaic virus (ALMV)

5. *Production of disease free and disease resistant plant:* Following method of breeding for disease resistance plants are commonly used: selection, introduction, mutation, hybridization, somaclonal variation, and genetic engineering. A comparison of normal and diseased tissues of various plants can be made by tissue culture. Which is mostly depends on strain of host and nutritional and physical environments. Changes in host and media can minimize chances of infection. Plants free from pathogens can be developed from infected plant's shoot tips or growing buds as pathogens infect almost all part except growing buds. These meristematic tissues can be utilized to developed disease free plant. Plants grown from tissue culture usually pass trough callus phase and show many variations. These show some agronomic characteristics like tolerance to pests, diseases, etc.

6. *Germplasm storage:* Generally most of the plants are stored in the form of seeds or plantlets. But some seeds fail to grow into plantlets. This problem can be overcome by raising identical clones in form of seeds, buds, protoplasts, shoot tips. This material is then stored in a minimal medium and with low light intensity and temperature or cryopreserving (storage at low temperature using liquid nitrogen) without affecting its viability. This is called germplasm storage which is then used to develop whole plant.

7. *Embryo rescue:* In many plants normal fertilization occurs but ovule fails to develop into a mature seed. In such cases, fertilized egg or immature embryo is removed and cultured to generate hybrids with few new characters. This is called embryo rescue. When it is not feasible to isolate embryo due to smaller size whole ovule or ovary can be cultured and it is called ovule or ovary culture.

8. *Somaclonal modification:* Generally clones from tissue culture bear uniformity in their characters but some times few clones show variations. This variant clones express new characters which are absent in their parent cells. Thus formation of variant clone cell from cultured callus tissue is called somaclonal variation which may desirable or not. Desirable clones are useful for crop improvement by testing their resistance to herbicide, temperature or heavy metals and further testing its productivity.

9. *Production of haploids:* Haploid plants are characterized by presence of only single set of chromosomes in their cells. Anther. Ovule or pollen grain culture mostly utilized to produce haploids which are very useful for detection and selection of recessive mutants for few characters. Thus very useful for crop improvement.

10. *Production of artificial seeds:* An artificial seed is synthetic seed which is made up of somatic embryo surrounded by the nutrient medium and this as a whole protected by a thin synthetic membrane. In comparison to natural seeds, these are smaller in size. They are identical and contain only somatic embryos of known strain. It can be stored even for a period of 1 year without any loss in viability. Seeds encapsulated in a synthetic gel like membrane made up of polyoxyethylene, carragenin, gel-rite, gelatin, sodium alginate or polyacylamide gel. Calcium salts, calcium chloride, potassium or ammonium chloride are commonly used as complexing agent. The pattern of germination is same as natural seeds. It can be directly sown in soil without need of hardening in green house. Disadvantage is high cost of production.

11. *Clonal propagation:* It involves propagation through techniques of cell, tissue or organ culture. Advantage: rapid multiplication of superior clones, Maintenance of genetic uniformity, multiplication of sexually derived sterile hybrids. In this technique shoot tips or auxiliary buds are utilized for propagation on culture media without intervention of callus phase.

12. *Micro propagation:* It is common method being utilize both at research and commercial level. It can be employed for the mass production of plant including nursery stock species, ornamental plants, vegetables and field crops.

Plant	Drug	Technique used
Atropa belladona	Atropine	Hairy root culture
Rauwolfia serpentina	Ajmaline	Cell suspension culture
Cephalis ipecacuanha	Emetine	Cell immobilisation

13. *Mutant selection:* It is an important tool for crop improvement. Cells are subjected to mutagenic treatments and subsequently mutants are selected. Selection of mutant cells is usually performed by addition of toxic substances to cells followed by isolation of resistant cells. In this manner cell lines of potato resistant to 5-methyltryptophan were selected and

this cultures permitted accumulation of free phenyl alanine, tryptophan and tyrosine. Induction of polyploidy Introduction of genetic variability

14. ***Somatic hybridization:*** Production of hybrid plants through the fusion of protoplasts of two different plant species/varieties is called somatic hybridization, and such hybrids are known as somatic hybrids. The technique of somatic hybridization involves the following four steps:
    - ➢ Isolation of protoplasts,
    - ➢ Fusion of the protoplasts of desired species/varieties,
    - ➢ Selection of somatic hybrid cells, and
    - ➢ Culture of the hybrid cells and regeneration of hybrid plants from them.

15. ***Cloning:*** A clone of cells consists of all the cells derived through mitosis from a single cell and the process of obtaining a clone is called cloning. The process of asexually producing a group of independent organisms or cells, all genetically identical, from a single ancestor. Therefore, all the cells of a clone are expected be identical with each other in their genotype and chromosome constitution, and other attributes, except for the changes that may arise afresh during and after cloning. Cloning is based on single cells separated from tissues and cultured in a manner to allow separate recovery of the cell mass derived from them.

16. ***Production of secondary metabolites:*** Most of the secondary metabolites are accumulated after certain age or maturity of the plant. It is difficult to increase the area under plantation and growth of the plants takes its own time. To meet the ever increasing demand (Example: Vincristine) the natural sources are not sufficient. The world political scenario may also affect the supply of a particular raw material. To overcome the all these hurdles the industry requires alternative methods of assured supply of uniform material throughout the year. Plant tissue culture techniques offer an excellent alternative through cell culture, organ culture, endophytes, genetic manipulations and now-a-days the hairy root culture is also became very popular method of producing secondary metabolites from plant roots. E.g.: cardiac glycosides: 1 mg/ml of suspension. Morphine codeine: 1.5 mg/gm of dry weight of *Papaver*um species. As several metabolites released in cell vacuoles not in medium and to release this constituents cell viability should be kept constant. The major advantages of a cell culture system over the conventional cultivation of whole plants are as follows:
    - ➢ Useful compounds can be produced under controlled conditions independent of climatic changes or soil conditions.
    - ➢ Cultured cells would be free of microbes and insects.
    - ➢ The cells of any plants, tropical or alpine, could easily be multiplied to yield their specific metabolites.
    - ➢ Automated control of cell growth and rational regulation of metabolite processes would reduce labor costs and improve productivity.
    - ➢ Organic substances are extractable from callus cultures.
    - ➢ Production can be more reliable, simpler, and more predictable.
    - ➢ Isolation of the phytochemical can be rapid and efficient, when compared with extraction from complex whole plants.
    - ➢ Compounds produced in vitro can directly parallel compounds in the whole plant.

> Interfering compounds that occur in the field-grown plant can be avoided in cell cultures.

> Tissue and cell cultures can yield a source of defined standard phyto-chemicals in large volumes.

> Tissue and cell cultures are a potential model to test elicitation.

> Cell cultures can be radiolabeled, such that the accumulated secondary products, when provided as feed to laboratory animals, can be traced metabolically.

3.7 Edible Vaccines

Vaccine are playing important role in preventive therapy of number of life threatening diseases. Unfortunately, many disadvantages of present animal and microbial originated vaccines, which relates to complexity (production, storage, delivery), rigid purification requirement, skilled personnel, expensiveness, toxicity and poor mucosal response limit their uses. Therefore, plant originated vaccine called as edible vaccine concept emerged as safer and cost effective alternative.

Methods of gene transfer

- **Chemical Method**
  - Heat shock
  - Calcium phosphate
  - Liposomes and polymers
  - Nanoparticles
- **Physical Method**
  - Electroporation
  - Biolistics
  - Microinjection
  - Sonoporation
  - Photoporation
  - Magnetofection
  - Hydroporation
- **Agrobacterium Method**
- **Viral delivery Method**
  - RNA-based viral vectors
  - DNA-based viral vectors

Concepts of gene transfer

A vector is a DNA molecule used as a vehicle to artificially carry foreign genetic material into another cell, where it can be replicated and/or expressed (e.g. plasmid, cosmid, Lambda phages). A vector containing foreign DNA is termed recombinant DNA. The four major types of vectors are plasmids, viral vectors, cosmids, and artificial chromosomes. Of these, the most commonly used vectors are plasmids

Modern artificially-constructed vectors contain essential components found in all vectors, and may contain other additional features found only in some vectors:

➢ **Origin of replication**: Necessary for the replication and maintenance of the vector in the host cell.

➢ **Promoter**: Promoters are used to drive the transcription of the vector's transgene as well as the other genes in the vector such as the antibiotic resistance gene. Some cloning vectors need not have a promoter for the cloned insert but it is an essential component of expression vectors so that the cloned product may be expressed.

➢ **Cloning site**: This may be a multiple cloning site or other features that allow for the insertion of foreign DNA into the vector through ligation.

➢ **Genetic markers:** Genetic markers for viral vectors allow for confirmation that the vector has integrated with the host genomic DNA.

➢ **Antibiotic resistance**: Vectors with antibiotic-resistance open reading frames allow for survival of cells that have taken up the vector in growth media containing antibiotics through antibiotic selection.

➢ **Epitope**: Some vectors may contain a sequence for a specific epitope that can be incorporated into the expressed protein. It allows for antibody identification of cells expressing the target protein.

➢ **Reporter genes**: Some vectors may contain a reporter gene that allow for identification of plasmid that contains inserted DNA sequence. An example is lacZ-α which codes for the N-terminus fragment of β-galactosidase, an enzyme that digests galactose. A multiple cloning site is located within lacZ-α, and an insert successfully ligated into the vector will disrupt the gene sequence, resulting in an inactive β-galactosidase. Cells containing vector with an insert may be identified using blue/white selection by growing cells in media containing an analogue of galactose (X-gal). Cells expressing β-galactosidase (therefore doesn't contain an insert) appear as blue colonies. White colonies would be selected as those that may contain an insert. Other commonly used reporters include green fluorescent protein and luciferase.

➢ **Targeting sequence:** Expression vectors may include encoding for a targeting sequence in the finished protein that directs the expressed protein to a specific organelle in the cell or specific location such as the periplasmic space of bacteria/plant.

➢ **Protein purification tags**: Some expression vectors include proteins or peptide sequences that allows for easier purification of the expressed protein. Examples include polyhistidine-tag, glutathione-S-transferase, and maltose binding protein. Some of these tags may also allow for increased solubility of the target protein. The target protein is fused to the protein tag, but a protease cleavage site positioned in the polypeptide linker region between the protein and the tag allows the tag to be removed later.

Examples of Recombinant Vaccines Expressed in Plants		
Year	**Vaccine antigen**	**Species**
1992	Hepatitis virus B surface antigen	Tobacco
1995	Malaria parasite antigen	Virus particle
1995	Rabies virus glycoprotein	Tomato
1995	*E. coli* heat-labile	Tobacco, enterotoxin, potato
1996	Human rhinovirus 14 (HRV-14) and human immunodeficiency virus type (HIV-1) epitopes	Virus particle
1996	Norwalk virus capsid protein	Tobacco, potato
1997	Diabetes-associated autoantigen	Tobacco, potato
1997	Hepatitis B surface proteins	Potato
1997	Mink enteritis virus epitope	Virus particle
1997	Rabies and HIV epitopes	Virus particle
1998	Foot and mouth disease virus VP1 structural protein	*Arabidopsis*
1998	*E. coli* heat-labile enterotoxin	Potato
1998	*E. coli* heat-labile enterotoxin	Potato
1998	Rabies virus	Virus particle
1998	Cholera toxin B subunit	Potato
1998	Human insulin-cholera toxin B subunit fusion protein	Potato
1999	Foot and mouth disease virus VP1 structural protein	Alfalfa
1999	Hepatitis B virus surface antigen	Yellow lupin, lettuce
1999	Human cytomegalovirus glycoprotein B	Tobacco
1999	Dental caries (*S. mutans*)	Tobacco
1999	Diabetes-associated autoantigen	Tobacco, carrot
2002	Respiratory syncytial virus	Tomato

Production

Introduction of gene encoding from pathogenic microorganism (Bacteria, virus, parasite) to plant: Two options are generally available to introduce pathogenic gene:

➢ Introduction of entire gene into plant transformation vector between 5' and 3' regulatory elements

➢ Introduction of DNA fragment encoding antigen epitope through plant viruses (Example: TMV, CMV)

There are chemical, mechanical and biological methods of introduction of foreign DNA into plants, which are discussed previously in transgenic plant development topic. However, Gene gun and *Agrobacterium tumefaciens* methods are more preferred in edible vaccine production. Each single antigen expressed in plants must be tested for its proper assembly and can be verified by animal studies, Western blot; and quantified by enzyme-linked immunosorbent assay (ELISA). Production of transgenic plants is species dependent and takes 3-9 months. Multicomponent vaccines can be obtained by crossing two plant lines harboring different antigens. Adjuvants may also be co-expressed along with the antigen in the same plant. Overcoat technology permits the plant to produce the entire protein, whereas epicoat technology involves expression of only the foreign proteins.

Plants of choice: any edible plant growing throughout year with good vegetative yield are suitable for edible vaccine production. **Example:** Banana, potato, tomato, tobacco, lettuce, rice, maize, soyabeans, wheat

Advantages:

➢ Easy to scale up

➢ Cheaper than traditional vaccines

➢ Enhance compliance, especially in children because of oral administration

➢ Eliminate the need for trained medical personnel

➢ Sidestepping demands for purification

➢ Do not require capital-intensive pharmaceutical manufacturing facilities.

➢ Good genetic stability

➢ Heat-stable

➢ Non-requirement of syringes and needles also decreases chances of infection.

➢ Fear of contamination with animal viruses - like the mad cow disease, which is a threat in vaccines manufactured from cultured mammalian cells - is eliminated, because plant viruses do not infect humans.

➢ These vaccines activate both mucosal and systemic immunity, as they come in contact with the digestive tract lining. This dual effect would provide first-line defense against pathogens invading through mucosa

➢ Administration of edible vaccines to mothers might be successful in immunizing the *fetus-in-utero* by transplacental transfer of maternal antibodies or the infant through breast milk. role in protecting infants

➢ Multiple antigens may also be delivered

Challenges

➢ Regulatory concerns would include lot-to-lot consistency, uniformity of dosage and purity.

➢ Due to low accumulation of foreign proteins high dose is require

➢ Dose determination depends on plant size and patient's age, weight

➢ Accurate dosing in infant is challenging due to spitting or throwing

➢ Chances of resistance to GM foods are more

➢ Quality assurance, efficacy and environmental impact need to be addressed

➢ Regulated controlled greenhouse facilities

➢ It is still unclear whether the edible vaccines would be regulated under food, drugs or agricultural products and what vaccine component would be licensed - antigen itself, genetically engineered fruit or transgenic seeds.

➤ Promoter is present in most commercially grown GM crops today and is especially unstable and prone to horizontal gene transfer, recombination or mutations by random insertion.

➤ Horizontal gene transfer/recombination, genetic engineering may contribute to emergence and re-emergence of infectious, drug-resistant diseases, rise of autoimmune diseases, cancers and reactivation of dormant viruses.

➤ Transgenic contamination is unavoidable. Besides pollen, transgenes may spread horizontally by sucking insects, transfer to soil microbes during plant wounding/breakdown of roots/rootlets and may pollute surface and ground water.

➤ Bacteria may take up transgenic DNA in food in human gut. Antibiotic resistance marker genes can spread from transgenic food to pathogenic bacteria, making infections very difficult to treat.

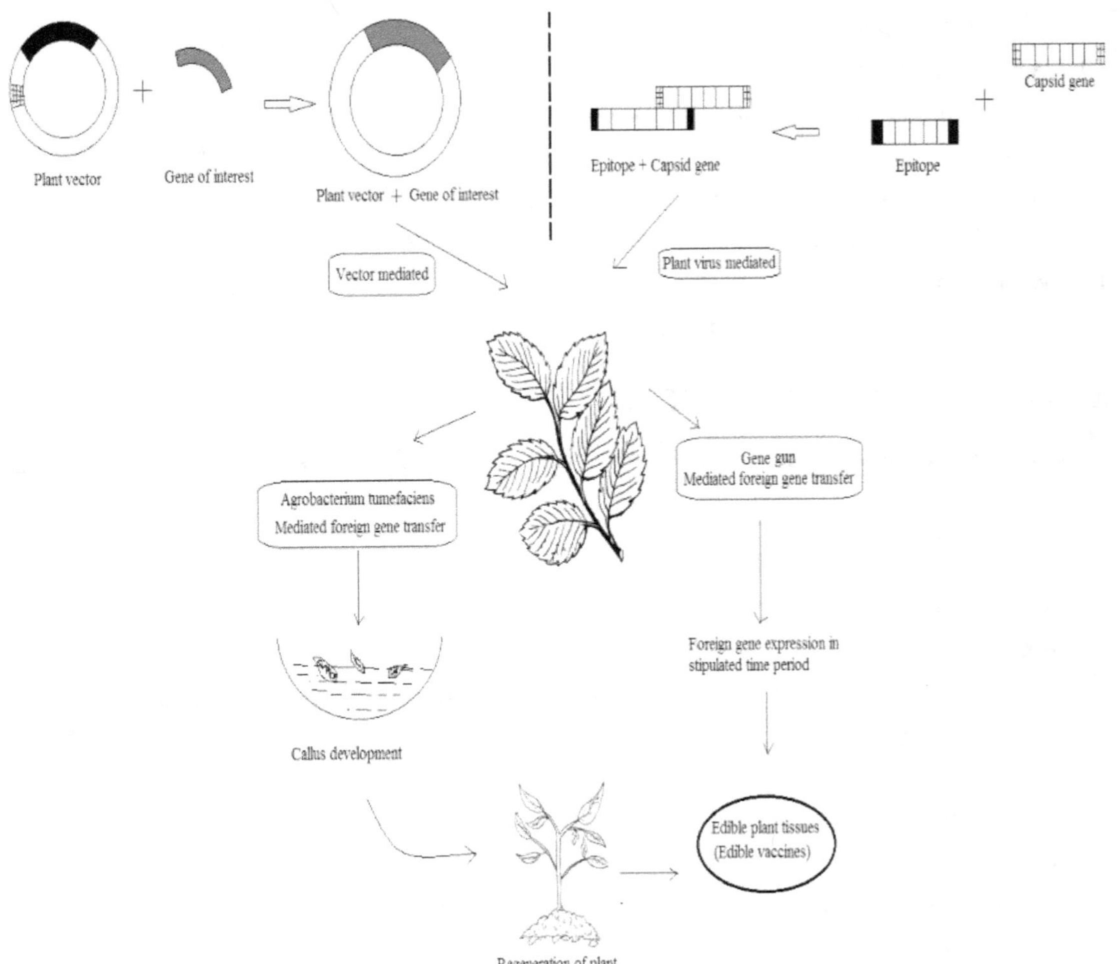

Fig. 3.6 Edible vaccine production

Subjective Questions

1. Define plant tissue culture?
2. Explain terms- totipotency, callus and explant?
3. Write a note on historical developments of plant tissue culture.
4. What are different nutritional requirements of plant tissue culture?
5. What are different types of plant tissue culture?
6. Write a note on applications of plant tissue culture.
7. What do you mean by edible vaccine?
8. What is GM crop?
9. What is protoplast?
10. What is Hairy root culture?
11. Which are hormones responsible for shooting and rooting in plant tissue culture?
12. What is biotransformation? Explain with examples?
13. What is elicitor? How it plays role in tissue culture growth?
14. How different Medias differ in their composition and applications?
15. What is synthetic seed?
16. Differentiate organogenesis and embryogenesis?

Multiple Choice Questions (MCQs)

1. The hypothesis of plant cell cultivation on artificial medium was first time put forward in 1902 by
   a. Robbins
   b. Haberlandt
   c. Kotte
   d. White

2. In 1934, successful continuous culture of tomato root tips was first time achieved by
   a. Haberlandt
   b. Kotte
   c. White
   d. Robbins

3. Liquid culture of *Nicotiana tobaccum* was first reported by Muir et al.,in
   a. 1955
   b. 1954
   c. 1956
   d. 1957

4. Naphthalene acetic acid (NAA) and 2,4-dichlorophenoxy acetic acid (2,4-D) are used to induce cell division in culture medium in molar concentration of
    a. 10^{-7} to 5×10^{-7}
    b. 10^{-7} to 5×10^{-5}
    c. 10^{-7} to 5×10^{-10}
    d. 10^{-7} to 5×10^{-9}

5. Which one of the following plant growth hormone is used to induce callus formation in culture medium
    a. Kinetin
    b. Benzyladenine
    c. Only a
    d. Both a and b

6. Surface sterilizing agent, Sodium hypochlorite should be used in concentration
    a. $0.1 - 1\,\%$
    b. $1\text{-}2\,\%$
    c. $10 - 12\,\%$
    d. $1\,\%$

7. Which one of the following is used as surface sterilizing agent in plant tissue culture?
    a. Hydrogen peroxide
    b. Sodium hypochlorite
    c. Mercuric chloride
    d. All of the above

8. For induction of shooting, auxin to cytokinin ratio should in proportion of
    a. 5: 1
    b. 6: 1
    c. 4:1
    d. 7:1

9. For induction of shooting, auxin to cytokinin ratio should in proportion of
    a. 100:1
    b. 1: 100
    c. 50:1
    d. 1: 50

10. Which part of plant is used in tissue culture to develop virus free plants?
    a. Root tip
    b. Shoot tip
    c. Meristem tip
    d. All of the above

11. Hairy root culture development involves incorporation of " Ri-DNA" from
   a. *Agrobacterium rhizhogens*
   b. *Agrobacterium tumefacines*
   c. *Escherichia coli*
   d. None of the above

12. P^H of culture medium should be
   a. 5-6
   b. 5.5 – 5.7
   c. 7-7.5
   d. 4-5

13. In tissue culture medium, sucrose or glucose is used as most suitable carbon source in concentration
   a. 1-2 per cent
   b. 2-3 per cent
   c. 3-4 per cent
   d. 2-4 per cent

14. The concentration of potassium and nitrate in culture medium should be at least
   a. 20 -25 mM each
   b. 25 -30 mM each
   c. 30 -35 mM each
   d. 10 - 20 mM each

15. The process in which tissue callus or cells are induced to form shoots and roots by manipulating plant growth hormones is known as
   a. Micro-propagation
   b. Harvesting
   c. Hardening
   d. Organogenesis

16. By using hairy root culture technique, significant amount of............................... Metabolites can be enhanced
   a. Primary
   b. Secondary
   c. Tertiary
   d. Quaternary

17. The formation of embryoids from the pollen grains in the tissue culture medium is due to

    a.   Organogenesis
    b.   Micro propagation
    c.   Cellular totipotency
    d.   Double fertilization

18. Which one of the follwing is main application of embryo culture?

    a.   Clonal propagation
    b.   Induction of somaclonal barriers
    c.   Production of embryoids
    d.   overcoming hybridization barrier

19. Edible vaccines are

    a.   Mucosal targeted vaccines
    b.   Antigen targeted vaccines
    c.   Both a and b
    d.   None of the above

20. Type of vaccine in which the selected genes are introduced in to the plants or transgenic plant to manufacture the encoded protein known as

    a.   Transgenic vaccine
    b.   Edible vaccine
    c.   food vaccine
    d.   Both a and b

Answer Key

1. b	2. c	3. c	4. b	5. d	6. b	7. d	8. c	9. a	10. c
11. a	12.b	13. d	14. a	15. d	16. b	17. c	18. a	19. a	20. b

Unit 4

4.1 Pharmacognosy in Various Systems of Medicine

4.1.1 Pharamacognosy and Allopathy

Allopathy term was coined in 1810 by the inventor of homeopathy, Samuel Hahnemann.The terms "allopathic medicine" and "allopathy" are drawn from the Greek prefix állos, "other," "different" + the suffix páthos, "suffering".As used by homeopaths, the term allopathy has always referred to the principle of treating disease by administering substances that produce other symptoms (when given to a healthy human) than the symptoms produced by a disease. Allopathic medicine is commonly considered as Western European and North American evidenced-based conventional medicine. This "technomedicine" rests on tangible data. Standardized protocols objectively test its hypotheses and offer pragmatic clinical approaches. Building on its several thousand-year-old Greek and Latin foundations, it has become increasingly scientific over the last centuries. Its methodology and findings are objectively verifiable using statistically valid and reliable parameters.

The term pharmacognosy as a constituent scientific discipline of pharmacy has been in use for nearly 200 years, and it refers to studies on natural product drugs. During the last half of the 20th century, pharmacognosy evolved from being a descriptive botanical subject to one having a more chemical and biological focus. At the beginning of the 21st century, pharmacognosy teaching in academic pharmacy institutions has been given new relevance, as a result of the explosive growth in the use of herbal remedies (phytomedicines) in modern pharmacy practice, particularly in western Europe and North America.

In turn, pharmacognosy research areas are continuing to expand, and now include aspects of cell and molecular biology in relation to natural products, ethnobotany and phytotherapy, in addition to the more traditional analytical method development and phytochemistry. The systematic study of herbal remedies offers pharmacognosy groups an attractive new area of research, ranging from investigating the biologically active principles of phytomedicines and their mode of action and potential drug interactions, to quality control, and involvement in clinical trials. Traditional Chinese Medicine (TCM) and Indian medicine (Ayurveda) are the two most established medical systems in Eastern medical traditions.

Examples of promising bioactive compounds presently available in market:		
Plant Name	**Family**	**Used Drugs**
Ammi majus	Umbelliferae	Xanthotoxin
Ananas comosus	Bromeliaceae	Bromelain
Atropa belladonna	Solanaceae	Atropine
Capsicum species	Solanaceae	Capsicum Oleoresin
Carica papaya	Caricaceae	Papain
Cassia acutifolia	Leguminosae	Sennosides A + B
Cassia angustifolia	Leguminosae	Sennosides A + B
Cathuranthus roseus	Apocynaceae	Leurocristine (vincristine)
		Vincaleukoblastine (Vinblastine)
Cinchona species	Rubiaceae	Quinine
Citrus limon	Rutaceae	Pectine

Contd...

Colchicum autumnale	Liliaceae	Colchicine
Digitalis lanata	Scophulariaceae	Digitoxine, Lanatoside C, Acetylligitoxin
Digitalis purpuria		Digitoxine
		Diosgenine
Dioscorea species	Dioscoreaceae	Atropine, Hyoscyamine, Scopolamine
Duboisiamyoporoides	Solanaceae	Ephedrine, Pseudoephedrine
		Sitosterols
Ephedra sinica	Ephedraceae	Opium, Codeine, Morphine
Glycine max	Leguminaceae	Noscapine, Papaverine
Papaver somniferum	Papaveraceae	Phytostigmine (Eserine)
		Pilocarpine
Physostigmavenenosum	Leguminosae	Podophyline
Pilocarpusjaborandi	Rutaceae	Prune concentrate
Podophyllum peltatum	Berberadaceae	Reserpine, Deserpidine, Reserpine,
Prunus domestica	Rosaceae	Rescinamine
Rauwolfia serpentine	Apocynaceae	Casanthranol
Rauwolfia vomitoria	Apocynaceae	Ricinoleic Acid
		Veratrum viride
Ricinus communis	Euphorbiaceae	Cryptennamine
Veratrum viride	Liliaceae	

4.1.2   Ayurveda System

It is about 5000 year old system of medicine native to India. It is holistic system of medicine which considers whole body while treating disease and not just a diseased part of body. Ayurveda has thousands year's evidence based history so it can be just complete system rather alternative system or complementary system. Ayurveda is a Sanskrit word which means (*Ayur*-life and *veda* – to gain knowledge or science) science of life. Ayurveda deals with different types of plants, minerals and animal products. Charaksamhita by Charak includes the principle components or theory of Ayurveda. Sushrutsamhita edited by Sushrut is about the surgical treatments in Ayurveda.

It is assumed that Sushruta was born in the Eastern part of India near Bihar (which was famous for sacred schools and universities at that time). Sushruta was a physician by occupation. In Mahabharata, he is represented as a son of Rishi Visvamitra.

His Samhita, divided into six volumes, compromises all aspects of general medicine. However, due to an extraordinary accuracy and detail of surgery in his work, he is also considered as the father of surgery.

These six volumes contain 184 chapters describing 1120 illness, 700 medical plants, 64 drugs prepared from minerals, and 57 from animal sources. It also discusses different surgical techniques suitable for different body parts along with 14 different types of bandages. Mostly, the Samhita focuses on surgery and midwifery, but it also deals with topics such as genetics, mental illness, embryology, anatomy, geriatric illness, and diabetes.

It has 300 surgical procedures and it classifies surgery into five subheadings such as

- Aharya (extraction of solid bodies),
- Bhedya (excising),
- Chhedya (incising),
- Eshya (probing),
- Lekhya (scarifying),
- Sivya (suturing),
- Vedhya (puncturing), and
- Visravaniya (evacuating fluids).

It describes more than 300 kinds of operations that call for 42 different surgical processes and 121 different types of instruments. For the purpose of anesthesia, he advised the use of wine with the incense of cannabis and this is the oldest form of anesthesia used with no world record before that. The instruments used for surgeries were constructed after the shape of beasts and birds and named after them like the crocodile forceps and hawk's bill forceps.

The Sushruta Samhita is best known for its approach and discussions of surgery. It was one of the first in human history to suggest that a student of surgery should learn about human body and its organs by dissecting a dead body. It describes haemorrhoidectomy, amputations, plastic, rhinoplastic, ophthalmic, lithotomic and obstetrical procedures.

Theory and principles: Ayurveda involves following fundamental principles:

Pancha Mahabhuta	*Prithvi* (earth) *Apa* (water) *Tej* (fire) *Vayu* (air) *Akash* (sky)
Panchshil theory	*Rasa* : Therapeutically active substances *Guna* : Quality *Virya* : Active principle and potency *Vipaka* : The end product of digestion *Prabhava* : Actual effect of drug on body.
Sapta Dhatu theory	*Rasa* (Plasma) *Raktam* (Blood) *Mansa* (Muscles) *Meda* (Fat) *Asthi* (Bone) *Majja* (Bone marrow and nerves) *Shukra* (Reproductive fluid or Semen)
Tridosha theory	*Vatta = Vayu + akash =* respiration and mobility *Pitta = Agni =* digestion and metabolism *Kapha = Prithvi + apa =* lubrication of joints and stability.
Triguna	*Satva* (good) *Raja* (aggressive) *Toma* (dullness)
Ama	a Sanskrit word meaning "uncooked" or "undigested" is used to refer to the concept of anything that exists in a state of incomplete transformation.

Diagnosis: The non-equilibrium between any of above principles causes to person suffers from diseases. Mental, physical, social and spiritual welfare of human beings is considered by Ayurveda to cure the disease cause. Observation of body color, tongue, nail, eyes, pulse and investigation of blood, urine and fecal matter is criteria of diagnosing actual cause of disease.

Treatment: Panchkarma is an important treatment in Ayurveda which includes Snehan (massage), Swedan (steam), Vaman (vomit), Virechan (expulsion) and Basti (medicated enemas). The medicines are given in the form of powder (churna, bhasma), liquid (asava, arishta and taila), semisolid (leha or paka) and tablets (gutika, vati). Treatment of ayurveda involves use of drugs obtained from plant, animal and mineral sources. Ayurveda also focuses on exercise, yoga, and meditation. One type of prescription is a Sattvic diet.

Dosage forms of Ayurveda are powders (churna), bhasma (metal oxides), asava and arishtha (alcohol containing liquids), quath (extracts), gutika (pills), lep (ointment) or taila (Medicated oils).

There are eight branches of Ayurveda:

1. Kayachikitsa (internal medicine)
2. Kumarbhritya (pediatrics)
3. Trachchikitsa (psychology medicine)
4. Shalakya Tantra [ear, nose and throat]
5. Shalya Tantra (surgery)
6. Agada tantra (toxicology)
7. Rasayana tantra (geriatrics)
8. Vajikaran tantra [gynecology]

4.1.3 Siddha System

Sidha system of medicine is one of the oldest medical systems known to mankind even before ayurvedic system which was flourished in Vedic culture, Dravidian culture and Indus Valley Civilization. Tamil traditional medicine is origin of Siddha system and hence most of literature of this system is given in Tamil Language. 18 "Siddhas" (Spiritual persons) developed this system so it is called as Sidha. Sage Agathiyar is considered the guru of all Sidhas.

According to Palm Leaf manuscript, it is believed that it was first described by Lord Shiva to his wife Parvathy and then to their son Lord Muruga. Then he passed this knowledge to his disciple sage Agasthya. Agasthya educated 18 Siddhars. Human beings got this knowledge from 18 Siddhars. Siddhars have to get Siddhi means attainment of supernatural powers.

Theory and principles: Generally the basic principles of Siddha and Ayurveda medicine are almost similar. But siddha system explains in detail about various basic treatments of diseases while surgery like modern treatments are practiced and written in detail in Ayurveda. Like Ayurveda, Siddha medicine also, classifies physiological components of the human beings as vata (air), pitta (fire) and kapha (earth and water). Siddha system is based on 96 principles and out of these Triguna theory, i.e., vatta, pitta and kapha is more prominent. Under normal conditions, the ratio between Vatta, Pitta, and Kapha is 4:2:1, respectively.

Siddha deals with thousands of herbs, animal, mineral and metals. Siddha system believes that health is perfect state of physical, mental, social, moral and spiritual component. It is based on AndapindaThathuvam means relationship between universe and human body. Siddhas are called as Vaithiyars.

Diagnosis: A Siddha physician studies eight important things of body i.e. nadi (pulse), varna (colour), na (tongue), mala (faeces) kan (eyes), swara (voice), sparisam (touch), and neer (urine).

Guna	Personalities	Complications
Vata	Stout, black, cold and inactive healthy	Increased *Vata* shows arrogant behaviour, paralysis, heart attack.
Pitta	Lean, whitish complexion and perfectionist	Increased *Pitta* shows graying of hair, anemia and instability.
Kapha	Well built, good complexion and well behaved	Increased *Kapha* causes jaundice, heart attack.

Treatment: Siddha medicines are divided into three categories: Thavaram (Herbal), Thadu (inorganic) and Janganam (animal). Internal as well as external medicines are divided into 32 categories each separately. Pressure or massage techniques are also part of treatment and called as Thokkanam. There are 108 varma points for pressure techniques.

Treatment is classified into three categories:

➢ **Devamaruthuvum (Divine method):** The medicines prepared from metals and minerals come under this topic. The speciality of these medicines is a very small dose brings quick recovery even from chronic ailments. These are highly potent. Most of these medcines has no expiry date that is they can be preserved life-long. In this method use of metals and minerals medicines like parpam, chendooram, guru, kuligai made of mercury, sulphur and pashanamsrecommended.

➢ **Manudamaruthuvum (Rational method):** In this method herbal medicines like churanam, kudineer, vadagam are used. They are herbal medicines which have short definite life span. Dose may vary accordingly. They comprise of 34 types – 22 Internal medicines and 12 External medicines

➢ **Internal medicines:** Charu (juice), Surasam (boiling the extracted juice), Kudineer (decoction), Karkam (Raw materials prepared into paste) etc.

➢ **External applications:** Vedhu (Steam- therapy), Pattru (Pasting proceed raw drugs on diseased part), Ottradam (Formentation), Kattu (Like Bandaging)

➢ **Asura maruthuvum (surgical method):** use of surgical method, incision, excisions, use of heat or leech

Treatment in this system emphasizes preparation of fresh medicine. It is then prepared and administered with some Pathya (some restriction). Example- Day time sleeping is not allowed or some food material is restricted like chicken, mango, coconut, mustard, groundnut, almond, tobacco etc. Medicine can be kashayam (extract), churnam (powder), tailams (medicated oil), gulligai (pills), chenduram (metal), bhasmam (calcination product) and or ghritam (medicated ghee).

4.1.4 Unani System

This system is also called asUnani-tibb or Yunani Medicine. Arab and Persian physicians such as Rhazes, Avicenna (Ibn Sena), Al-Zahrawi, and Ibn Nafis developed this system.

Book: Ibn Sina's the Canon of Medicine. First book, "On General Means of Treatment" describes that treatments are done in three ways: "one of them is regimen and nutrition; the second, application of drugs; and the third, manual treatment, i.e., surgery". The second book gives rather detailed pharmacological and pharmacotherapeutic characteristic of 811 drugs, among which those of vegetable kingdom constitute 594 (73.7%), of animal kingdom 118 (14.5%) and of mineral origin 99 (12.2%).

Theory and principles: Unani medicine involves concept of the four humours (akhlat) i.e. Phlegm (Balgham), Blood (Dam), Yellow bile (Safra) and Black bile (Sauda). These "humors" and a open air blood sedimentation test exhibits close relation where a dark clot at the bottom resembles black bile, a layer of unclotted erythrocytes resembles blood, a layer of white blood cells resembles phlegm and a layer of clear yellow serum resembles yellow bile. Abnormality in humor leads to disease condition in body.

Diagnosis: The human body is considered to be made up of seven components i.e. 1. Elements (Arkan) 2. Temperament (Mijaz). 3. Humors (Aklat) 4. Organs (Aaza) 5. Faculties (Quwa) 6. Spirits (Arwah). 7. Functions (Afaal) which have direct bearing on the health status of a person and considered by the physician for diagnosis and treatment.

In diagnosis Unani Physican (Hakim) asks a detail history and decides treatment.

Treatment: After diagnosing the disease, treatment involves either to eliminate cause (Izalaesabab), normalize humors (Tadeeleakhlat) or to normalise tissues or organs (Tadeeleaza). Method of treatment involves modification of essential pre-requisites of health (Ilaj- Bil-Tadbeer) or Panchkarma like in Ayurveda (Ilaj-Bil-Tadbeer) or pharmacotherapy (Ilajbiladvia) or surgery (Ilaj-Bil-Yad).

➢ Regimental therapy (Ilajbiltadbeer) – Use of exercise, climate change, massage, venesection, leaching, cupping, diet therapy etc.

➢ Pharmacotherapy (Ilajbildava) – use of plant, animal and mineral origin drugs, either alone or in combination.

➢ Surgery (Ilajbil Yad) – Surgical intervention in treatment

As far as possible Unani medicine therapy attempts to use simple physical means to cure a disease. Some of the techniques used in Ilajbil- Tadbir (Regimental therapy) include Hijamah (Cupping), Fasd (Venesection), Tareeq (Sweating), Idrar-e-Baul (Diuresis), Hamam (Turkish Bath), Dalak (Massage), Kai (Cauterization), Ishal (Purging), Qai (Vomiting), Riyazat (Exercise) and Taleeq (Leeching).

Unani dosage forms are-

➢ Solid dosage forms [Example: (Habb (pills), quers (tablet), safoof (powder)]

➢ Liquid dosage forms [Joshnda (decoction), Khisanda (Infusion), Arq (Distillate), Sharbat (Syrup), Qutur (Drops)]

➢ Semi-solid dosage forms [Huqna (enema) and tila (liniment)].

4.1.5   Homeopathy System

Homeo means similar and Pathos means suffering so homeopathy is the "system of similar suffering". German physician Samuel Hahnemann first stated the basic principle of homeopathy in 1796, known as the "law of similars" (let like be cured by like.")

This system was developed by Dr Samuel Hahnemann in Germany. Dr Samuel had written a book *The Curative Powers of Drugs and Some Examinations of Previous Principles* which was based on his study of effect of *cinchona* on his own body where he actually found "law of similars" which indicates similarity between drug and disease.

Theory and principle: Homeopathy emphasises the root cause of the disease and the nature's law of its cure that is 'like cures like'. Thus, homeopathy deals with the following seven principles which are outlined below:

➢ ***Individualisation*** : No two individuals in the world are alike, i.e. the disease affecting two individuals cannot be similar though they may share common symptoms. So the medicines used to cure the same disease in different individuals are different.

➢ ***Principle of similiar*** : Use of the medicine will produce similar symptoms of disease in an healthy individual. For example, watery eyes and burning nose caused by an onion hence an attack of hay fever with watering eyes and a burning nose can be cured homeopathic remedy made from onion.

➢ ***Principle of simplex***: Only one single simple medicine at one time and no combination is allowed.

➢ ***Minimum dose*** : Minimum medicine at a time

➢ ***Law of proving***: Medicine should have the capacity to produce disease state in a healthy individual.

➢ ***Law of dynamisation***: Medicine should preserve the normal state of healthy body.

➢ ***Vital force:*** Medicine should have the capacity to arouse sufficient energy to maintain a healthy body.

Diagnosis: It involves knowing of complete hereditary history as well as observation of moods, habits, skin, eyes, tongue, blood, urine etc of patients.

Treatment:

Not considering imponderabilia, the source materials for homeopathic medicines may consist of the following:

➢ **plant material such** as: roots, stems, leaves, flowers, bark, pollen, lichen, moss, ferns and algae;

➢ **microorganisms** such as: fungi, bacteria, viruses and plant parasites;

➢ **animal materials** such as: whole animals, animal organs, tissues, secretions, cell lines, toxins, nosodes, blood products;

➢ **human materials such** as: tissues, secretions, cell lines and endogenous molecules such as hormones;

➢ **minerals and chemicals.**

When the symptoms picture matches with the drug picture, the physician always attempts to identify a single medicine. Homeopathic preparation involves "dynamisation" or "potentiation", whereby a substance is diluted with alcohol or distilled water and then vigorously shaken in a process called "succussion". Three logarithmic potency scales are in regular use in homeopathy for dilution. Hahnemann created the "centesimal" or "C scale", diluting a substance by a factor of 100 at each stage.Inert substance like sugars, typically lactose, is used to prepare homeopathic pills and then a drop of liquid homeopathic preparation is placed on pills.Hahnemann began to test what effects substances produced in humans, a procedure that would later become known as "homeopathic proving".

Imponderabilia: Homeopathic medicines prepared from energy, emanating from natural and physical reactions. It means "not weighable", i.e. which have no perceptible weights. They are energy forms such as sunlight (Sol), magnetic fields (Magnetis Polus Australis), radiation (X-ray).

Mother solution (also called solution): the most concentrated solution prepared from a substance of mineral or chemical origin by dissolving it in alcohol or purified water. It may also be prepared by exposing alcohol or purified water to an energy source (see Imponderabilia).

Mother tincture (also called tincture): The initial homeopathic preparation made from source material that can be further potentized (also called "liquid stock"), sometimes used as homeopathic medicines, is regarded as the most concentrated form of a finished homeopathic medicine. Mother tinctures are obtained classically by maceration or percolation (sometimes also by digestion, infusion, decoction or fermentation) techniques from source materials according to a procedure prescribed by a recognized homeopathic pharmacopoeia. Sometimes a mother tincture corresponds to the first decimal dilution, "1D" or "1X" (10-1), mostly when dry plant material is used as starting material.

Nosodes: Homeopathic medicines prepared from disease products from humans or animals; from pathogenic organisms or their metabolic products; or from decomposition products of animal organs.

Sarcodes: Homeopathic medicines made from healthy animal tissues or secretions. In Greek, sarcode means fleshly.

Potency: The denominated degree of serial trituration or dilution and succession that is reached for each homeopathic medicine. The degrees of dilution or potencies are normally indicated by the letters D, DH or X for successive 1 to 10 (decimal) dilutions, the letters C, CH or K or CK for successive 1 to 100 (centesimal) dilutions while Q or LM denote successive 1 to 50 000 (Hahnemannian quinquagintamillesimal) dilutions.

Dilution by 1 to 10 denotes 1 part processed with 9 parts of diluent (Hahnemannian decimal), dilution by 1 to 100, 1 part processed with 99 parts (Hahnemannian or Korsakovian centesimal), and so on.

The number preceding the letters (e.g. D, C or LM) normally indicate the number of dilution steps employed.

As a consequence of different views in various approaches in homeotherapy and because the notion of these terms may depend on the nature of the starting materials, the terms "high potency" and "low potency" cannot be defined unambiguously.

Potentization (also called dinamization): The combined process of serial dilution and succussion or trituration at each step in the manufacture of homeopathic medicines from stocks. (According to the tenet of homeopathy, potentization represents the process by which the activity of a homeopathic medicine is developed.)

The potentisation steps in a potency row can be performed in different dilution ratios:

D or X: 1:10

C or CH: 1:100

LM 1:50,000.

So, for example, D4 means potentised four times in the ratio 1:10. The higher the number of potency the lower the concentration.

4.1.6   Chinese System

Traditional Chinese Medicine (TCM) is older than 2,000 years have been developed in China. Historical physicians in TCM include Zhang Zhongjing, Hua Tuo, Sun Simiao, Tao Hongjing, Zhang Jiegu, and Li Shizhen.

Book: Yellow Emperor's inner Canon, Treatise on Cold Damage

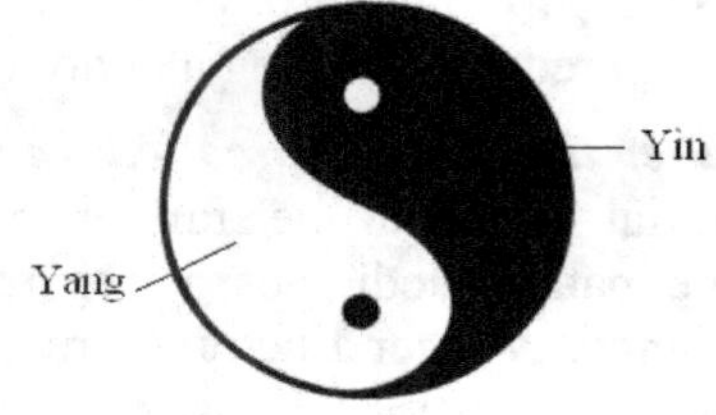

Fig. 4.1 Yin and Yan Symbol of Chinese system

Theory and principles: Chinese medicine involves concept of Yin and Yang. Yin means negative, dark, water, moon, female, inside, cold or moist. Yang means positive, bright, sun, fire, male, outside, hot or dry. Yin dominating body shows inactivity, cold or lethargy while yang dominating body shows fever, hyper-activity. Five element theory of TCM (wood-germination, water-decay, fire-growth, earth-ripening and metal-nourishment) relates to five body organs (wood-liver, fire-heart, water-kidney, earth-spleen and metal-lung) and symolises man and nature relationship. TCM believes that *qi* means energy, blood and water are three essential substances for body's normal health.

Chinese medicine views the body as an energetic system in dynamic balance.

> ➤ *Chi* or *Qi*, which can be **translated as energy or life force** which flows in a regular pattern through a system of channels or **meridians to all parts of the body**.
> ➤ Xue: The red liquid running in the blood vessels.
> ➤ Jinye: body fluids like tears, sputum, saliva, gastric acid, joint fluid, sweat, urine, etc
> ➤ Zàng refers to the five entities considered to be yin in nature–Heart, Liver, Spleen, Lung, Kidney
> ➤ Fǔ (refers to the six yang organs–Small Intestine, Large Intestine, Gallbladder, Urinary Bladder, Stomach and Sānjiaō (Hollow space in human body)

Diagnosis: Diagnosis is based on "pattern of discrimination" i..e valuation of the present signs and symptoms. Underlying disharmony pattern is studied based on "Eight Principles" or causes like internal, external, heat, cold, vacuity (deficiency), repletion (excess), yin and yang from examination of pulse and tongue.

Treatment: Treatment includes

1. **Acupuncture**: The acupuncture points located in skin are opened and closed by a stainless steel needle for 20-40 minutes to adjust proper blood circulation.Acupuncture can either be used to fortify a weakness or release/reduce an excessive condition.Acupuncture works quicker than moxibustion; however, the effect of moxibution lasts longer. Clinically, they are often used together.

2. **Moxibustion**: Moxibustion uses burning moxa or moxa cones (moxa refers to the Chinese mugwort herb) above the skin to warm or heat certain designated points. These designated points are called acu-points in both acupuncture and moxibustion. The chosen points and locations will vary according to the disease. The methods activate the flow of qi (vital energy) and removes blockages in the meridians, so that the body can reach a new balance through its self-healing processes.

3. **Herbal Medicine**: Specific herbs and their combinations are used to cure diseases.

4. **Diet**: Herbal supplements are given as a part of diet to fortify the body constituents.

5. **Exercise**: For healthy individuals as well as for patients, exercise is properly planned in the Chinese system.

6. **Massage**: It is an important part of the Chinese system to harmonize body climate.

7. **Gausha**-abrading the skin with pieces of smooth jade, bone, animal tusks or horns or smooth stones; until red spots then bruising cover the area to which it is done.

8. **Qìgōng-Qi is** air, breath, energy, or primordial life source that is neither matter or spirit. While Gong is a skillful movement, work, or exercise of the qi

4.2   Introduction to Secondary Metabolites

4.2.1 Alkaloids

The term "alkaloids" or "pflanzenlkalein" was coined by Meissner, a German pharmacist in 1819. The term alkaloids derived from the word "alkali like." Ladenburg defined alkaloids "as naturally occurring plant compounds having a basic character and containing at least one nitrogen in a heterocyclic ring" But now due to advancement in knowledge in chemistry alkaloids are defined as **"physiologically active basic compounds of natural origin, in which at least one nitrogen atom forms part of a cyclic system."**

Exceptions to the above definition of alkaloids

Cholines, Ephedrine	N-atom in side chain not in ring.	Ephedrine

Contd…

Piperine	a compound from black pepper neither basic nor possessing any potent physiological activity, still it is included in the list of alkaloids.	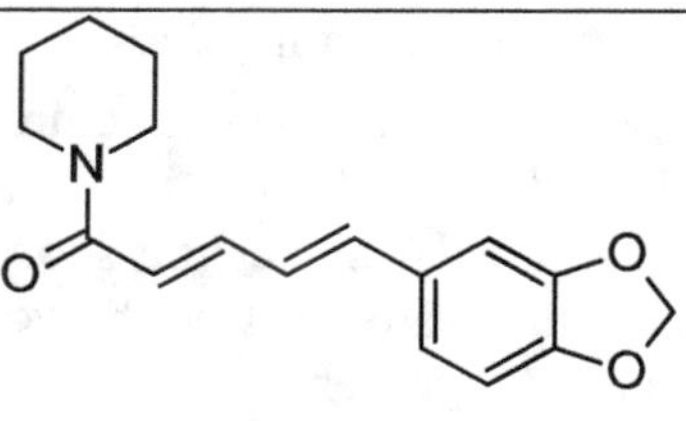 Piperine
Colchicine	Neither basic nor it contains N-atom in heterocyclic ring but possesses distinct pharmaco-logical activity.	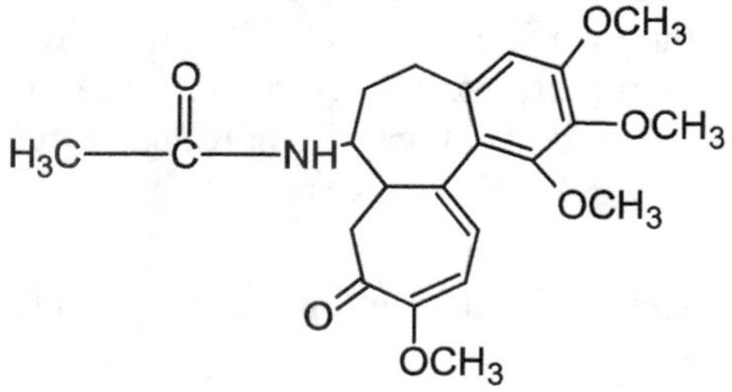 Colchicine
Thiamine	It has heterocyclic nitrogenous base, but it is universally distributed in living matter.	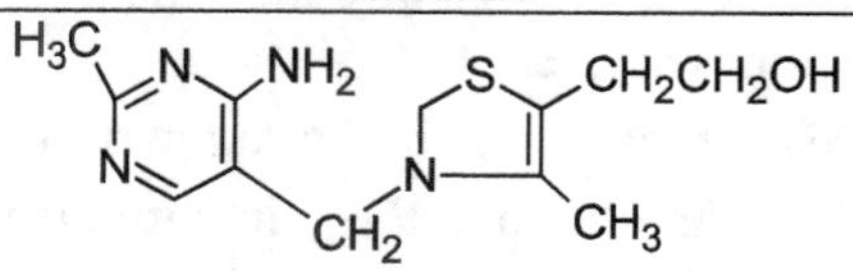 Thiamine

Occurrences	➤ Alkaloids are found to be distributed in plant and animal kingdom but **absent in algae and in the lower groups of plants** with the exception of one or two families of fungi (Example: ergot alkaloids). Dicotyledons family like *apocynaceae, rubiaceae, rutaceae, ranunculaceae, papaverace, solonaceae, papilionaceae are prominent alkaloid containing families and* labiatea and rosaceae do not contain alkaloids. Alkaloids are less frequently found in monocotyledons plants of families *amaryllidaceae, liliaceae* ➤ The concentration of alkaloids in plants depends upon the season, age and its locality. ➤ It also observed that different genera of the same family contain same or structurally related alkaloids. Example: seven different genera of the family solanaceae contain hyoscyamine. ➤ It is also found that simple alkaloid are often found in different plants where the complex alkaloids in one species or genus of family. ➤ Nearly 300 alkaloids belonging to more than 24 classes are known to occur in the skins of amphibians along with other toxins. They include the potent neurotoxic alkaloids of frogs of the genus phyllobates, which are among some of the most poisonous substances known.
Nomenclature	Generally all alkaloid's name must end with suffix *–ine.* From the generic name of plant producing them: Atropine from A. belladona From specific name of plant yielding them: Belladonine from A. belladona From common name of drug producing them: Ergotamine from C. Purpurea From their specific physiological activity: Emetine from Hedera helix, Morphine from P. somniferum From the name of discoverer: Pelletierine
Physical properties	➤ Alkaloidal salts are soluble in polar solvent and insoluble in organic solvent while all alkaloidal bases are soluble in the organic solvent and insoluble in the polar solvent.

Contd...

	➤ They are generally **bitter** in taste. Most of the alkaloids are generally colorless, crystalline solid compound. However some alkaloids are liquid in nature like nicotine, coniine, sparteine and few alkaloids are colored (Berberine is yellow in color, sanguinarine is copper red in color) ➤ Alkaloids are optically active and majority being a levorotatory. There is considerable difference in pharmacological activities of different isomers of alkaloids. However few are exceptions like (-) and (+) quinine both are pharmacologically active, (+) tubocurarine is more potent than (-) tubocurarine
Chemical properties	➤ In plants alkaloids, due to their basic nature, generally exist as salts of organic acid like acetic acid, oxalic acid, citric acid, malic acid, lactic acid, tartaric acid, tannic acid. ➤ Example: opium alkaloids like morphine are found in the salts form of meconic acid, Cinchona alkaloids are found with quinic acid and Aconite alkaloids with aconitic acid. ➤ Some alkaloids like narceine and nicotine are occurring free in nature. ➤ A few alkaloids also occur as glycosides of sugars like glucose, rhamnose and galactose. E.g. alkaloids of solanum. Most of the alkaloids contain one or more N atoms usually in the tertiary state in a ring system.

Chemical Tests

Name of test	Procedure	Inference
Dragendorff's reagent (potassium bismuth iodide solution)	Mix 2 ml of reagent with 2 ml of filtrate of plant drug extract.	Reddish brown precipitate
Modified Dragendroff's reagent or Kraut's reagent (potassium bismuth iodide solution containsing Nitric acid in place of Glacial acetic acid))	Mix 2 ml of reagent with 2 ml of filtrate of plant drug extract.	Precipitation
Hager's reagent (solution of picric acid)	Mix 2 ml of reagent with 2 ml of filtrate of plant drug extract	Yellow colour
Mayer's reagent (Potassium mercuric iodide solution)	Mix 2 ml of reagent with 2 ml of filtrate of plant drug extract.	Cream coloured precipitate
Wagner's reagent (Iodine – Potassium iodide solution)	Mix 2 ml of reagent with 2 ml of filtrate of plant drug extract.	Reddish brown precipitate
Marme's reagent (Potassium cadmium iodide)	Mix 2 ml of reagent with 2 ml of filtrate of plant drug extract.	Precipitation
Sonneschein's reagent (Phosphomolybdic acid)	Mix 2 ml of reagent with 2 ml of filtrate of plant drug extract.	Pale yellow to pink to colourless.
Bertrand's reagent (Silicotungustic acid)	Mix 2 ml of reagent with 2 ml of filtrate of plant drug extract.	Bluish to purple colour
Schiebler's reagent (Phosphotungustic acid)	Mix 2 ml of reagent with 2 ml of filtrate of acidified plant drug extract.	Yellow to orange precipitate

Classification

1. **Simple classification:** In this classification following classes of alkaloids are considered

Class	Biogenesis Precursors	N-Hetrocyclic ring	Identification tests	Examples
True alkaloids	Amino acid	N-Hetrocyclic ring	Positive	Morphine, emetine, hyoscyamine.
Proto/Amine alkaloids	Amino acid	N-Side chain	Positive	Mescaline, colchicines, ephedrine
Pseudo alkaloids	Other than amino acid	N-Hetrocyclic ring	Positive	Caffeine, solasodine.

2. **Biosynthetic classification:** This method gives significance to the precursor from which the alkaloids are bio-synthesized in the plant. Hence, the variety of alkaloids with different taxonomic distribution and physiological activities can be brought under same group, if they are same precursors.

Alkaloid Type	Biosynthetic Origin
Tropane and Pyrrolizidine alkaloids	Ornithine
Piperidine, Quinolizidine, Indolizidine alkaloids	Lysine
Pyridine alkaloids	Niconitic acid
Tetrahydro isoquinoline, Benzyltetra-hydro isoquinoline, Phenthyl isoquinoline alkaloids	Tyrosine
Indole, Quinoline alkaloids	Tryptophan
Quinazoline and Acridine alkaloids	Anthranilic acid
Imidazole alkaloids	Histidine
Amine alkaloids	Phenylalanine /Acetate
Terpenoid alkaloids	Monoterpenes
Steroid alkaloids	Steroids
Purine alkaloids	Purine

3. **Pharmacological classification:** Depending on the physiological response or use, the alkaloids are classified under various pharmacological categories. Within the same drug, the individual alkaloids may exhibit different pharmacological action. E.g. cinchona contains quinine and quinidine. In which quinine acts as anti-malarial, while quinidine acts as anti-arrthmic agent.

Pharmacological action	Example
Narcotic analgesic	Opium
Respiratory stimulant	Lobelia, Tobacco, Areca
Expectorant	Vasaka, Ipecac
Anti-cancer	Vinca, Podophyllum, Taxol
Anti-cholinergic	Belladonna, Datura, Nux-vomica, Ephedra, Cocca
Para-sympathomimetic	Pilocarpus, Tea, Physostigma, Tobacco

4. Taxonomic classification: This classification is done **according to the family.** Thus alkaloids may be described as solanaceous or papilionaceous **without reference to the chemical type of alkaloids present.** Since, both families contain alkaloids of several types. It is more usual to describe alkaloids according to the genus in which they occur. E.g. ephedra, cinchona.

Solanaceae	Tropane, pyridine, steroidalalkaloids
Papilionaceae	Quinolizidine and pyrrolidine alkaloids
Liliaceae	Steroidal alkaloids
Rubiaceae	Qinoline alkaloids

5. Chemical classification: This is the most accepted way of classification of alkaloids. The main criteria for the chemical classification of alkaloids are the type of fundamental (normally heterocyclic) ring structure present in the alkaloids. They are broadly categorized into two divisions.

➤ *Heterocyclic*: - divided into different groups according to the nature of their heterocyclic ring.

➤ *Non heterocyclic*: Proto alkaloids or biological amine.

Chemical Classification of Alkaloids

- **True alkaloids:** Pyrrolidine, Piperidine, Pyrrolizidine, Tropane, Indole, Quinoline, Iso-quinoline, Quinazoline, Aporphine, Imodazole
- **Proto alkaloids:** Amine
- **Pseudo alkaloids:** Steroid, Purine

Fig. 4.2 Classification of alkaloids

True alkaloids	
Fundametal Chemical Moiety	**Examples**
Pyrrolidine	Hygrine, *Erythroxylon coca*, Erythroxylaceae

Contd...

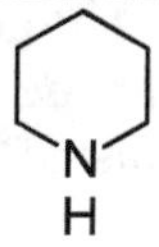 Piperdine	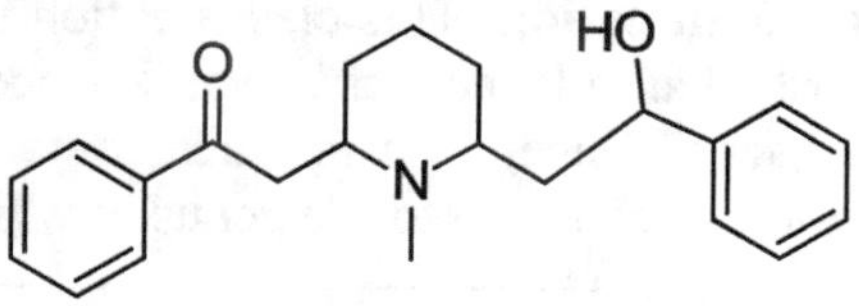 Lobeline, *Lobelia inflata*, Lobeliaceae (Respiratory Stimulant) 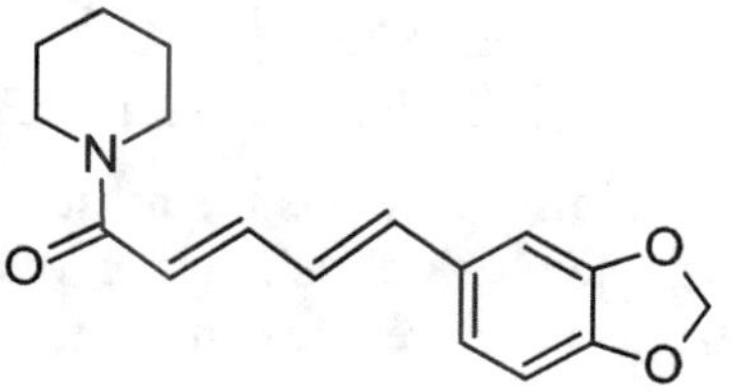 Piperine (Bioavailability enhancer)
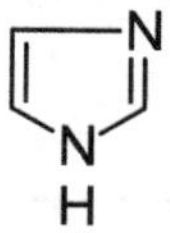 Imidazole	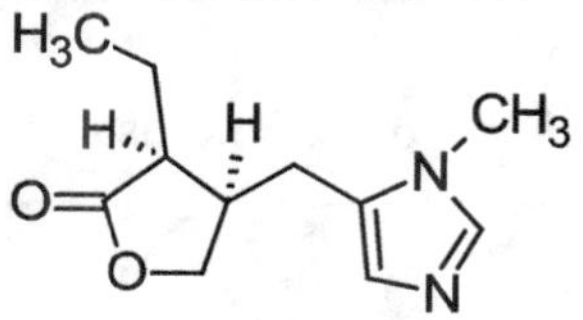 Pilocarpine, *Pilocarpus jaborandi*, Rutaceae To treat dry mouth and eye issues. (Eye drops it is used to manage angle closure glaucoma until surgery can be performed, ocular hypertension, primary open angle glaucoma, and to bring about constriction of the pupil following its dilation.)
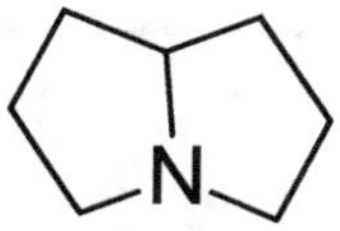 Pyrrolizidine	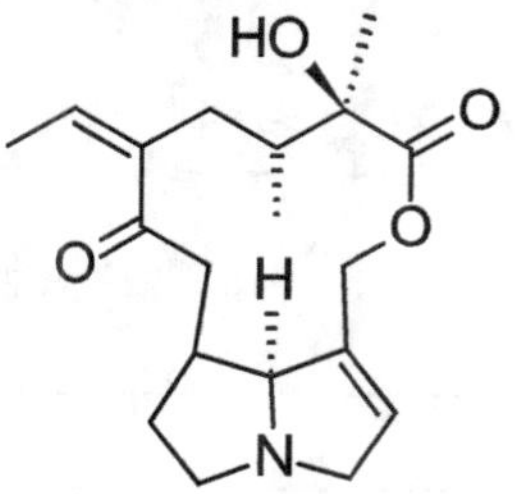 Senecionine, *Senecio brasiliensis*, Asteraceae (It is used as arrow Poision)
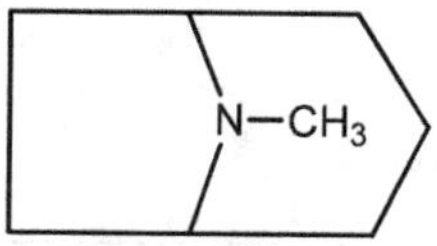	Atropine, *Atropa belladonna*, Solanaceae (Atropine is indicated for the treatment of bradycardia associated with hypotension, second- and third-degree heart block, and slow idioventricular rhythms. Atropine is the initial drug of choice in acute organophosphate poisoning.)

Contd...

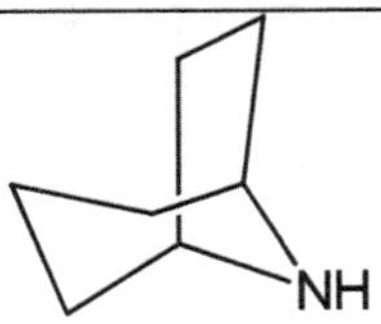 Tropane	
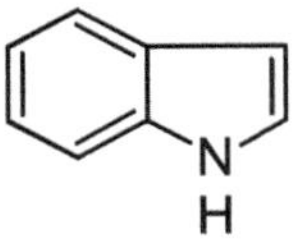 Indole (Benzpyrrole) Vinca, Raulwoflia, Nux vomica	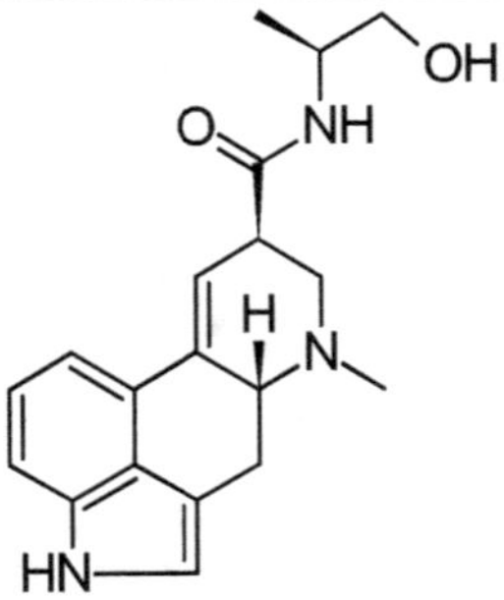 *Ergot alkaloids, Clavicepus purpurea,* Clavicepataceae (Ergometrine is Oxytocic, Ergotamine is use to treat migraine or cluster headache)
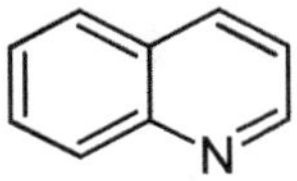 Quinoline	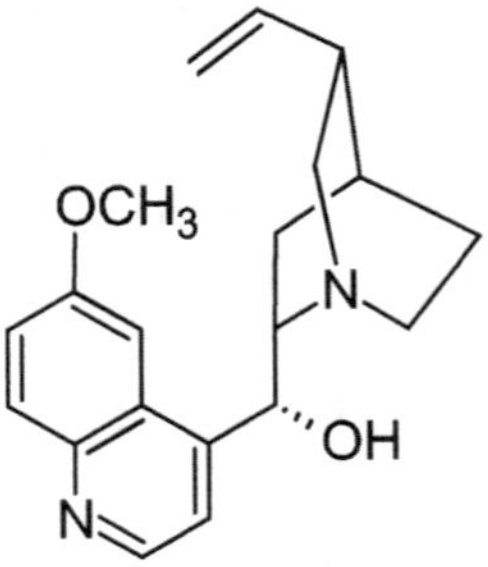 Quinine, *Cinchona officinalis*, Rubiaceae (Anti-malarial)
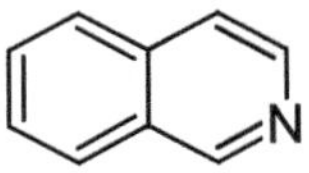 Isoquinoline	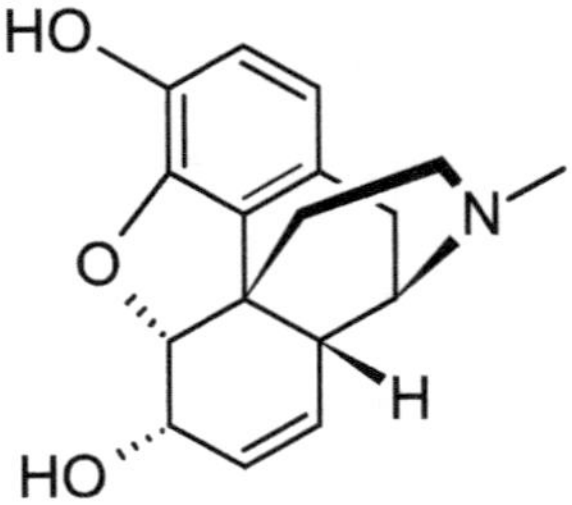 Morphine, *Papaverum somniferum*, Papaveraceae (Narcotic sedative)

Contd...

Quinazoline	Vasicine , *Adhatoda vasica, Acanthaceae* (Expectorant and bronchodilator. weak cardiac stimulant)
Aporphine	Boldine, *Peumus boldus*, Monimiaceae (Antioxidant, Hepatorpotective, neuroprotective)
Pseudo alkaloids	
Purine/Xanthine	Caffeine, *Thea sinensis*, Theaceae CNS Stimulant
Steroid	Solasodine, *Solanum species, Solanaceae*

Contd...

Diterpene	Aconitine *Aconitum napellus*, Ranunculaceae (Potent Poision- 0.028 mg/kg. In small doses as pain relief caused by trigeminal and intercostal neuralgia, rheumatism, migraine, and general debilitation)
Proto or amine alkaloids	
Amines	Ephedrine from *Ephedra gerardiana*, ephedraceae (Bronchodialator to treat cough)

Alkaloid containing crude drugs				
1. Indole Alkaloids				
Sr. No.	**Name of drug and synonym**	**Biological source**	**Active constitutents**	**Uses**
1	Ergot, Ergot of rye, Ergota	A fungal sclerotium of *Claviceps purpurea* in ovary of rye plant *Secale cereale*. Family of fungus- Clavicipitaceae; family of rye Graminae.	Indole alkaloids which are derivatives of lysergic acid, Laevorotatory alkaloids like Ergometrine (Water soluble), Ergotamine, Ergosin, Ergocristine, Ergocryptine, Ergocornine etc. (Water insoluble). Dxtrorotatory alkaloids Ergometrinine, Ergotaminine, Ergosinine, Ergocristinine, Ergocryptinine, Ergocorninine.	Oxytocic, prevents postpartum haemorrhage; used in treatment of migraine
2	Nux vomica, Crow Fig, Semen strychni, Nux vomica seed.	Dried ripe seeds of *Strychnos nux vomica* Linn., Family- Loganiaceae.	Bitter indole alkaloids, Strychnine, brucine, vomicine, alpha- colubrine, pseudostrychnineandstrychnicine. Isostychnine, N-oxystrychnine, protostrychnine, beta-colubrine, andnovacine. Glycoside viz. loganin, chlorogenic acid and fixed oil.	CNS stimulant, bitter stomachic, tonic

Contd...

3	Phystigma, Calabar beans, ordeal bean	Dried ripe seeds of *Physostigma venonosum* Balfour, Family - Loganiaceae.	Indole alkaloids Physostigmine, eserine, physovenine, eseramine, geneserine, calabatine, calabasine, isophysostigmine, and N-8-norphysostigmine.	Cholinergic, (ophthalmic) in Glaucoma. Physostigmine is a cholinesterase inhibitor used to treat glaucoma. It is also an antidote for Atropa belladonna, datura or atropine poisoning.
4	Rauwolfia, Sarpagandha, Rauwolfia root, Serpentina root, Chhotachand	Dried roots and rhizomes of the plant *Rauwolfia serpentina* Benth, Family-Apocynaceae.	Indole alkaloids, Indoline alkaloids, Indolenine alkaloids, Oxyindole alkaloids, Pseudo indoxy alkaloids, Reserpine, rescinnamine, oleo-resin, Phytosterol, fatty acids, alcohol and sugars. Other alkaloids presents areajmaline, ajmalicine, rauwolfinine, rescinnamine, reserpinine, yohimbinine, serpentine and serpentinine.	Hypotensive tranquilliser
5	Vinca, Catharanthus, Periwinkle,	Whole herba of *Catharanthus roseus*, Family-Apocynaceae	Indol alkaloids, Vincristine, vinblastine, ajmalicine, lochnerine, serpentine, and tetrahydro-alstonine .	Anticancer (treatment of Hodgkin's diseases andleukemia)

2. Isoqunoline Alkaloids

Sr. No.	Name of drug and synonym	Biological source	Active constitutents	Uses
6	Berberis	Roots and rhizomes of *Berberis aristata*, and other berberis species, Family-Berberidaceae	Berberine	Astringent in inflammation of mucous membrane
7	Curare, South American arrow poision	Dried extract of stem and leaves of *Chondrodendron tomentosum* Family-Menispermaceae	d-tubocurarine chloride, curine, curarine, isochodrodendrin, cycleaninechondrocurine, tomantocurine.	Skeletal muscle relaxant
8	Hydrastis , Golden seal, yellow root.	Roots and rhizomes of *Hydrastis Canadensis*, Family- Berberidaceae	Berberine,hydrastine	To control uterine haemorrhage
9	Ipecacunha, Ipecac.	Dried roots and rhizomes of *Cephaelis ipecacuanha* and *C. acuminate*, Family-Rubiaceae	Isoquinoline alkaloid Emetine, cephaeline, psychotrine, o-methyl psychotrine and emetamine, ipecacuanhic acid Glycoside ipecacuanhin, starch and calcium oxalate.	Antiamoebic, emetic, expectorant

Contd...

10	Opium, Raw opium	Dried latex from the capsules of *Papaveum somniferum* Linn., Family-Papaveraceae.	Morphine, Codein, Narcotine, Papaverine, Heroin.	Narcotic analgesic, in diarrhoea
3. Tropane alkaloids				
11	Belladonna Herb, Deadly night shade leaf, Belladonna Leaf, Belladonae Folium	Dried and flowering tops of *Atropa belladonna*, Family-Solanaceae	l-hyoscyamine, Atropine (Racemic mixture of l- hyoscyamine), Belladonine, Scopoletine, Hyoscine, pyridine and n-methyl pyroline, homatropine,	Anticholinergic, antispasmodic
12	Coca, Coca leaves	Dried leaves of *Erythroxylon coca*, Family-Erythroxylaceae	Cocaine, Cinnamyl-Cocain, Alpha-truxillline, Tropocaine, Benzoyltropine, Dihydroxytropane, ecgonine and Benzoylecgonine.	Local anaethetic
13	Duboisia, Cork-tree, cork wood.	Dried leaves of *Duboisia myoporoides*, Family-Solanaceae	Scopolamine, Atropine, l-hyoscymine, nor hyoscymine, Tigloidine, Valtropine, tiglyoxitripine.	Anticholinergic
14	Datura herb, Angel's trumpet.	Dried leaves and flowring tops of *Dhatura metel* var. Fastuosa, Family-Solanaceae	Scopolamine, hyoscamine, atropine	Anticholinergic, in duodenal ulcers
3. Tropane alkaloids				
Sr. No.	**Name of drug and synonym**	**Biological source**	**Active constitutents**	**Uses**
15	Hyoscymus, Henbane, Hyoscymus herb, Hyoscymus leaves.	Dried leaf and flowring top of *Hyoscymus niger*, Family- Solanaceae	l-hyoscyamine, Hyoscine.	Anticholinergic, antispasmodic
16	Stramonium Leaf, Thornapple leaves.	Dried leaves and flowring tops of *Datura stramonium*, Family-Solanaceae	l-hyoscymine, hyoscine and atropine	Anticholinergic, mydriatic, control motion, sickness
4. Quinoline alkaloids				
17.	Camptotheca, Cancer tree	*Camptotheca acuminata*, Family-Nyssaceae	Camptothecin, 10-hydroxy campothecine, 10 methoxy-campothecine.	Antitumour
18.	Cinchona , Peruvian bark, Jesuit's bark	Dried root or stem bark of *Cinchona calisaya, C.officinalis, C.ledgeriana, C.succirubra*, Family-Rubiaceae	Quinine, Quinidine, Cinchonine, cinchonidine, Cupreine, hydroquinine,	Antimalarial, bitter tonic.
5. Pyridine alkaloids				
19.	Areca nut, betal nut.	Dried ripe seeds of *Areca catechu*, Family- Palmae	arecoline, arecaidine, Guvacine, Gevacoline, Lipids, Volatile oils, tanins, Gum.	Respiratory stimulant

Contd…

20	Lobelia, Indian tobacco, Asthma weed.	Dried leaves and tops of *Lobelia nicotianefolia*, Family- Campanulaceae	Lobeline, lobelanedine, Lobelanine, Isolabalinine, Pungent volatile oil,Renin, Gum and fix oil	Respiratory stimulant

6. Imidazole alkaloids

21	Jaborandi, pilocarus	Dried leaves of *Pilocarpus jaborandi*, Family-Rutaceae	Pilocarpine, pilosine, isopilocarpine, pilocarpidine, psudopilocarpine, isopilocine.	Cholinergic (ophthalmic), use in the treatment of glaucoma.

7. Quinazoline Alkaloids

22	Vasaka, adulasa, Adhatoda, Mulabar nut	Leaves of *Adhatoda vasaka*, Family- Acanthaceae	Vasicine and vasicinone, 6 hydroxyvasicine, volatile oil, betain , Vasakin, Adhatodic acid ,Vasicol, Adhatodine	Anti- tussive expectorant

8. Purine alkaloids

Sr. No.	Name of drug and synonym	Biological source	Active constitutents	Uses
23	Cocoa seed , cocoa beens	Seed of *Theobroma cacao*, Family-Sterculiaceae	Theobromine, cocoa butter, Volatile compound, Polyphenol and caffeine, etc	Diuretic
24	Coffee, Coffee bean, Coffee seed.	Dried ripe seed of *Coffea arabica*, Family-Rubiaceae	Caffine, trigonelline, Tannin, Fixoil, proteins, Clorogenic or caffeotannic acid, and sugars in the form of dextrin, glucose etc.	Stimulant, to counter over dosage of CNS depressant
25	Tea, thia, Camellia thea	Leaves leaf buds of *Thea sinensis* Family-Theaceae	Caffeine theobromine-theoromine, theophylline	CNS stimulant and diuretic

9. Steroidal Alkaloids

26	Ashwagandha, Asgandha, Withania root, winter cherry.	Dried roots of *Withania somnifera*, Family-Solanaceae	Withanine, somniferine, withanolide, (Steroid), Somnine, somniferinine, psudowithanine, tropine, Psudotropine, 3-alpha gloyoxytropane,choline, cuscohygrine, isopelletierine, Anaferine and anahydrine, di isopelletierine, sitoindoside VII and VIII, Withaferine A, Withanolide D. and E to N	Sedative and also as antirheumatic.
27	Kurchi, Hollarrena	Dried bark of *Hollarrhena antidysentrica*, Family-Apocynaceae	Conessine, isoconessine, norconessine, dioxiconessine, conessimine, hollarridine, hollarrine,	Antiamoebic
28	Veratrum, White and green hellebore.	Dried rhizomes of *Veratrum album* and *V. viride*, Family- Liliaceae.	Germidine, Protoveratrine, veratrine, Germetrine, Cevadine, Psudojervijne, Veratrosine, Veratrosine, etc Protoveratrine A and B	Hypotensive, cardiac depressant.

Contd...

10. Amino alkaloid (Proto alkaloids)				
Sr.	Name of drug and synonym	Biological source	Active constitutents	Uses
29	Aconite, Monkshood, Aconite root, Bachnag, Monkshoot	Dried roots of *Aconitum napallus*, Family-Raunanculaceae	Aconitine, neopelline, Aconine, Hypaconitine, Napelline, Neoline, and Traces of Sparteine, Ephedrin, Aconitic acid Succinic acid	In treatment or rheumatism sciatica
30	Colchicum , Meadow Saffron seed, Autumn, crocus	Dried ripe seed and corm of *Colchicum autumnale* Linn. and C. luteum Baker. Family-Liliaceae	Colchicine, demecolcine, Tropolone or cycloheptatrien-ol-one ring structure.	Treatment of gout, induction of polyploidy
31	Ephedra, Ma huang	Dried stem of *Ephedra gerardiana, E.equeisetina, E. sinica,* Family-Ephedraceae	Ephedrine, nor ephedrine, n-methyl ephedrine, Pseudoephedrine (Alkaloidal amines)	Sympathomimetic, Antiasthmatic, Treatment of hay fever.
32	Glorisa, Glory lily	Dried rhizome and roots of *Glorisa superba,* Family-Liliaceae	Colchicine, Colchicine derivatives.	In the treatment of gout and cancer.

4.2.2   Volatile (Essential) Oils

Introduction	➢ Odorous volatile principles of plant and animal origin are known as essential oils/ etheral oils or volatile oils." ➢ Plants containing essential oils are known as Aromatic plants. ➢ They all produce characteristic flavors and or odors due to presence of compounds that are volatile in nature ➢ Essential due to fact that it represents essence or active principle of plant.
Occurrence	➢ Majority of terpenoids are present in the plant kingdom more particularly among phanerograms. Commonly found in labiatae, rutaceae, piperaceae, zinziberaceae, umbelliferae, myrtaceae, lauraceae.
Physical properties	➢ Always volatile, characteristic flavour and or odour, colorless liquids when fresh, immiscible with water, high refractive indices, optically active
Chemical properties	➢ Chemically these are derived from isoprene units (terpenes) and their oxygenated compounds (terpenoides), unsaturated, open chain, or cyclic, with one or more carbon atom in the ring. CH_3 / H_2C OOP — **IPP** IPP Isomers — Isoprene synthesis → **Isoprene** (H_3C, H_2C, CH_2) H_3C / H_3C OOP — **DMAPP**

Contd...

	➢ Only mono and sesquiterpenoids are volatile in nature. Further higher terpenoids (diterpenoids, sesterterpenoids, triterpenoids, tetraterepnoids, polyterpenoids) are non-volatile in nature. ➢ They easily undergo addition reactions with hydrogen and halogen, polymerization, dehydrogenation and oxidation

Methods of analysis	➢ **Physical properties**: Optical rotation, refractive index, specific gravity
	➢ **Chemical testing**:
	  o To the section of the drug add alcoholic solution of **Sudan red-III**, the **red color** obtained by globules indicate the presence of volatile oil.
	  o To the thin section of the drug, add the drop of the **tincture of the alkana, red color** indicates the presence of the volatile oil.
	  o Most of the volatile oils are **soluble in the organic solvent**. (90 %) ethanol.
	  o Volatile oils (monoterpenoids) do **not leave any translucent spot** on the filter paper when applied but fixed oils leaves greasy spot on the paper.
	➢ **Gas chromatography (GC) or GC-MS (Mass spectroscopy) analysis**
	➢ **Thin layer chromatographic (TLC) analysis**

Analytical standards for few volatile oils

Sr. No.	Type of oil	Specific gravity	Optical rotation	Ref. Index
1	Anise	0.978 - 0.988	+1 to -2	1.553-1.560
2	Black pepper	0.898- 0.900	-3 to -5	1.4539-1.4977
3	Camphor	0.875-0.90	+9 to +27	1.465-1.470
4	Cassia cinnamon	1.045 – 1.063	-1 to +1	1.6020-1.6060
5	Chenopodium	0.970 – 0990	-3 to -8	1.474-1.480
6	Cinnamon	1.00 - 1.030	0 to -2	1.562-1.582
7	Citronella	0.895 - 0.900	-2 to -5	1.468-1.473
8	Clove	1.038-1.06	-0° to -2°	1.527-1.535
9	Coriander	0.863-0.875	+8 to +15	1.462-1.472
10	Cubeb	0.905-0.925	20 to -40	1.4800-1.5020
11	Cummin	0.900 - 0.935	+4 to +8	1.4950-1.5090
12	Dill	0.900-0.915	+70 to +80	1.481-1.492
13	Eucalyptus	0.870-0.912	0 to +10	1.457-1.469
14	Fennel	0.953 - 0.973	+12 to +24	1.526-1.538
15	Gaultheria	1.180 - 1.187	0 to -1	1.537-1.539
16	Lemon peel	0.849-0.855	+57 to +65	1.4742-1.4755
17	Lemon-grass	0.88700 – 0.89900	-3 to +1	1.4808-1.4868
18	Palmarosa	0.885 - 0.896	+1.4 to -2	1.4760-1.4805
19	Peppermint	0.808-0.908	-16 to -30	1.4590-1.4650
20	Rosemary	0.894 - 0.912	-5 to 10	1.464-1.476
21	Sandal wood	0.973 to 0.985	15 to 20	1.500-1.510
22	Spearmint	0.930-0.940	48 to -59	1.4820-1.4900
23	Turpentine	0.860-0.875	-25° ~ -31°	1.467-1.477
24	Vetiver	0.990 - 1.032	+15 to +45	1.512-1.523

Classification of Terpenoids based on number of isoprene units

Class	Isoprene unit	Molecular formulae	Examples
Hemiterpene /isoprene	1	C_5H_8	*Hamamelis japonica* leaf
Monoterpenes (Geranyl pyrophosphate)	2	$C_{10}H_{16}$	Limonene, cineole, menthol
Sesquiterpenes (Farnesyl pyrophosphate)	3	$C_{15}H_{24}$	Eugenol, zingiberine, santonin
Diterpenes (Geranyl geraniol pyrophosphate)	4	$C_{20}H_{32}$	Taxol, forskolin, abietic acid
Triterpenes (Squalene)	6	$C_{30}H_{48}$	Glycyrrhizin, azadirachtin.
Tetraterpenes (Carotenoids)	8	$C_{40}H_{64}$	Crocetin, bixin, b-carotene
Polyterpenes	n	(C_5H_8) n	Rubber

Classification of Volatile oil (mono and sesqui terpenoids) based on functional group

Functional Group		Phytoconstituents	Plant	
Hydrocarbon	C_5H_8	Pinene	Turpentine	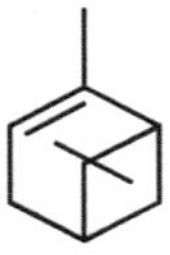 (+) α-pinene
Alcohol volatile oil	C−OH	Linalool, menthol	Coriander, pepermint	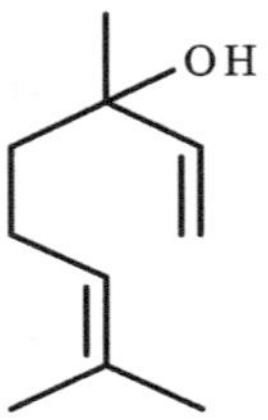 Linalool
Aldehyde volatile oil	CHO	Citronellal, cinnamic aldehyde	Citronella, cinnamon	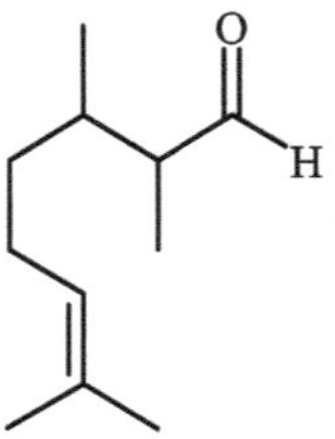 Citronella

Contd...

Ester volatile oil	−HC=O	Borneol acetate, gualtherin	Lavender, gaultheria	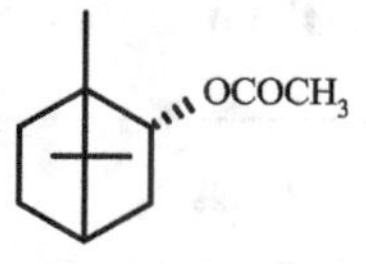 Bomyl acetate
Ketone volatile oil	C=O	Carvone, camphor, menthone	Caraway, camphor, spearmint	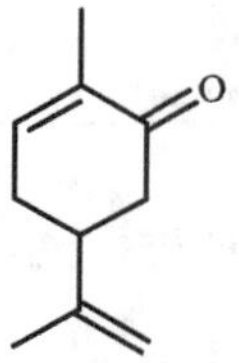 Carvone
Ether	R-O-R'	Cineol, myristicin	Eucalyptus, jayphal	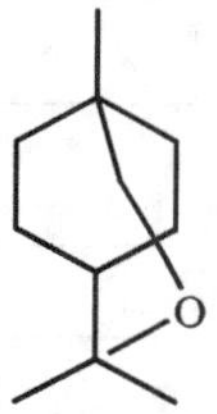 Cineol
Peroxide volatile oil	R−O−O−R'	Ascaridole	Chenopodium	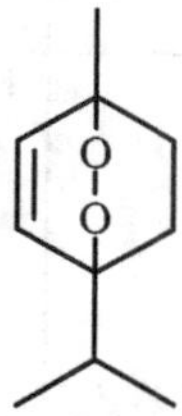 Ascaridole
Phenol volatile oil	Ar−OH	Eugenol, thymol	Clove, cinnamon	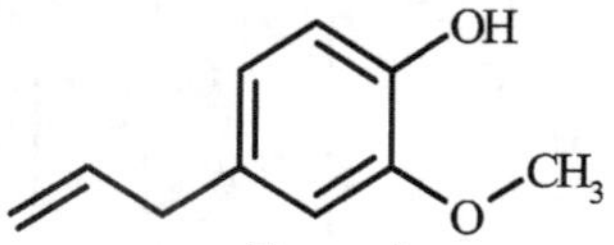 Eugenol
Glycoside derived	R-Sugar	Allylisothiocynate, methyl salycilate	Wintergreen, mustard	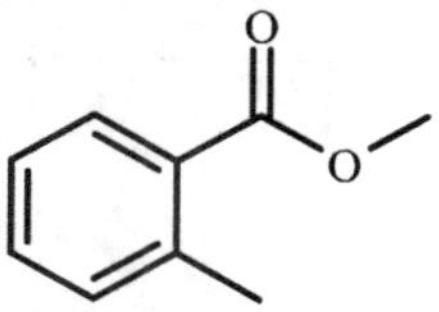 Methylsalicylate

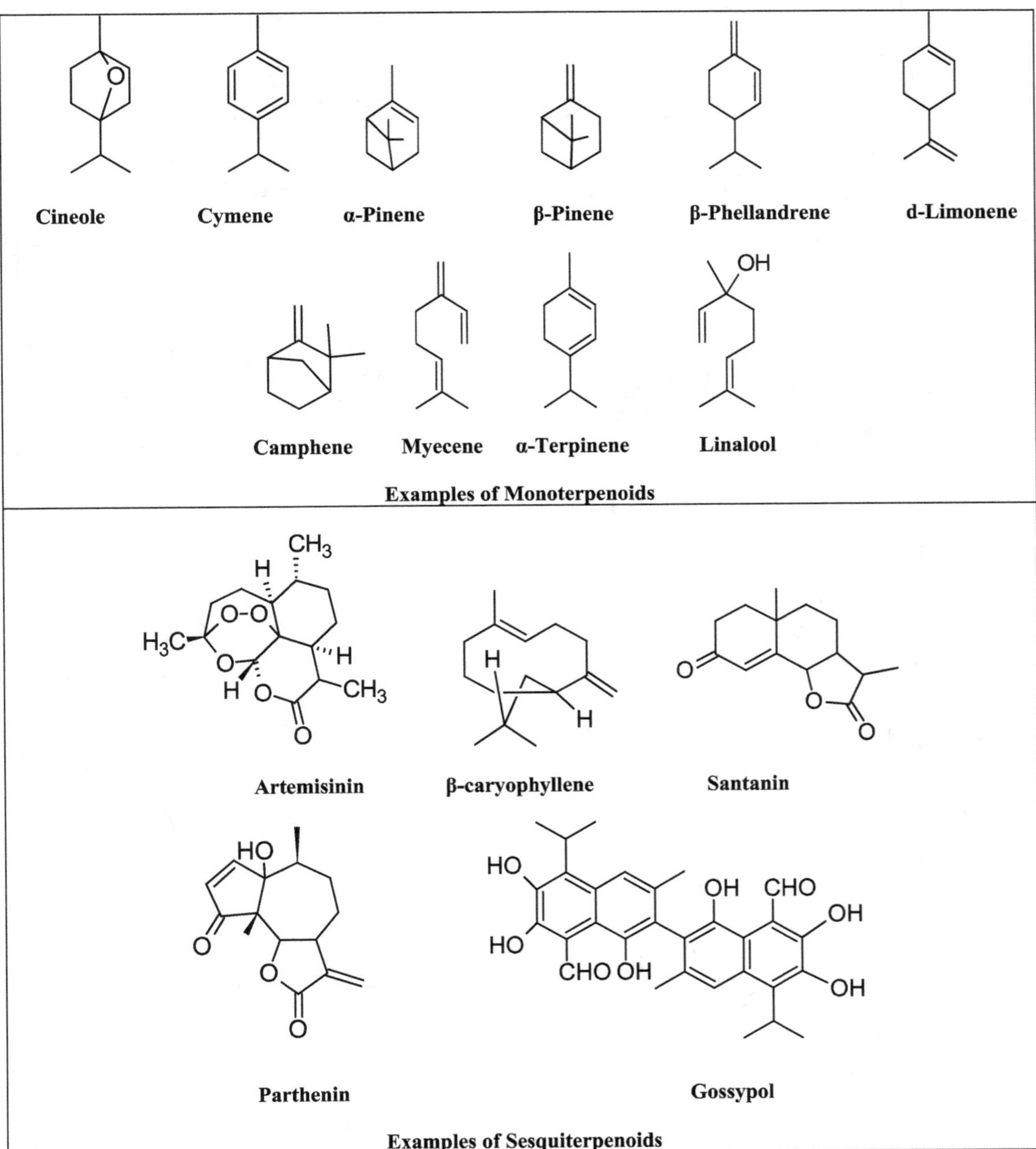

Examples of Monoterpenoids

Examples of Sesquiterpenoids

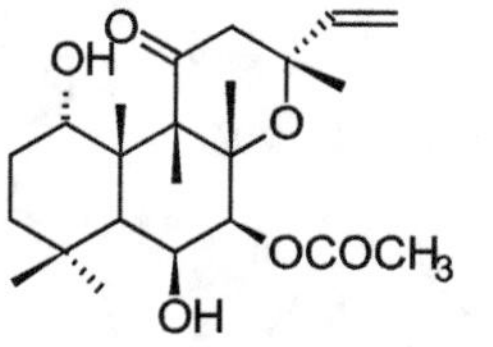

Forskolin

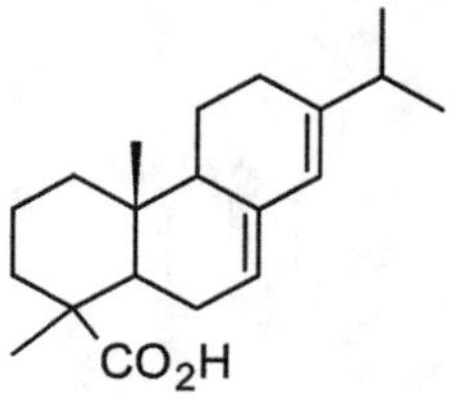

Abletic acid

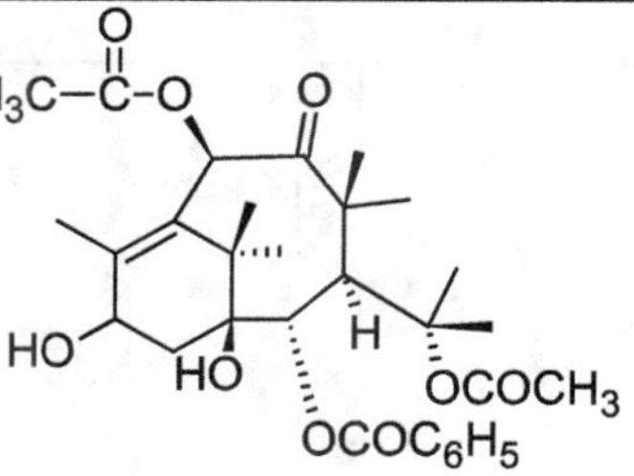

Baocatin III

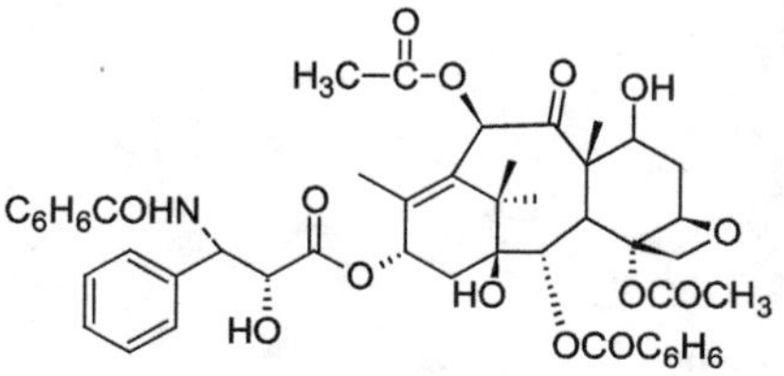

Taxol

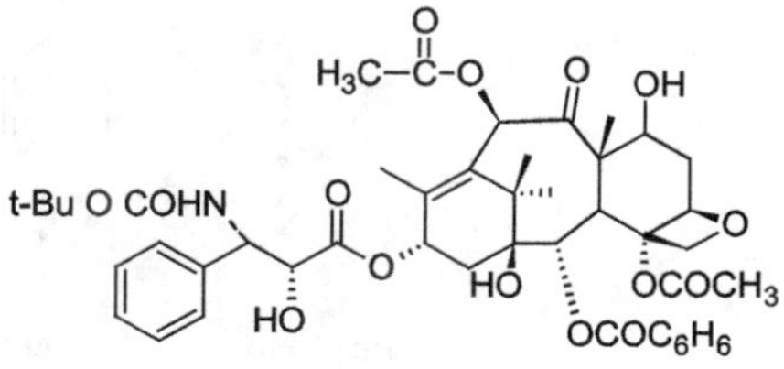

Taxotore

Examples of Diterpenoids

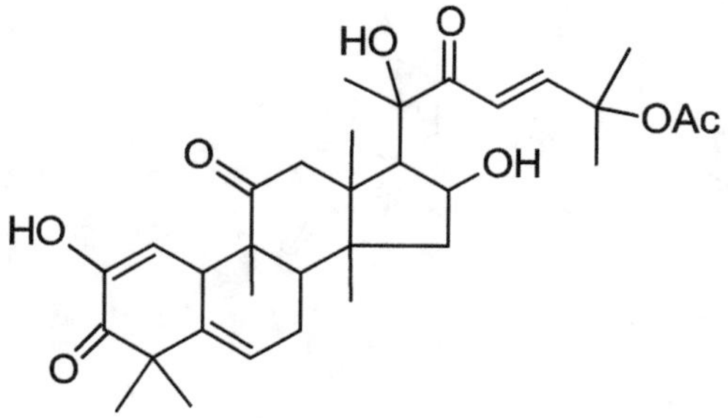

Cucurbitacin E

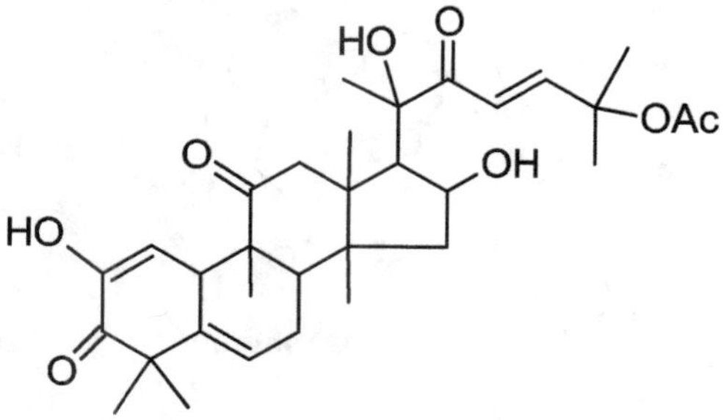

Cucurbitacin B

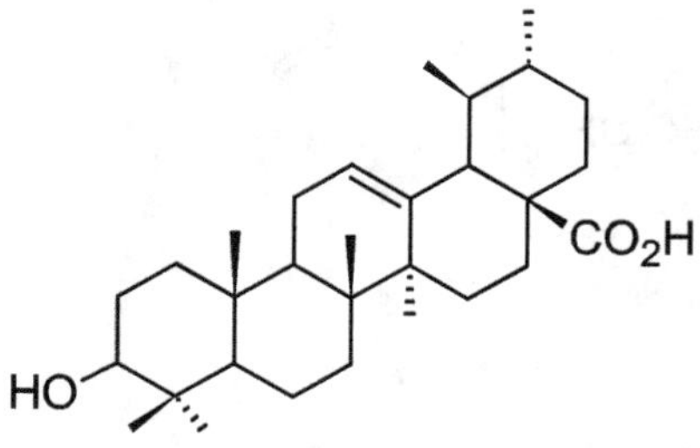

Soyasapogenol B

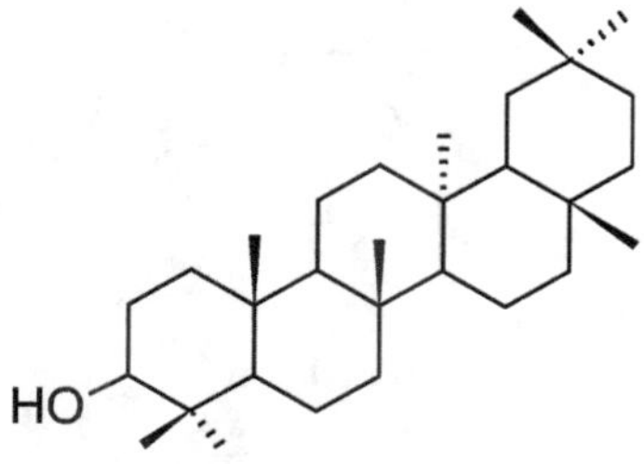

Taraxerol

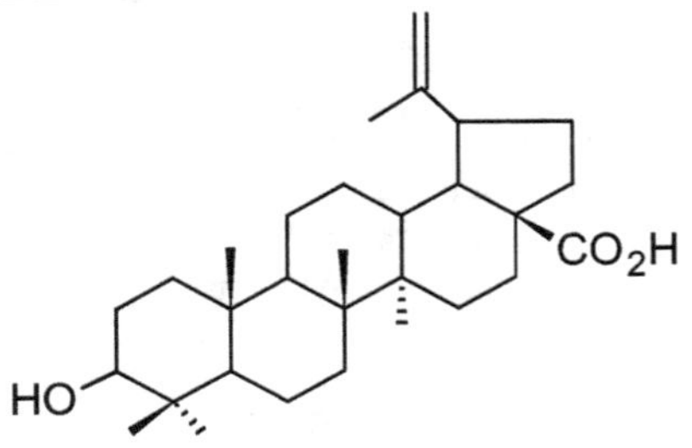

Betullic acid

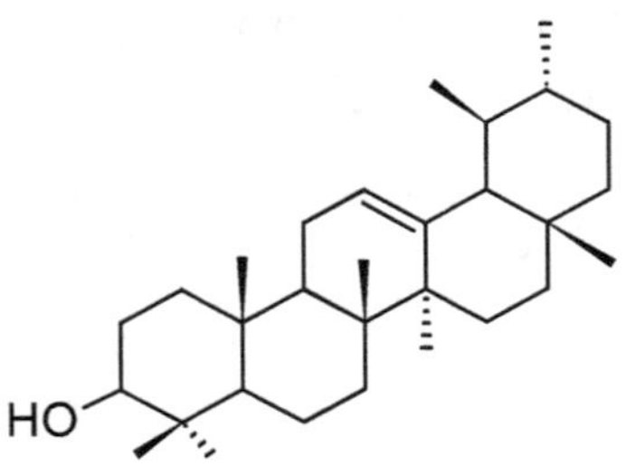

Ursollic acid

Examples of Triterpenoids

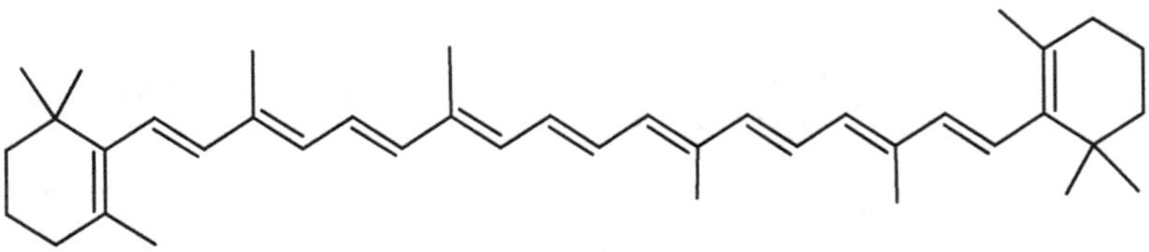

α- carotene

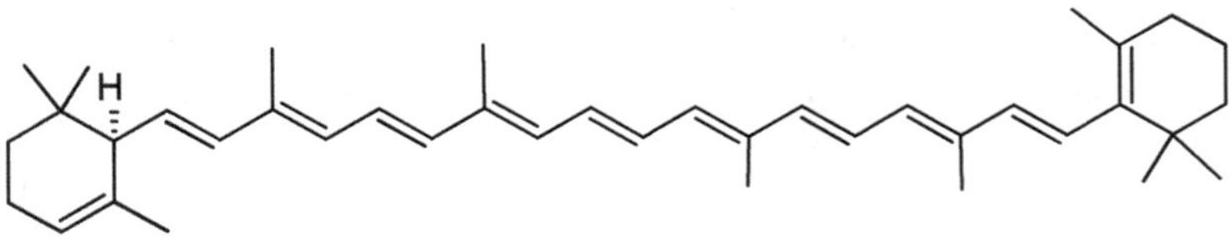

β- carotene

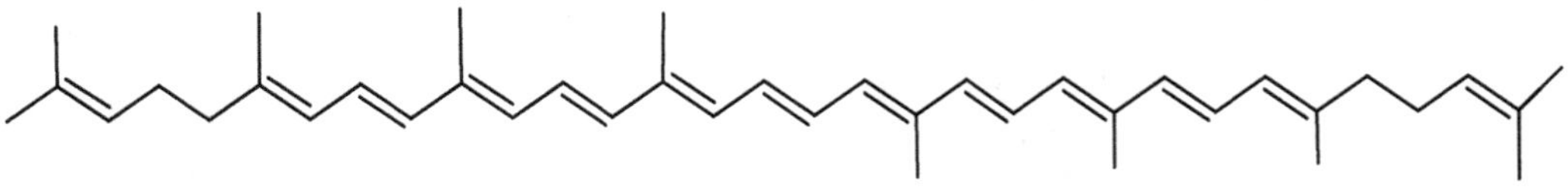

Lycopene

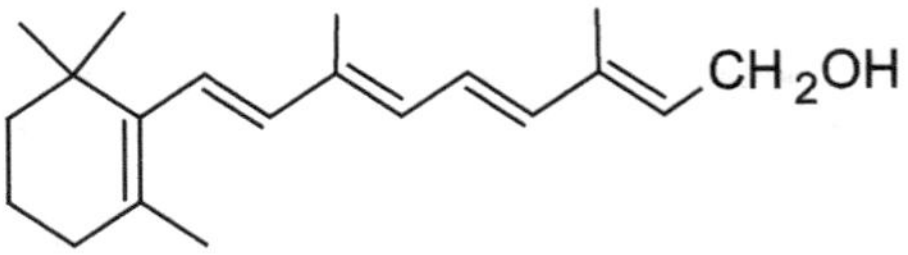

Retinol (Vitamin A)

Examples of Tertaterpenoids

Essential oil containing crude drugs				
Alcohol				
Peppermint oil	Mentha oil, Oleum mentha piperites, Colpermin	Obtained by steam distilation of the fresh flowring tops of the plant, *Mentha piperita* Family-Labiatae	Menthol, pulegone menthone, menthofuram, Jasmone, methyl isovalerate, Methyl acetate, Limonene, Isopulegone, Cineol , Pinene, Camphene	Carminative, stimulant, flavour, antiseptic and perfumes
Name of crude drug	**Synonyms**	**Biological name and family**	**Active constituent**	**Uses**
Cinnamon	Kalmi-Dalchini, Cinnamon bark Ceylon cinnamon	Dried inner bark of the shoots of coppiced trees of Cinnamomum zeylanicum, Family- Lauraceae	Eugenol, benzaldehyde cuminaldehyde, Cinnamaldehyde, Phellandrene, Pinene, Cymene, Caryophyllene Starch, Mucilage, Mannitol	Carminative stomachic, Flavour, Stimulant, aromatic, antiseptic, Astringent
1) Drugs containing monoterpenoids				
Aldehyde				
Cassia cinnamon	Cassia bark, Chinese cinnamon	Dried stem bark of the plant *Cinnamomum cassia*, Family-Lauraceae	Mucilage, Coumarin, Cinnamic aldehyde Eugenol Cinnamyl acetate Starch and tannins	Carminative,st imulant, flavour, stimulant, flavour, aromatic, spices
Lemon grass oil	East-Indian lemon grass oil, Indian Melissa oil	Obtained by the steam distillation from the leaves and aerial parts of the plants *Cymbopogon flexuausus* Family-Graminae`	Citral, nerol, citronella, methyl heptenol Dipentene geraniol	Flavour
Orange peel	Orange cortex	Dried or fresh outer part of *Citrus aurantium,* Family-Rutaceae	Pectin, Aurantiamarin and aurantianic acid, Hesperidin, Isohesperidin, Neohesperidin, Vit-C, Limonene, Citral	Stomachic, aromatic carminative carminative, flavour
Oxides				
Chenopodium	American wormseed oil, chenopodiol chenoposom	Obtained by steam distillation from the fresh flowering and fruiting plants *Chenopodium ambrosioides*, Family-Chenopodiaceae	Asconidole p-cymene myrcene 1-limonene and camphor	Anthelmintic, to expel hook worms and intestinal amoebae

Contd...

Eucalyptus oil	Dinkum oil eucalyptus Lemon gum tree	Obtained by the distillation of the fresh leaves of *Eucalyptus globulus* Family-Myrtaceae	Cineole camphene phellandrene Geranyl acetate Eucalyptol Pinene	Counter-irritant, antiseptic, expectorant, used in cough, chronic bronchitis
1) Drugs containing monoterpenoids				
Ketone				
Cummin	Jira	Dried ripe fruits of Cuminum Cyminum Family-Umbelliferae	Cuminaldehyde, alpha-pinene, beta-pinene, Phellendrene Volatile oil, fixed oil, proteins Phellandrene Cuminic alcohol Hydro-cuminine	Stimulant, carminative and used in diarrhoea and dyspepsia
Caraway	Carum, caraway seed	Dried ripe fruits of *Carum carvi,* Family-Umbelliferae	Carvone, carvacrol, Dihydrocarvone, Caravacrol,	Aromatic, stimulant, carminative, flavour
Name of crude drug	**Synonyms**	**Biological name and family**	**Active constituent**	**Uses**
Dill	European dill, Dill fruits, Anethum	Dried ripe fruits of *Anethum graveolens,* Family-Umbeliferae	Dill-apiole, carvone, Dihydrocarvone, D-limonene, Phelandrene,	Aromatic, Stimulant, Carminative flavour, used in gripillo
Fennel	Fennel fruits, Fructus foeniculum	Dried ripe fruits of *Foeniculum vulgare,* Family-Umbeliferae	Fenchone, anethol, ketone, phellandrene, limonene, Methyl charvicol, Anisicaldehyde	Carminative, flavour, aromatic, stimulant, expectorant
Coriander	Coriander fruits	Dried ripe fruits of *Coriandrum sativum,* Family-Umbeliferae	Pinene, Geraniol, Coriandrol, Coriandryl acetate, L-borneol, cineol	Aromatic, Flavour, Carminative,S timulant
1) Drugs containing monoterpenoids				
Phenol				
Tulsi	Sacred basil, holy basil	Fresh and dried leaves of *Ocimum sanctum,* Family-Labiate	Eugenol, Methyle eugenol, Carvacrol, Caryophyllin Vitamin C Traces of maleic Citric and tartaric acid	Antibacterial, insecticidal, stimulant, aromatic, anticatarrhal, spasmodic, diaphoric, antiperiodic, stomachic, good immunomodul atory agent

Contd...

Name of crude drug	Synonyms	Biological name and family	Active constituent	Uses
Ether				
Nutmeg	Myristicci Nux-Moschata	Dried kerrnel of seed of *Myristica fragrans,* Family-Myristicaceae	Myristicin, Palmitic acis, Oleic acid, Lauric acid, saffrole, elimicin	Aromatic, flavour, stimulant, carminative used in soap industry, treat rheumatism
Ester				
Garlic	Allium	Consist of bulbs of the plant *Allium sativum,* Family-Liliaceae	Allicin, alliin, iron, phosphorus, copper, propyl disulphide Diallyl disulphide Albumin Fat, mucilage and Volatile oil	Carminative, expectorant, stimulant, disinfectant, condiment, rubefacient, anthelmintic
Mixtures				
Turpentine	Oleum terbinthae	Obtained by distillation from oleoresin of *Pinus roxburghii* Family-Pinaceae	Alpha pinene, Beta-pinene, Camphene, limonene, Beta phelandrene, turpentine, delta 3 carene	Counter irritant, rubefacient, expectorant, antiseptic
Ajowan	Carum copticum, Hieren, Trychyspermum copticum	Dried ripe fruits of *Trachyspermum ammi,* Family-Umbeliferae	Tymol, Dipentenes, Tannin, Glycoside, Volatile oil, Protein, Carbohydrate, thymol, p-cymene, terpinen	Antispas-modic, Stimulant, Carminative,Antiseptic, Anti-fungal, insecticide, Anthelminitic
Rosemary	-	Obtained from fresh flowering tops of the plant *Rosmarinus officinalis* Lab. Family-Labitae	Volatile oil, resins, borneol, ursolic acid, bornyl acetate Camphor eucalyptol Pinene d-camphene, cineol and terpenes	Carminative, Flavour, stimulant, rubefacient
Lavender	Common Lavender	Obtained by steam distillation of fresh flowering tops of *Lavandula officinalis,* Family-Labiateae	Esters linalyl acetate linalool, pinene, geraniol, cineol	Aromatic, carminative, flavour in perfumary

Contd...

Gaultheria	Bectula oil, oil of wintergreen Sweet birch oil Tea berry oil	Obtained by steam distillation from the leaves the *Gaultheria procumbens*, Family-Ericaceae	Gaultherin, methylsalicylate Gaultherase Enanthic alcohols	Rheumatism, flavour, vermicide (Hook worms)
Palmarosa	Rosha oil, Geranium oil Motia-variety	Obtained from leaves and tops of *Cymbopogon Martini*, Family-Graminae	Gereniol, Linalool, Citronella dipentene	Flavour, Treatment of Rheumatism and skin Diseases
Camphor	Formosa oil Rectified oil of camphor	Obtained from the wood by steam distillation of *Cinnamomum camphora* Family-Lauraceae	Safrole, d-pinene acetaldehyde, dipentene cineol Camphor eugenol Eucalyptol and phellandrene	Flavour, rebefacient counter irritant

Name of crude drug	Synonyms	Biological name and family	Active constituent	Uses
Thyme	Garden thyme, mother of thyme Red thyme French thymes	Consist of dried or partially dried leaves and flowering tops of the plant *Thymus vulgaris* Family-Labiateae	Thymol, Linalool, Carvacrol, caffeic acid, labiatic acid Ursolic acid, resins and tanninss	Carminative, Antispas-modic, flavour, expectorant

1) Drugs containing monoterpenoids

Mixtures

Geranium	Algerian geranium Moroccan geranium oil	Obtained from fresh leaves and stems of *Pelargonium graveolens*, Family-Geraniaceae	Geraneol, Citronellol Geranyl acetate Geranyl-tiglate Citranellyl formate and citranellyl acetate	Flavouring agent
Spearmint	Mentha viridis Mint Spearmint leaves Common spearmint	Dried leaves and flowering tops of the plant *Metha spicata*, Family-Labiatae	l-carvone, Carvone Linalool, Pinene Cineole, Phellandrene Resin Tannins	Flavouring agent

Name of crude drug	Synonyms	Biological name and family	Active constituent	Uses
Kapur kachari	Spiked ginger lily	Dried sliced rhizomes of the plant *Hedychium spicatum*, Family-Zingiberaceae	Paramethoxy cinnamic acid ester, Cineol, Limonene 8-caryophyllene Ethyl cinnamate Cinnamic aldehyde	Stomachic, carminative, stimulant tonic, flavour preparation of ABIT

Contd...

Black pepper	Pepper	Dried unripe fruit of perennial climbing *Piper nigrum*, Family-Piperaceae	Piperine, starch piperidine, l-phellandrone, Caryophyllene	Aromatic, stimulant, stomachic, carminative, condiment, stimulant the taste buds with gastric juice

1) Drugs containing monoterpenoids

Mixtures

Musk	Kasturi moschus	Dried secretion obtained from the preputial follicles of musk dear *Moschus moschiferus*, Family-Cervidae	Musckone, Cholesterin, albuminoidsand resins Volatile oil, fat, wax	Perfumary used in treatment of hysteria

Name of crude drug	Synonyms	Biological name and family	Active constituent	Uses
Artemisia annua	Quinghao, Sweet annie	Chinese traditional herb *Artemisia aannua*, Family-Asteraceae	Sesquiterpene lactone, Artemicinin, deoxy artemicinine, Artemicinic acid, Arteannuin A and B , Amyrin,Luteolin, Beta sitosterol, Stigma stero, Artemisia alcohol, Artemisia ketone, Camphor, Caryophyllin and Myrecene	Antimalerial
Davana oil	-	Steam distillation of flowring herbs *Artemisia pallens*, Family-Compositae	Davanone, artemone, nondavanone, Cineol, Borneol, Geraneol, Linalool, Eugenol	Perfume, flavour
Arnica	Arnica flower, Mountain tobacco, Wolf's bane, Leopards bean	Dried flower heads of *Arnica Montana*, Family-Compositae	Volatile oil, flavonoids, terpenoids, Dehydrohelenanin, Epoxy helanin, Arnicin, Apegenin, Querecetin, Tricin, Kemoferol,Tymol, 4-hydroxy thymol diethyl ether	Counter-irritant, cosmetic, rheumatism, spinal paralysis and blindness
Sandal wood oil	East indian sandal wood oil	Distillation from the heart wood of *Santalam album*, Family-Santalaceae	Alpha, beta-santalol, santene, santenone, teresantol, santalone, santalene	Treatment of dysuria, used in perfume

Contd...

Name of crude drug	Synonyms	Biological name and family	Active constituent	Uses
Clove	Clove-flower, Clove-buds, Caryophyllum	Dried flower buds of *Eugenia caryophyllus,* Family-Myrtaceae	Eugenin, Eugenol acetate, Caryophyllin, Ester, ketone and alcohol, Eugenol, ester eugenin	Dental analgesic, carminative, flavour, stimulant, aromatic and antiseptic

4.2.3 Glycosides

Glycosides can be defined as "organic compounds which on hydrolysis give one or more sugar moieties along with nonsugar moiety. The nonsugar component is known as the aglycone. The sugar component is called the glycone".

Classification of Glycosides based on <u>Linkage</u>	
C-glycoside (Uncommon in higher plants) Example- Aloin from aloe, cascarosides from cascara Glycone-OH + HC-aglycone → glycone-C-aglycone + H_2O	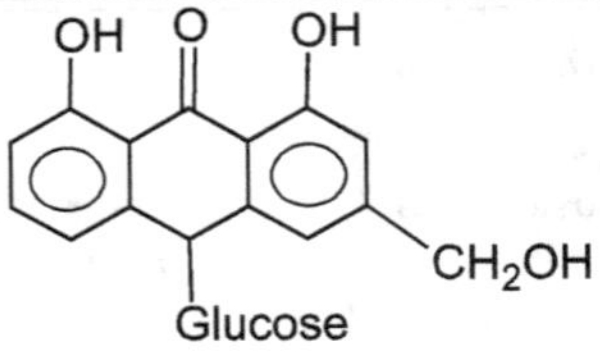 OH O OH CH_2OH Glucose **Barbaloin**
O-glycosides (Common in higher plants) Example- Sennosides from Senna, cascarosides from cascara Glycone-OH + HO-aglycone → Glycone-O-aglycone + H_2O	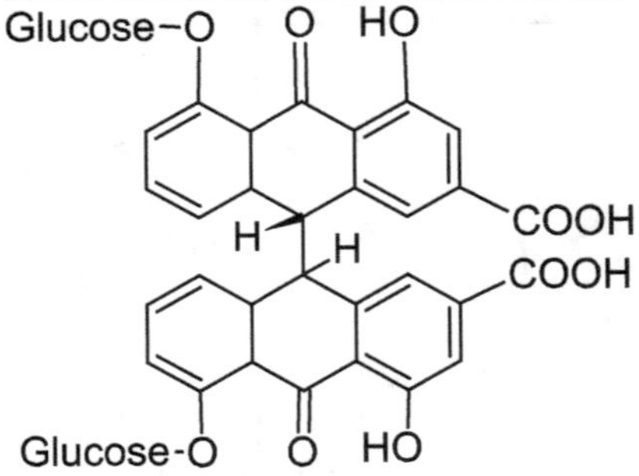 Glucose–O O HO H H COOH COOH Glucose-O O HO **Sennoside-A**
S-glycosides from sulfhydryl group Example- Sinigrin from black mustard Glycone-OH + HS-glycone → glycone-S-aglycone + H_2O	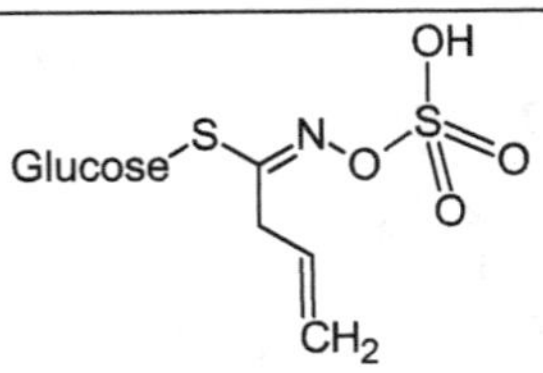 OH Glucose–S–N–O–S=O CH_2 **Sinigrin**

Contd...

N-glycosides Example- Nucleosides Glycone-OH + HN-glycone → glycone-N-aglycone + H_2O	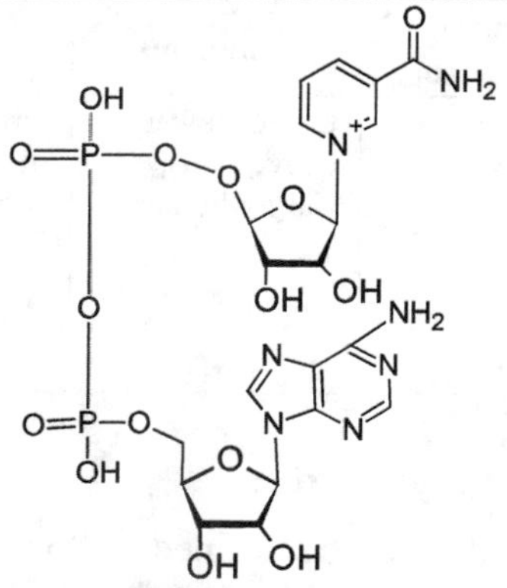 **Nicotinamide Adenine Dinucleotide**

Classification of Glycosides based on <u>aglycone</u> moiety	
Class with example	**Basic Moiety**
Anthraquinone ➢ Sennoside A, B, C, D from senna ➢ Palmidin A, B, C, D from rhubarb ➢ Aloin, Barbaloin from aloe ➢ Cascarosides from Cascara	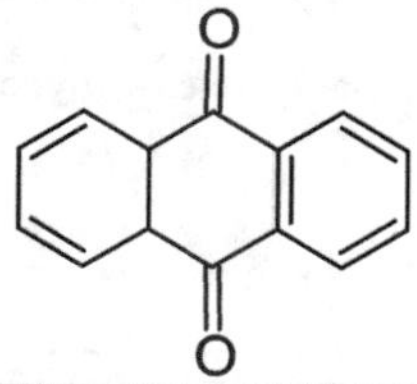
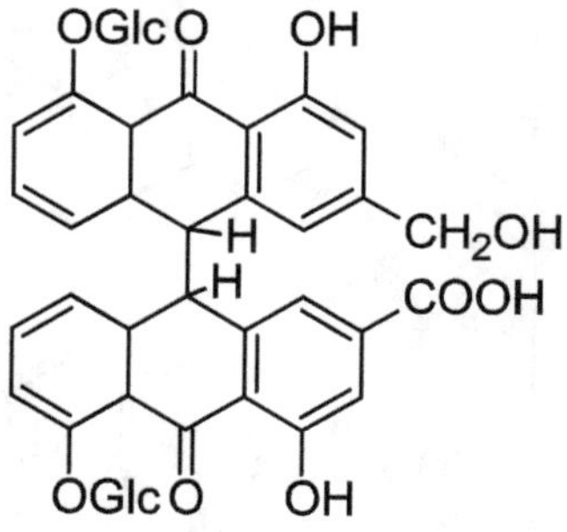 **Sennoside A (meso)**	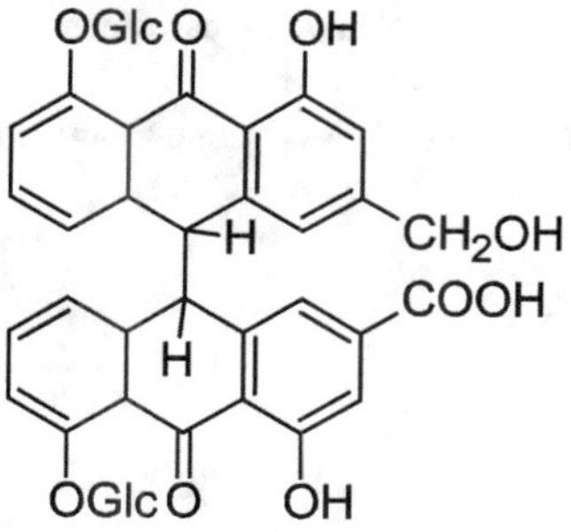 **Sennoside B (trans)**
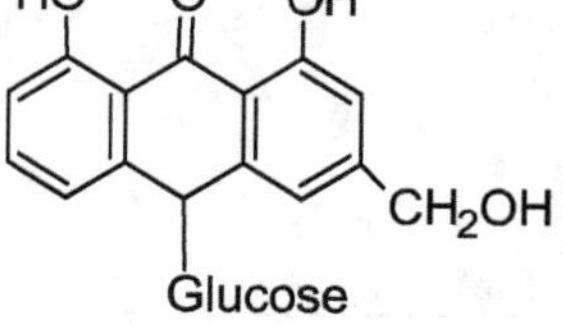 **Aloin** 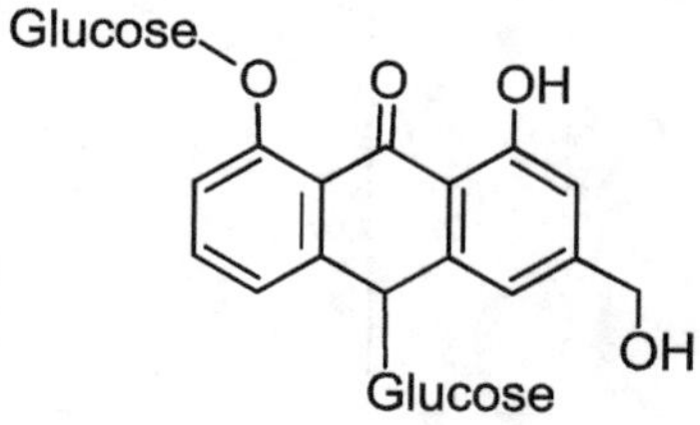 **Cascaroside A**	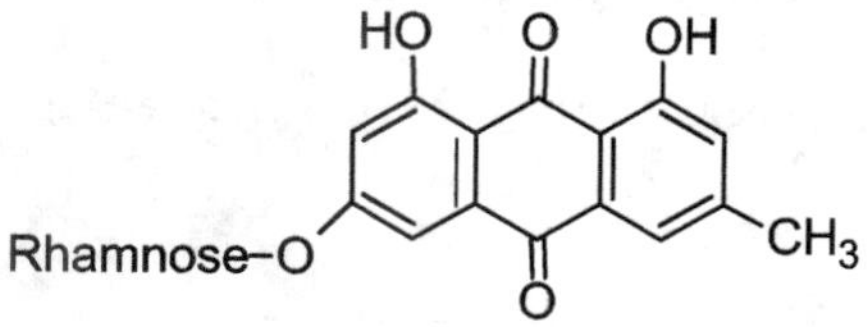 **Frangulin A**

Contd...

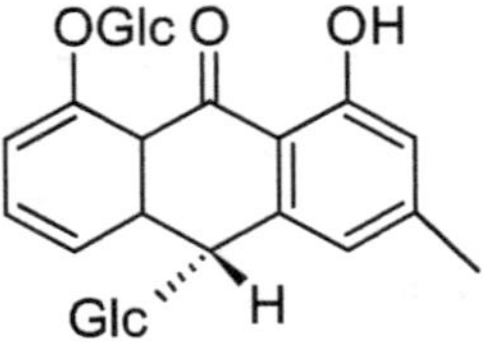

Cascaroside A

Cascaroside C

Cascaroside B

Cascaroside D

Anthraquinone aglycones

Aglycones	R1	R2
Rhein	COOH	H
Aloe-emodin	CH_2OH	H
Chrysophanol	CH_3	H
Emodin	CH_3	OH
Physcion	CH_3	OCH_3

Dianthrone aglycones

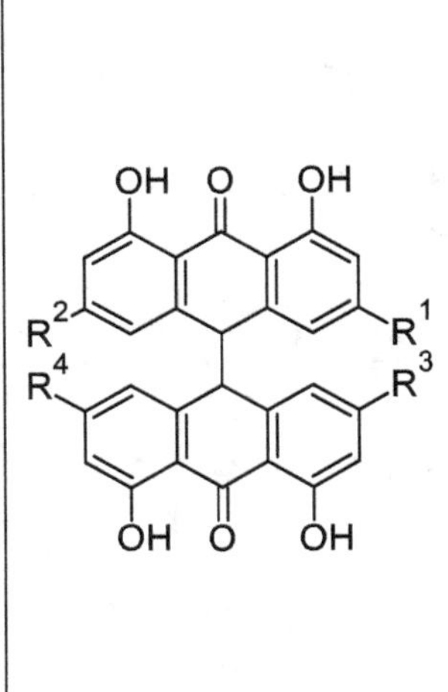

Homodianthrones	R1	R2	R3
Aloe-emodin dianthrones	CH_2OH	H	CH_2OH
Chrysophanol dianthrones	CH_3	H	CH_3
Emodin dianthrones	CH_3	OH	CH_3
Physcion dianthrones	CH_3	OCH_3	CH_3
Sennidin A,B	COOH	H	COOH
Heterodianthrones	**R1**	**R2**	**R3**
Palmidin A	CH_3	OH	CH_2OH
Palmidin B	CH_3	H	CH_2OH
Palmidin C	CH_3	H	CH_3
Palmidin D	CH_3	H	CH_3
Rheidin A	CH_3	OH	COOH
Rheidin B	CH_3	H	COOH
Rheidin C	CH_3	OCH_3	COOH
Sennidin C,D	CH_2OH	H	COOH

Contd...

Flavonoid ➤ Hesperidin from citrus fruits ➤ Rutin from Buckwheat	**Flavonoid**
Sterol ➤ Cardenolide digitoxin, gitoxin, digoxin from digitalis ➤ Cardenolide K-stropanthin and G-stropanthin from stropanthus seeds ➤ Cardenoide thevetin-A, thevetin-B from thevetia seeds ➤ Bufadienolids scillaren A from Squill	**Cardenolide** **Bufadienolide**
Saponin ➤ Steroidal saponins diosgenin from dioscorea ➤ Steroidal saponins ginsenosides from ginseng ➤ Triterpenoidal saponins glycyrrhizin from licorice ➤ Triterpenoidal saponin senegin from senega	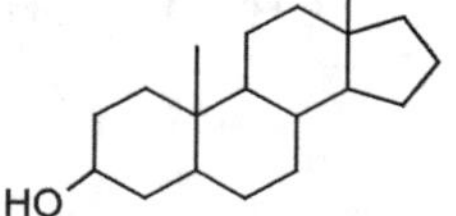 **Triterpenoid saponin**　　**Steroid saponin**

Contd...

Types of triterpenoid saponins

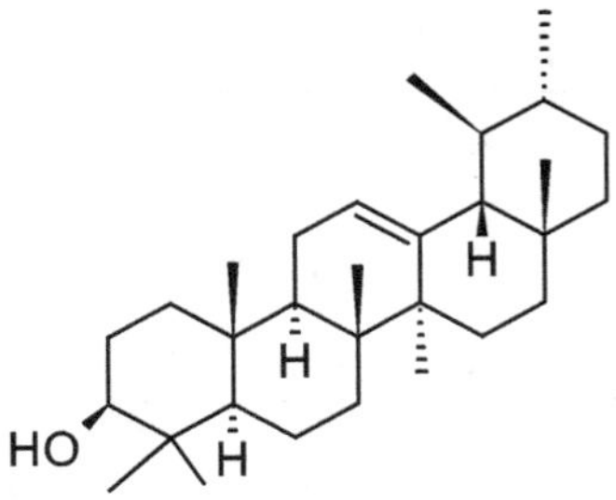

Alpha-amyrin 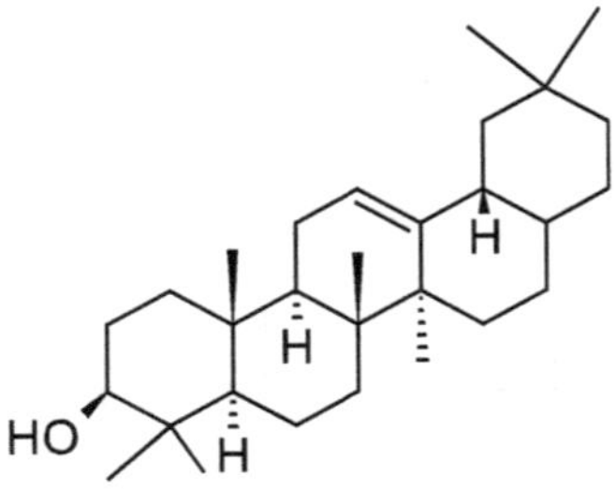   **Beta-amyrin** 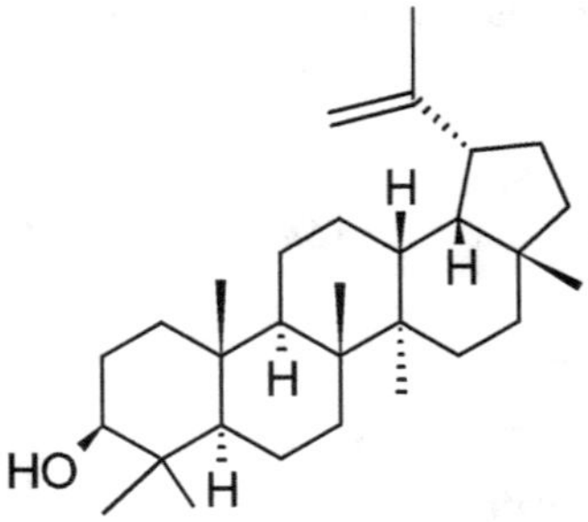   **Lupeol**

Types of steroid saponins

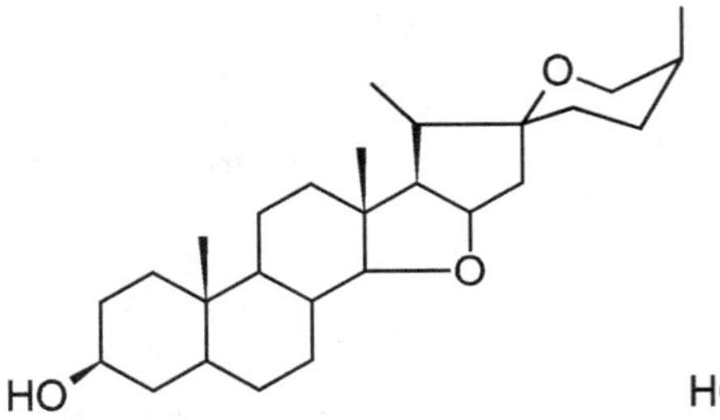

Spirostanol 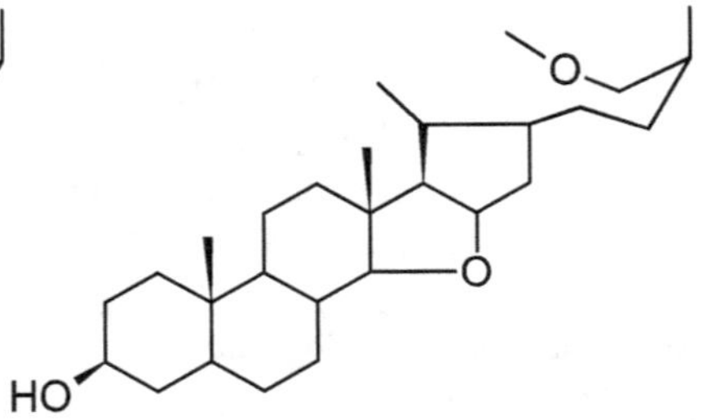   **Furostanol**

Coumarin ➤ Khellin, visnagin from Visnaga ➤ Bergapten, xanthotoxin from Ammi ➤ Psoralen from Psoralea	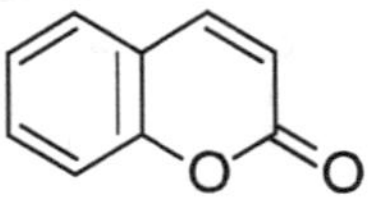
Isothiocynate ➤ Sinigrin from black mustard ➤ Sinablin from white mustard	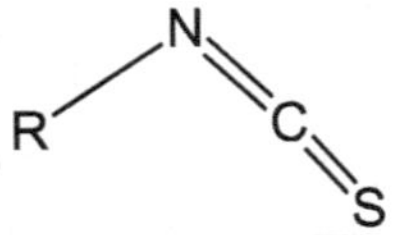
Mandelonitrile or cyanaogenetic ➤ Prunacin from wild cherry bark ➤ Amygdalin from bitter almond	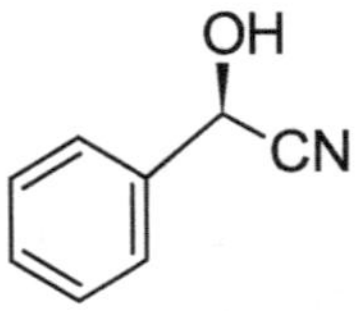
Phenol ➤ Arbutin from bearberry	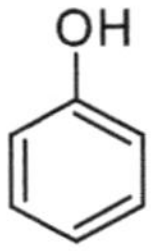

Contd...

Aldehyde ➢ Glucovanillin from vanilla pods	(structure: formyl/carboxylic group — O double bond to C, C bonded to OH and H)
Alcohol ➢ Salicin from *Salix* species	(structure: R—C—OH with R above and H below)

Chemical tests

Test	Procedure	Inference
General Glycoside test	Solution A: Extract sample powder with alcohol or water, and then, add Fehling Solution. Solution B: Add sulfuric acid and then add Fehling Solution to water or alcoholic extract	If solution B has dark color than solution A (if sugar content is high in solution B than solution A), it indicates the presence of glycosides. Note: Acid hydrolyzes glycone and aglycone moiety and thus, sugar content is increased in solution B.
Cardiac Glycosides		
Kedde's test (methanolic solution dinitro benzoic acid)	Mix 1 ml of test solution with 2 ml reagent.	Blue to purple color
Baljet reagent	Mix 2–3 mg of sample in 2 ml sodium picrate solution.	Yellow and orange to deep red color
Keller-kiliani test for digitoxose sugar	To the alcoholic extract of sample, add 5 ml of water and 0.5 ml of strong solution of lead acetate. Filter and treat the clear filtrate with equal volume of chloroform, and evaporate to yield dry residue. Add glacial acetic acid, 0.5 ml of ferric chloride solution, and 2 ml of concentrated sulfuric acid.	The initial red-brown layer changes to blue green.
Legal's test (Cardenolides)	Mix 1 ml of test solution with 2 ml pyridine and sodium nitroprusside.	Pink or red color
Raymond test (alkaline meta dinitrobenzene)	Mix alcoholic extract of sample in 0.1 ml of Raymond's reagent and add 2-3 drops of 20% NaOH solution.	Violet color changes to blue
Flavonoid Glycosides		
Shinoda test	Add magnesium powder and a few drops of concentrated HCl or H_2SO_4 to 2 ml of sample solution.	• Flavones, flavonols and xanthones: Orange, pink, red, and purple. • Flavanones and flavononols: weak pink to magenta colors, or no color at all.

Contd...

Test	Procedure	Inference
Modified shinoda test	The procedure is same as above except the use of zinc powder instead of magnesium.	Flavanonols: Deep-red to magenta color
Sulphuric acid	Add 3 ml of H_2SO_4 in sample.	<ul><li>Flavones and flavonols: Deep yellow color.</li><li>Chalcones and aurones: Red or red-bluish.</li><li>Flavanones: Orange to red colors.</li></ul>
Lead acetate	Mix test solution with lead acetate.	Yellow precipitate
Alkali test	Treat test solution with increasing amount of NaOH.	Yellow coloration which decolorizes after addition of acid
Triterpenoid saponin glycosides		
Liebermann–Burchard test	Mix 2 ml test extract with 1 ml chloroform, 1 ml acetic anhydride, and add one drop concentrated H_2SO_4.	Blue-green to red-orange color. A bluish-green or blue color indicates presence of steroids, and a pink-violet color indicates terpenoids.
Noller's test	Mix 2 ml test extract with small quantity of tin and thionyl chloride.	Pink coloration indicates the presence of triterpenoids.
Sannie test	Mix 2 ml extract with stannous chloride, acetic acid and carbon tetrachloride (6:50:50). Heat at $100^{\circ}C$	Brown color
Steroidal saponin glycosides		
Liebermann test	Mix 2 ml test extract with 2 ml acetic anhydride. Boil and add 0.5 ml of H_2SO_4.	Blue color.
Zimmermann test	Mix 2 ml test extract with 1 ml of 2N KOH in alcohol and 1 ml 1% dinitrobenzene in alcohol. After 10 min add this mixture to 8 ml alcohol.	Violet color
Tschugaeff test	Mix 1 ml sterol solution with 2 ml glacial acetic acid, 0.5mg zinc chloride and 1 ml acetyl chloride.	Red color
Pinus test	Mix 2 ml of test solution with 2 ml of antimony trichloride in acetic acid.	Blue color
Salkowski reaction	Dissolve 1–2 mg of the sample in 1 ml of $CHCl_3$ and add 1 ml concentrated H_2SO_4.	Chloroform layer shows red color and acid layer shows green fluorescence
Saponin Glycosides		
Foam test	Shake aqueous solution of a saponin containing sample producing foam, which is stable for 15 minutes or more.	Foam lasts for more than 15 seconds

Contd...

Test	Procedure	Inference
Hemolysis test	Mix red blood sample with sufficient quantity of extract solution. Shake and observe.	Clear red solution
Anthraquinone Glycosides		
Borntrager's test	Take a little quantity of aqueous solution of sample; add H_2SO_4, then add CCl_4 or ether in it. Separate the organic layer and shake with dilute ammonia.	Rose pink color of ammonia layer.
Schonteten's test for anthranols	Take a little quantity of aqueous solution of sample and add sodium borate.	Green fluorescence
P-nitrosodimethylaniline test for anthrones	Take a little quantity of aqueous solution of sample and add P-nitrosodimethylaniline in it.	• Anthrones change color of solution. • Anthraquinones do not change color.
Modified anthraquinone test for C-glycosides	Take little quantity of aqueous solution of sample; add ferric chloride solution, HCl, and then add CCl_4 or ether. Separate the organic layer and shake with dilute ammonia.	Rose pink color of ammonia layer
Cyanogenetic Glycosides		
Sodium picrate test (guignard picrate test)	Take the aqueous test solution of sample in test tube and add dilute H_2SO_4; suspend sodium picrate treated filter paper.	Hydrogen Cyanide (HCN) turns the paper to brick red color due to formation of sodium iso-perpurate.
Mercurous nitrate test	Mix 2 ml test extract solution with 3% aqueous mercurous nitrate solution.	Formation of metallic mercury
Guaiacum test	Dip strip of paper in guaiacum resin, then, moisten with dilute $CuSO_4$ and exposed to cut surface of crude drug.	Paper turns to blue due to HCN.
Coumarin Glycosides		
Odour test	Take the odour of powder or extract.	Aromatic smell.
Alkali test	Mix the test solution with alkali.	Blue green fluorescence
Fluorescence test	Take the moist powder of drug in test tube, cover test tube with alkali moist filter paper. Heat the test tube and observe paper under UV light.	Yellow green fluorescence

4.2.4   Flavonoids

Flavonoids are secondary metabolites corresponding to polyphenols, which have a varied structure, found in the form of aglycones or glycosides in many plants. About 2 % of carbon photosynthesized by plants converted to flavonoides or closely related compounds. Flavonoids are found in nature either in free form or glycoside form. Flavonoid glycosides have flavonol **(flavous: yellow color) as** aglycone moiety. It is large group of glycosides. It is obtained from shikimic acid pathway, acetate pathway.

Occurrence and distribution

Most flavonoids are found in the vacuole of the plant cell of Pteridophyta, dicots, monocot and gymnosperms. Families like leguminoseae, polygonaceae, rutaceae, apiaceae are prominent for presence of flavonoids.

Flavon

Biosynthesis

Flavonoid glycosides are derived from chalcones through cinnamic acid formed in shikimic acid pathway.

Properties

Over 5000 naturally occurring flavonoids have been characterized from various plants. Generally, flavonoids are crystalline solids, and only a few of them are amorphous powders. Flavanones and flavanonols are colorless. Chalcones are yellow-orange color. Flavones, flavonols and their glycosides are yellow in color. Color of anthochyanidines are varies with pH ranges i.e. pH < 7 = red; pH = 8.5 = purple; pH > 8.5 = blue. All flavonoid glycosides are optically active due to presence of sugars. Flavonoid glycosides are soluble in water and methanol.

Functions

Flavonoids are one of the most studied phytochemicals due to their diverse health benefits. Flavonoids are the most important plant pigments for flower coloration producing yellow or red/blue pigmentation in petals designed to attract pollinator animals. In higher plants, flavonoids are involved in UV filtration, symbiotic nitrogen fixation and floral pigmentation. They may act as a chemical messenger or physiological regulator; they can also act as cell cycle inhibitors. In addition, some flavonoids have inhibitory activity against organisms that cause plant disease Example: Fusarium oxysporum. Flavonoids protects plant from attack by microbes and insects.

Chemistry

Flavonoids have a chemical structure of 15 carbons constituted by a common skeleton of phenyl-benzo-γ-pyran (C6–C3–C6), also known as nucleus flava, composed of two phenyl rings (A and B) and a ring heterocyclic (pyran) C. Two phenyl rings converted to 3-carbon bridge. Chalcone and dihydrochalcone showes 3- carbon bridge open. But in others it is part of heterocyclic ring involving phenolic group on adjacent ring.

Uses

Flavonoids are "nature's biological response modifiers" because of strong experimental evidence of their inherent ability to modify the body's reaction to allergens, viruses, and carcinogens. They have properties like antioxidant, antimicrobial, antiinflammatory, anticancer and heart disease, antidiabetic, hypolipidemic etc. Few flavonoids like hesperidine found to decrease capillary fragility.

Extraction: Take accurately weighed dried material. If flavonoid aglycones like isoflavones, flavonols, flavanones are present, then extract with non-polar or less polar solvents (Example: chloroform, diethyl ether or dichloromethane). If flavonoid glycosides are present then extract with polar solvents like alcohols or aqueous alcohols. Fractionation of alcoholic extract with ethyl acetate separates most of semi-polar to polar flavonoid from mixtures but non-polar flavonoid need to be separated by column chromatography. Anthocyanidines need to be extracted with acidic water or actone.

Chemical Tests

Shinoda test	Add magnesium powder and a few drops of concentrated HCl or H_2SO_4 to 2 ml of sample solution	➢ Flavones, flavonols and xanthones : Orange, pink, red, purple. ➢ Flavanones and flavonols: weak pink to magenta colours or no colour at all.
Modified Shinoda test for Flavanonols	Use zinc instead of magnesium	Flavanonols: Deep-red to magenta colour.
Sulfuric acid test	Add H_2SO_4 in sample	➢ Flavones and flavonols: Deep yellow colour. ➢ Chalcones and aurones: Red or red-bluish. ➢ Flavanones : Orange to red colours.
Lead acetate test	Mix test solution with lead acetate	Yellow precipitate
Alkali test	Treat test solution with increasing amount of NaOH	Yellow colouration which decolourises after addition of acid

Flavnoid classes and examples	
Class	**Example**
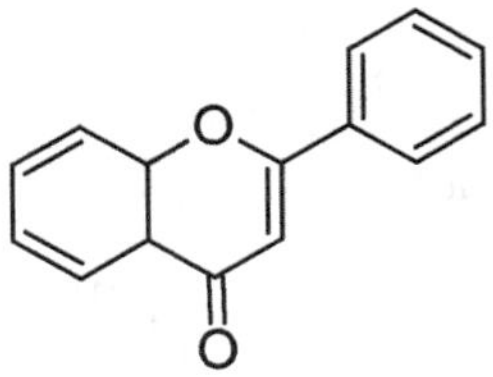 **Flavone**	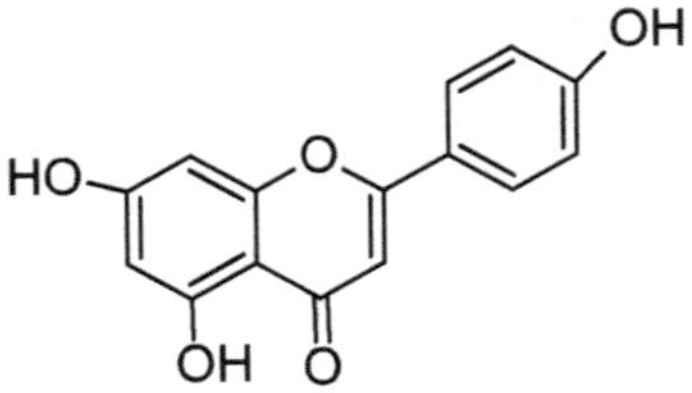 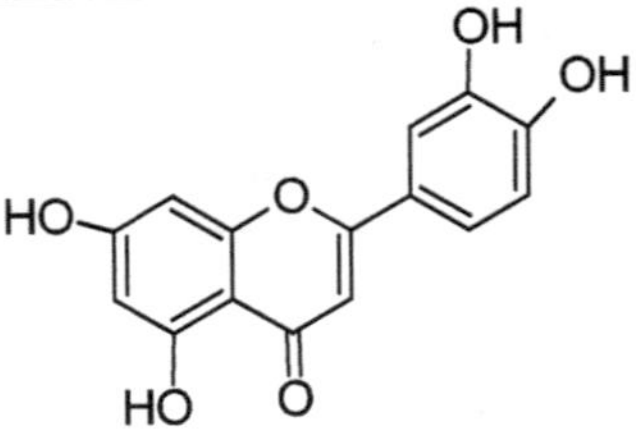 **Apigenin** **Luteolin**
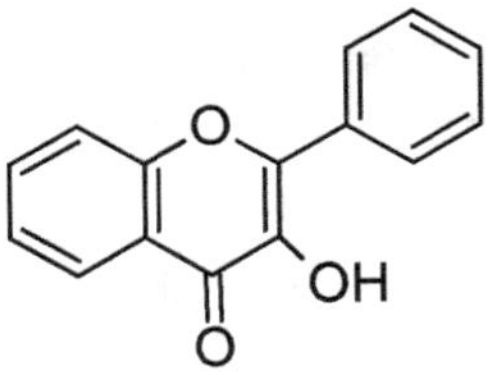 **Flavonol**	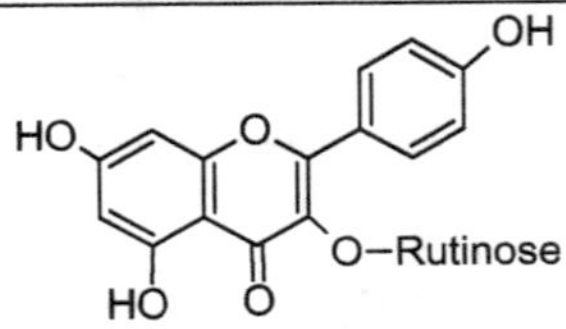 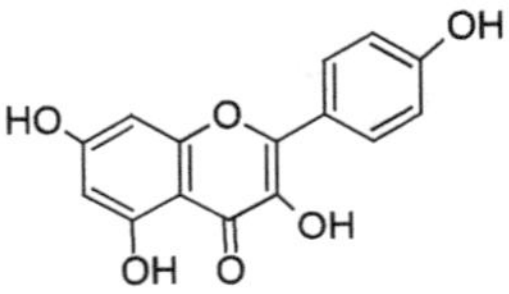 **Rutin (Sophorin)** **Kaemferol** 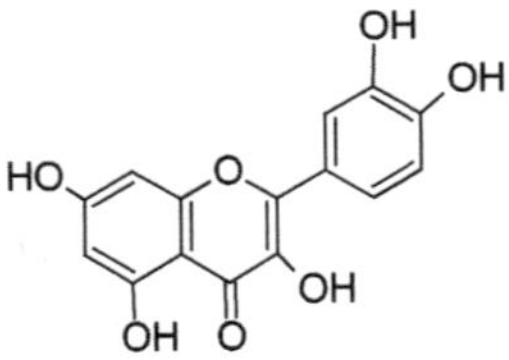 **Quercetin**
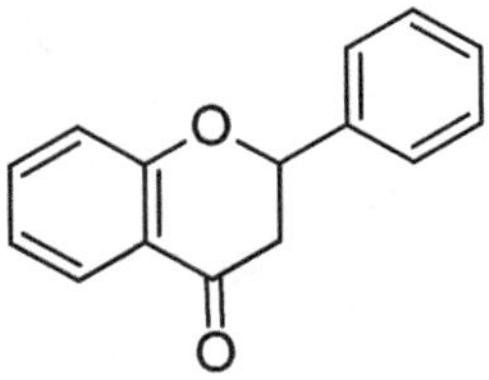 **Flavonone**	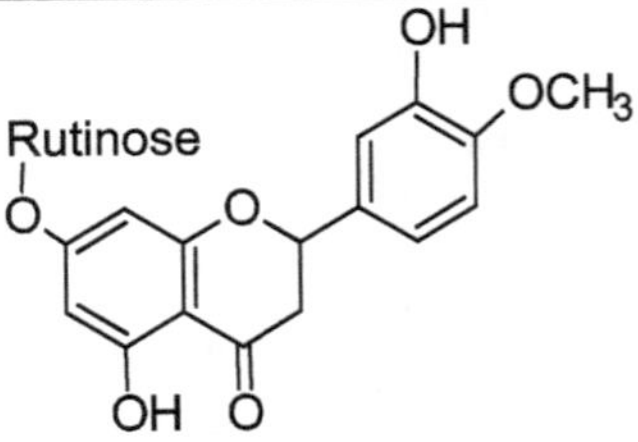 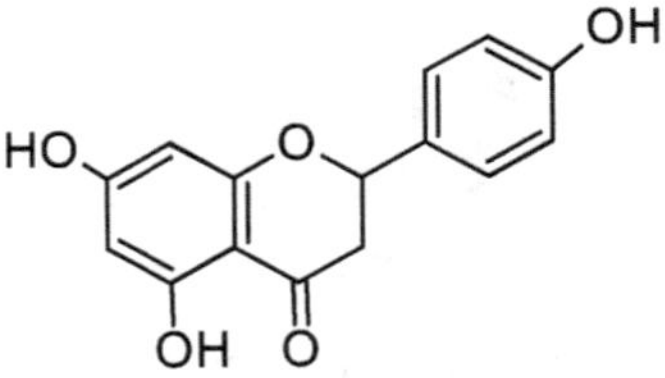 **Hesperidin** **Naringenin**
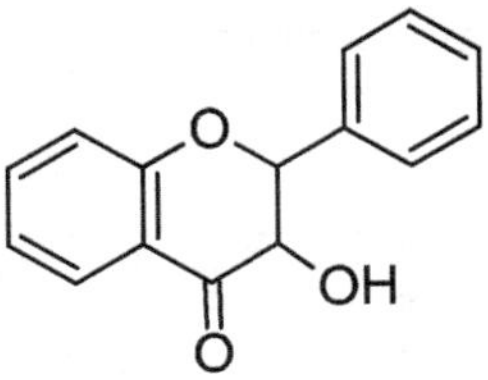 **Flavanol**	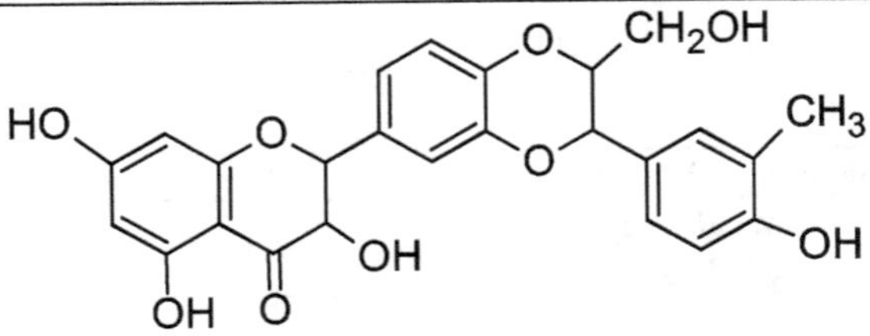 **Silibinin**

Contd...

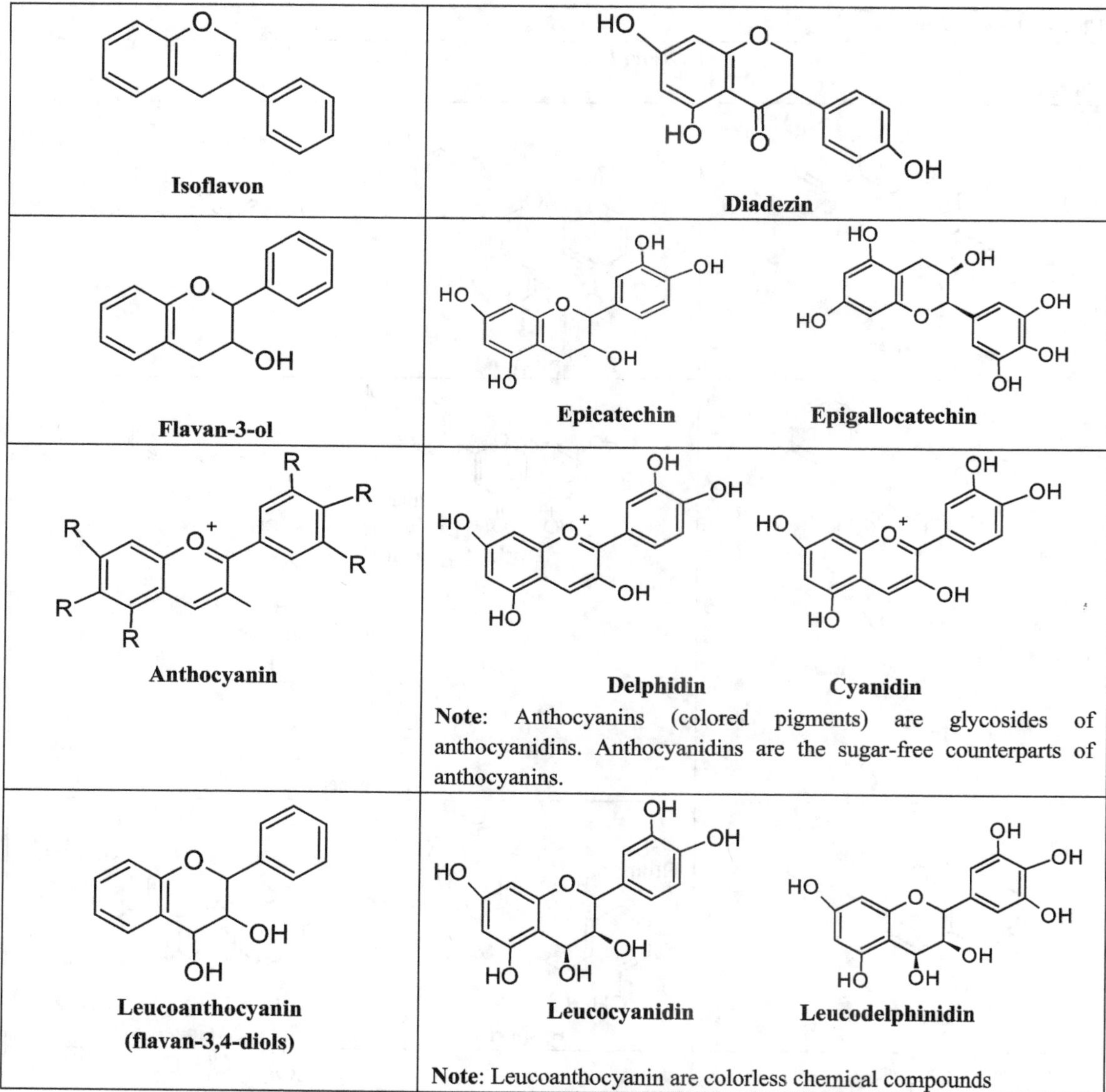

Note: Anthocyanins (colored pigments) are glycosides of anthocyanidins. Anthocyanidins are the sugar-free counterparts of anthocyanins.

Note: Leucoanthocyanin are colorless chemical compounds

Flavonoid containing crude drugs				
Sr. No.	Name of Drug and synonym	Biological source	Active constituent	Uses
1	Buck wheat	Dried fruits of *Fagopyrum esculentum*, Family-Polygonaceae.	Proteins and fat, Rutin (also from Ruta graveolens)	Treatment of capillary bleeding
2	Citrus-fruits	Rind of unripe, green *Citrus* fruits, Family - Rutaceae.	hesperidin	In capillary fragility

Contd...

Sr. No.	Name of Drug and synonym	Biological source	Active constituent	Uses
3	Gingko, Maiden hair tree, Knew tree.	Dried leaves of *Gingko biloba*, Family- Gingkoaceae.	Flavonol, Kaempferol, quercetin, isorhamnetin, Biflavones are ginkgetin, isoginkgettin, gingkolic acid and bilobetin, Gingkolide A, B, C and J, anthocyanins, sitosterol, catechins, organic acids like 4- hydroxyl- benzoic acid and shikimic acid.	Treatment of Metabolic and Vascular disorder.
4	Silymarin, Milk-Thistle, Marian Thistle, Our Lady's Thistle, The wild artichoke.	The ripe seeds of Milk thistle *Silybus marianum*, Family- Asteraceae.	Silybin, silycrystin and silydianin, dehydrosilybin, desosilycrystin, desoxy silydianin, silyharmin, neosilyharmin, silybinome and silandrin, betaine, apigenin and silybonol.	Liver disorder, hepatoprotective, hepatitis treatment.

4.2.5 Tannins

The term tannin refers to tanning animal hides into leather. However, the term "tannin" by extension is widely applied to any large polyphenolic compound containing sufficient hydroxyls and other suitable groups (such as carboxyls) to form strong complexes with proteins and other macromolecules. Tannins molecular weights ranges from 500 to over 3,000 (gallic acid esters) and up to 20,000 (proantho-cyanidins).

Tannins are classified as ergastic substances, i.e., non-protoplasm materials found in cells. Tannin is an astringent, bitter, plant polyphenolic compound that binds to and precipitates proteins and various other organic compounds including amino acids and alkaloids.

Occurrence

Tannins are distributed in species throughout the plant kingdom, soil and water. They are commonly found in both gymnosperms as well as angiosperms. Tannins are mainly physically located in the vacuoles or surface wax of plants. Tannins are found in leaf, bud, seed, root, and stem tissues. An example of the location of the tannins in stem tissue is that they are often found in the growth areas of trees, such as the secondary phloem and xylem and the layer between the cortex and epidermis. The most abundant polyphenols are the condensed tannins, found in virtually all families of plants, and comprising up to 50% of the dry weight of leaves.

Functions

Tannins are found to be active against plant predators. Tannins may help to regulate the growth of plant tissues.

Extraction

Extract the powder crude drug n-hexane or petroleum ether to remove impurities. Then extract marc with acetone. Add diethyl ether and separate acetone layer to get tannins. Extraction of tannins requires skills to separate other polyphenolic compounds too.

Chemistry and Classification

There are three major classes of tannins:

1. *Hydrolysable tannins,* as the name implies, these compounds are easily hydrolyzed in alkali, giving rise to a polyhydric alcohol and attached gallic acid moieties.

2. *Non-hydrolysable or condensed tannins* are essentially derived from the polymerization of the flavan-3-ols like catechin, epicatechin and their derivatives. The name pro-anthocyanidin is used alternatively for condensed tannins because on treatment with hot-acid, some of the C-C linking bonds are broken and anthocyanidin monomers are released.

3. *Pseudo tannins* are low molecular weight compounds associated with other compounds. They do not answer gold beater skin test unlike hydrolysable and condensed tannins.

Comparision between different classes of tannins			
Class	**Hydrolysable tannins (divided into simple gallotannins and complex ellagitannins)**	**Non-hydrolysable or condensed tannins or flavolans or proanthocyanidins**	**Phlorotannins**
Basic nucleus	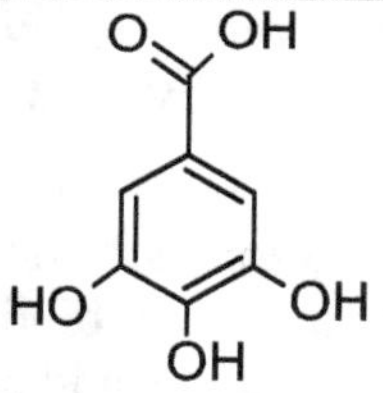 Gallic acid	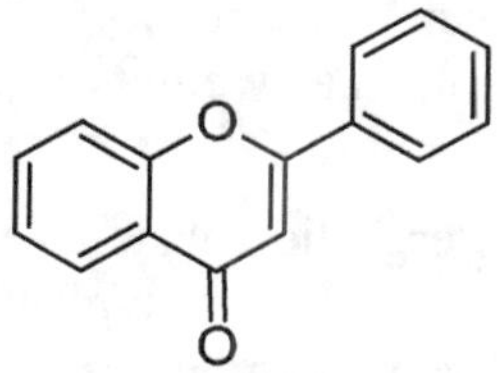 Flavan-3,4-Diols	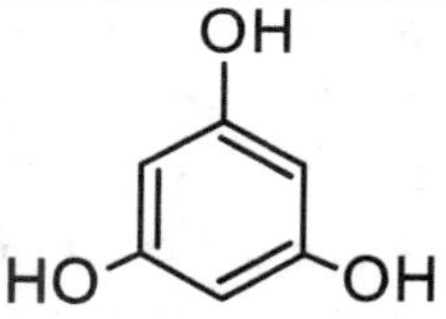 Phloroglucinol
Chemistry	Glucose linked gallic acid or ellagic acid in the form of galloylglucose depside or hexahydroxydiphenic acid	High molecular weight oligomers of catechins and flavan-3,4-diols	These are polymers of Phloroglucinol and restricted to be present in brown algaes
Sources	Dicots Plants	Plants	Algae

Uses

➤ Tannins are an important ingredient in the process of tanning leather.

➤ Tannins have been investigated for the production of wood adhesives too.

➤ Tannins appear to be able to substitute a high proportion of synthetic phenol in phenol-formaldehyde resins for wood particleboard.

➤ Tannins are used for production of anti-corrosive primer and rust inhibitors.

➤ Tannins are anticancer, antiviral, antibacterial and antiparasitic agents.

➤ Due to strong antioxidant potential i.e. free radical scavenging effects, tannins are found to be useful in treatment of cancer, diabetis, arthritis, obesity as well as neuroaging related diseases (due to neuroprotective effect).

Examples of hydrolysable and non-hydrolysable Tannins		
(+) Catechin	(-) Epicatechin	(-) Epigallocatechin
Condensed Tannins	(-) Epigallocatechin gallate Gallic acid	

Hydrolysable Tannins containing crude drugs

Sr. No.	Name of Drug and Synonyms	Biological source	Active Constituent	Uses
1	Amla, Indian goose berry, Emblica.	Dried as well as fresh fruits of *Emblica officinalis* Family- Euphorbiaceae.	Vitamin C, phyllemblin, tannins, mineral matters like phosphorus, iron and calcium, fat.	Diuretic, laxative, ingradient of Triphala and Chyavanprash.
2	Arjuna, Arjun bark, Arjun.	Dried stem bark of *Termanalia arjuna,* Family- Combretaceae.	Ellagic acid, beta-sitosterol, triterpenoid saponin arjunolic acid, arjunic acid, Calcium, aluminium and magnesium Salts, and sugars.	Cardiotonic, hypotensive.
3	Bahera, Beleric myrobalan, Baheda, Bibhitak.	Dried ripe fruits of *Terminalia belerica,* Family- Combretaceae.	Gallic acid, chebulagic acid, ellagic acid, phyllemblin, ethyl gallateandgalloyl glucose.	Astringent, ingredient of triphalachurna.
4	Myrobalan, Harda, Chebulicmyrobalan, Haritaki.	Dried mature fruits of *Termenalia chebula,* Family- Combretaceae.	Chebulic acid, Chebulagic acid, Gallic acid, Chebulinic acid, ellagic acid, glucose, sorbitol.	Astringent, stomachic, purgative, ingredient of triphalachurna.
5	Tannic acid, Tannin, Gallatonic acid, Acidumtannicum.	Fermented oak galls which are grown on young twings of *Quercus infectoria,* Family- Fagaceae.	Gallic acid, glucose.	Astringent for mucous membrane.

Condensed Tannins containing crude drugs				
Sr. No.	Name of Drug and synonym	Biological source	Active constituent	Uses
1	Ashoka, Ashoka bark	Dried stem bark of *Saraca asoca*, Family-Leguminosae.	Tannins, haematoxylin, Catechol, ketosterol, saponin, organic Calcium and iron compounds.	Uterine tonic, oxytocic, stimulant.
2	Black catechu, cutch, Kattha, Khadir-catechu.	Dried aqueous extract of heartwood of *Acacia catechu*, Family-Leguminosae.	Acacatechin, quercetin, catechin, catechol, gum, Catechu red, quercitrin.	Astringent for boils, skin eruptions, main used for commercial purposes.
3	Pale catechu, Gambier, Gambir, Catechu	Dried aqueous extract of leaves and young shoots of *Uncaria gambier*, Family-Rubiaceae.	Catechin, catechutannic acid, catechu red, quercetinandgambierfluorescin.	Astringent for treatment of diarrhoea.
4	Pterocarpus, Bijasal, Indian kino tree, Malbarkino.	Dried juice of the plant *Petrocarpus marsupium*, Family-Leguminosae.	Kinotannic acid, kinored, k-pyrocatechin, resin, gallic acid.	Hypoglycemic, powerful astringent.

4.2.6 Resins

Introduction	➢ **Resins** are complex hydrocarbon secretion different from sap, latex, or mucilage due to presence of volatile as well as non-volatile mixture of chemical compounds.
Functions	➢ Non-volatile part gives protection from herbivorous animals, insects, and pathogens ➢ Volatile part attracts insects for pollination
Biosyntheis	➢ Shikimic and mevalonate pathways ➢ Lignan, podophyllotoxin which presumably arises via an oxidative coupling of 2 cinnamic acid residues.
Properties	➢ Resins are hard, transparent or translucent brittle materials.
Actions	➢ Hard transparent resins, (copals, dammars, mastic and sandarac) are principally used for varnishes and cement Softer odoriferous oleo-resins (frankincense, elemi, turpentine, copaiba) and gum resins containing essential oils (ammoniacum, asafoetida, gamboge, myrrh, and scammony) are more largely used for therapeutic purposes and incense. Resin in the form of rosin is applied to the bows of stringed instruments (Example- violin, rebec, erhu, sarangi, etc.), because of its quality for adding friction to the hair Resin has also been used as a medium for sculpture by artists

Chemistry and Classification

Class	Composition	Example
Oleo resins	Mixtures of oil and a resin *Common Oil Compounds:* bicyclic terpenes alpha-pinene, beta-pinene, delta-3 carene and sabinene, the monocyclic terpenes limonene and terpinolene, and smaller amounts of the tricyclic sesquiterpenes, longifolene, caryophyllene and delta-cadinene. *Common Resin compounds:* resin acids are abietic acid (sylvic acid), plicatic acid contained in cedar, and pimaric acid	Turmeric, ginger, copaiba
Gum resins	Mixtures of gum or mucilaginous substances and a resin	Ammoniacum
Oleo-gum resins	Mixture of oil, gum and resin	Myrrh, asafoetida
Balsams	Mixture of benzoic acid, cinnamic acid or their esters and resin	Tolu balsam, peru balsam, storax

Examples of important resin moieties

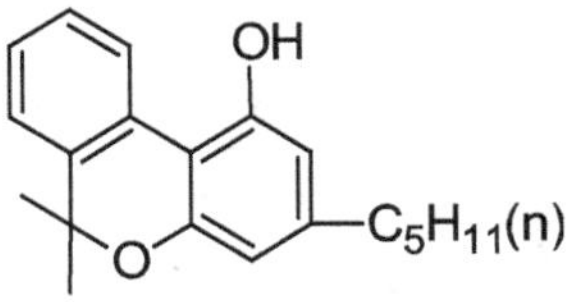

Cannabinol (CBN) — $C_5H_{11}(n)$

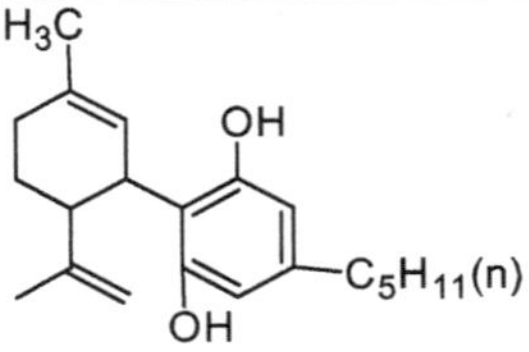

Cannabidiol (CBD) — $C_5H_{11}(n)$

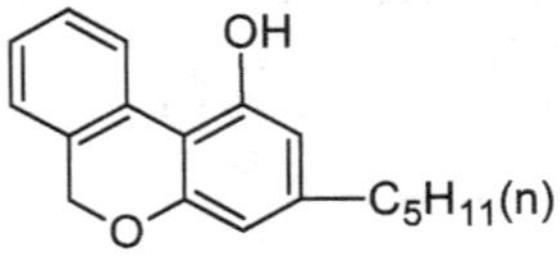

$\Delta 9 - THC$, $\nabla - THC$ — $C_5H_{11}(n)$

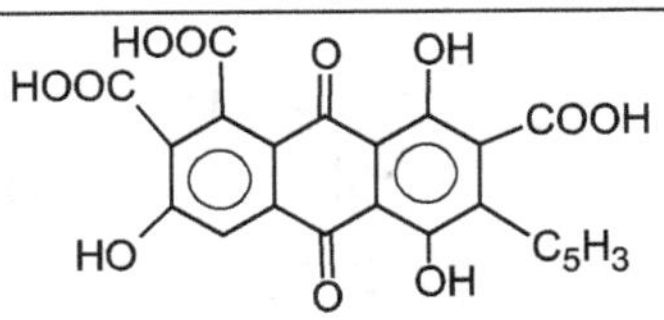

Laccaic acid

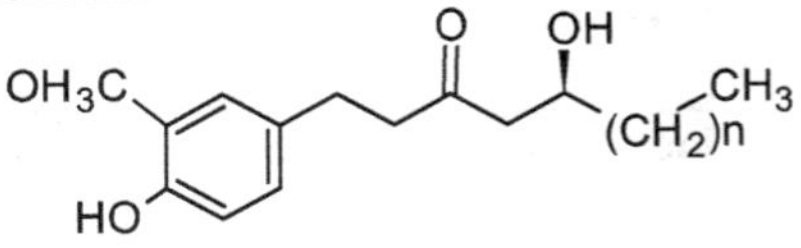

Gingerol [n= 4,6 or 8]

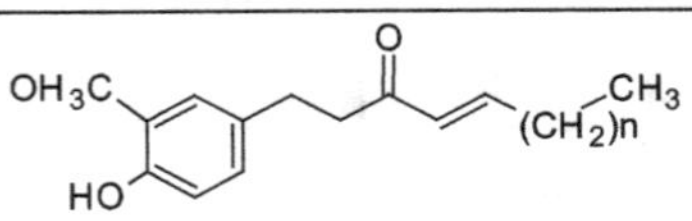

Shagoal [n= 4,6,,8]

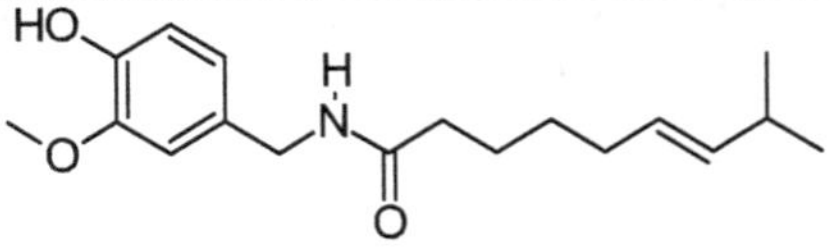

Capsaicin

Resin Classification based on functional group			
Class	Composition	Biological sources	Uses
Acid			
Asafoetida	Ferulic acid	Exudates from *Ferula foetida*, Family- Umbelliferae	Flavouring agent.
Colophony	Abietic acid	Exudates from *Pinus palustris* Family- Pinaceae	Manufacturing of varnishes and soaps
Copaiba	Capaivic acid	Exudates from Species of *Copaifera* of family- Leguminoseae.	Manufacturing of varnishes and paper

Contd...

Myrrh	Commiphoric acid	Stem of *Commiphora obyssinica* Family- Burseraceae.	Antiseptic, perfume
Shellac	Alleuritic acid	Secretion of insect *Laccifer lacca* Family- Coccidae.	Manufacturing of varnishes and inks
Ester			
Benzoin	Benzyl benzoate	*Styrax benzoin*, Family- Styraceae	Topical protecting agent
Peru balsum	peruresinotannol	From *Toluifer pereiare* of Family- Leguminoseae.	Protecting and rubefacient
Tolu balsum	Toluresinotannol cinnamate	From *Tolufera balsamum*, Family- Leguminoseae.	Perfumery, expectorant.
Alcohol			
Cannabis	Cannabinol, canabol	Exudates from Flowering tops of *Cannabis sativa*, Family- Moraceae.	Sedative, antidepressant, appetite stimulant, analgesic.
Ginger	Gingerol and shagoals	From Rhizomes of *Zingiber officinalis* Family- Zingiberaceae.	Carminative, aromatic
Resenes			
Bdellium	Oleo gum resin	From bark of *Commiphora mukul* Family- Burseraceae.	Antioxidant lowers cholesterol, treatment of arthritis.
Glycoresins			
Podophyllum	Podophyllotoxin	From Roots of *Podophylum hexandrum* Family- Berberidaceae.	Abortifacient, emetic, antihelmentic.
Jalap	Jalapin	From *Ipomea purga* Family- Convulalaceae	Purgative.
Lignan			
Guaiac	Guaiaretic acid	From Heartwood of *Guaiacum officinale* Family- Zygophyllaceae.	Expectorant, diaphoretic
Turmeric	Curcumin	From Rhizomes of *Curcuma longa* Family- Zingibereaceae	Condiment and colouring agent

Subjective Questions

1. Write a note on theory, principle, diagnosis and medicines used in system of Ayurveda/Siddha/Unanai/Homeopathy/Chinese?

2. Differentiate Yin and Yang?

3. Explain seven principles of Homeopathy?

4. How Ayurveda is different from Siddha system?

5. Differentiate primary and secondary metabolites?

6. Define alkaloids? Write in details about properties and classification of Alkaloids.

7. Define glycosides? Write in details about properties and classification of glycosides.

8. Define flavonoids? Write in details about properties and classification of flavonoids.

9. Define tannins? Write in details about properties and classification of tannins.

10. What is difference between hydrolysable and non-hydrolysable tannins?

11. Define resins? Write in details about properties and classification of resins.

12. Define volatile oils? Write in details about properties and classification of volatile oils.

13. How to identify alkaloids/glycosides/flavonoids/tannins/resins/volatile oils by chemical tests.

14. Write a note on old medicinal texts from different parts of world?

15. What are identification tests for alkaloids/glycosides/tannins/resins

16. Give the examples of polar, semi-polar and non-polar alkaloids and flavonoids?

17. Give the examples of liquid alkaloids

18. What is difference between cardenolides and bufadienolides?

19. Which terpenoids are volatile in nature?

20. Pilocarpine and physostigmine drugsbelongs to which class of Alkaloids?

21. What do you mean by rosin and balsams?

22. What is true, pseudo and proto alkaloids?

23. What are biosynthetic sources of quinoline and tropane alkaloids?

24. What is example of ester and ether class of volatile oil containing plants?

25. What are examples of acid and lignin class of resins?

26. What are volatile and non-volatile constituents of Ginger and turmeric?

27. What is difference between Bortrager's test and modified Borntrager's test?

28. What is Kedde's test?

29. What is difference between Shinoda and modified Shinoda test?

30. What is C-glycosides?

31. What is isothiocynate and mandelonitrile glycosides?

32. What is Bijasal?

Multiple Choice Questions (MCQs)

1. Which one of the following traditional system medicine is based on *yin* and *yang* theory?
    a. Chinese
    b. Korean
    c. Japanese
    d. both a and b

2. In which year AYUSH was established as the Department of Indian Systems of Medicine and Homeopathy?
   a. 1995
   b. 1996
   c. 2001
   d. 2003

3. Which one of the following is NOT among the tridoshas?
   a. Prithvi
   b. Vata
   c. Pitta
   d. Kapha

4. Unani system of medicine was first introduced in India by
   a. Portuguese
   b. Japanese
   c. Arabs
   d. Chinese

5. Which one of the following is NOT part of panchakarmas?
   a. Virechana
   b. Vaman
   c. Nasya
   d. Agada

6. Among tridoshas, *Pitta* dosha is related to
   a. Space and air
   b. Energy and liquid
   c. Liquid and solid
   d. Prithvi and Jal

7. Credit of Unani system of medicine goes to
   a. Aristotle
   b. Hippocrates
   c. Hahnemann
   d. Both a and b

8. " The organon of Medicine" was compiled by
   a. Aristotle
   b. Hippocrates
   c. Hahnemann
   d. Both a and b

9. Which one of the traditional system of medicine is based on hypothesis 'Like cures like'
   a. Unani
   b. Sidhha
   c. Ayurvedic
   d. Homeopathy

10. 'Arnica' belongs to
   a. Homeopathy
   b. Ayurvedic
   c. Siddha
   d. Unani

11. The literature of Sidhha system of medicine is documented mostly in ……………language
   a. Sanskrit
   b. Hindi
   c. Tamil
   d. English

12. In Sidhha system of medicine, Gomthai means
   a. *Datura stramonium*
   b. *Papaver somniferum*
   c. *Euphorbia nerifolia*
   d. *Nericum indicum*

13. In Sidhha system of medicine, diagnosis is done through
   a. Pulse reading
   b. Urine examination
   c. Colour of body
   d. All of the above

14. In which traditional system of medicine, the term 'Beheshajya –vigyan' is used for pharmacy?
   a. Sidhha
   b. Unani
   c. Homeopathy
   d. Ayurveda

15. Who is known as "Father of natural history"?
   a. Aristotle
   b. Hahnmann
   c. Hippocrates
   d. None

16. Panax ginseng is
    a. Ayurvedic medicine
    b. chinese medicine
    c. Unani medicine
    d. Japanese medicine

17. *Kampoh* is
    a. Traditional system of Japanese medicine
    b. Traditional system of Korean medicine
    c. Traditional system of Chinese medicine
    d. Traditional system of Unni medicine

18. Which one of the system is based on Hippocratic theory of four humors and Pythagorean theory of four proximate qualities
    a. Sidhha
    b. Unani
    c. Homeopathy
    d. Ayurveda

19. Authentic information on Ayurveda is compiled in
    a. Charaka
    b. Sushrutha
    c. Samhita
    d. Materia medica

20. Dosage forms like bhasma, avaleha, churna belongs to
    a. Traditional system of Ayurvedic medicine
    b. Traditional system of Chinese medicine
    c. Traditional system of Unani medicine
    d. Traditional system of Sidhha medicine

21. Which one of the following is first synthesized alkaloid in history? And in which year?
    a. Nicotine, 1806
    b. Papaverine, 1821
    c. Coniine, 1826
    d. Thebaine, 1835

22. Alkaloids are
    a. Chemically heterogeneous group of natural substances
    b. Comprise nitrogen containing organic compounds
    c. Both a and b
    d. Only b

23. True alkaloids normally present in plants in the form of
    a.   Salts of organic acids
    b.   Salts of inorganic acids
    c.   Salts of organic bases
    d.   Salts of inorganic bases

24. The alkaloids in which nitrogen is not present in heterocyclic ring are called
    a.   Proto alkaloids
    b.   Pseudo alkaloids
    c.   Amino alkaloids
    d.   Both a and c

25. Which one of the following is example of pseudo alkaloid?
    a.   Conessine
    b.   Caffeine
    c.   Both a and b
    d.   Shikonine

26. Berberine belongs to
    a.   Isoquinoline type of true alkaloids
    b.   Quinoline type of true alkaloids
    c.   Phenanthrene type of true alkaloids
    d.   Tropane

27. The organic compounds from plants or animal sources which on enzymatic or acid hydrolysis gives one or more sugar moieties along with non-sugar moiety are known as
    a.   Glycosides
    b.   Alkaloids
    c.   Flavonoids
    d.   Resins

28. The sugar moieties involved in glycosides are mostly
    a. $\beta - D$ sucrose
    b. $\beta - D$ glucose
    c. $\beta - D$ lactose
    d. $\beta - D$ fructose

29. Which types of glycosides are present in secondary metabolite, Serin which is found in mustard?
    a.   C- glycosides
    b.   S-glycosides
    c.   O - glycosides
    d.   N – glycosides

30. Sta otto method is used for isolation of
    a. Glycosides
    b. Flavanoids
    c. Volatile oils
    d. Resins

31. Anthracene glycosides are present in
    a. Aloe
    b. Digitalis
    c. Gokhru
    d. Psorelia

32. Which types of glycosides are present in *Prunus amygdalis*?
    a. Isothiocyanate glycosides
    b. Anthracene glycosides
    c. Cyanogenetic glycosides
    d. Furanocoumarin glycosides

33. The anthracene glycoside, Carminic acid is derived from
    a. Cascara
    b. Rhubarb
    c. Cochineal
    d. Aloe

34. Which types of glycosides are present in Safed musali?
    a. Cardiac glycosides
    b. Anthraquinone glycosides
    c. Aldehyde glycosides
    d. Saponin glycosides

35. Borntrager's test is used for identification of
    a. Alkaloids
    b. Glycosides
    c. Resins
    d. Carbohydrates

36. Flavanoid compounds are regarded as
    a. $C_6-C_3-C_6$ compounds
    b. $C_6-C_4-C_6$ compounds
    c. $C_6-C_5-C_6$ compounds
    d. $C_6-C_2-C_6$ compounds

37. Which one of the following is structure of quercetin?

a.

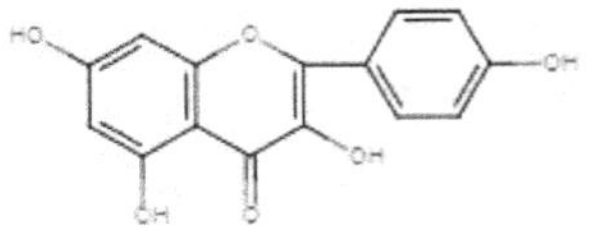

b.

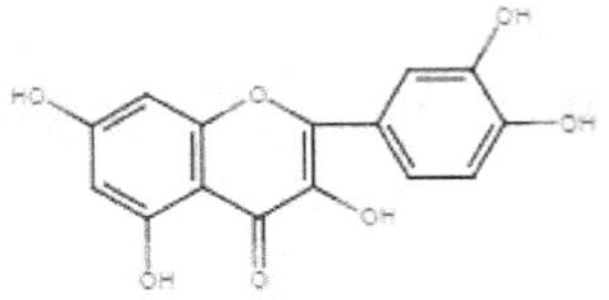

c.

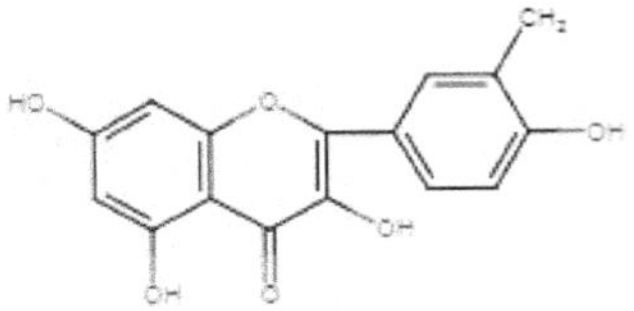

d.

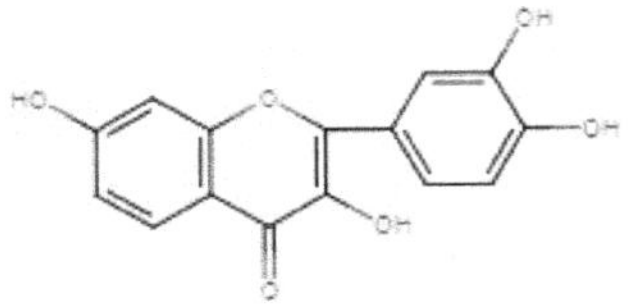

38. Goldbeater's skin test is used for identification of

    a.   Resins

    b.   Flavanoids

    c.   Tannins

    d.   Alkaloids

39. Which one of the following is example of pseudotannins?

    a.   Chlorogenic acid

    b.   Carmic acid

    c.   Ipecacuanhic acid

    d.   Both a and c

40. Effleurage method is used for extraction of

    a.   Resins

    b.   Lipids

    c.   Alkaloids

    d.   Perfumes

41. Liquid carbon dioxide is used for extraction of
    a.   Glycosides
    b.   Alkaloids
    c.   Volatile oil
    d.   Resins

42. Natural compounds which are composed of both isoprenoid and nonisoprenoid units are called as
    a.   Monoterpenoids
    b.   Tetraterpenoids
    c.   Diterpenoids
    d.   Sesquiterpenoids

43. Resins are amorphous mixtures of
    a.   Essential oils
    b.   Oxygenated products of terpene and carboxylic acid
    c.   Both a and b
    d.   None of the above

44. Which one of the following is example of acid resins?
    a.   Benzoin
    b.   Storax
    c.   Balsam
    d.   Myrhh

45. Alleuritic acid is also known as
    a.   Sandrac
    b.   Copaiba
    c.   Shellac
    d.   Myrhh

Answer Key

1. b	2. a	3. a	4. c	5. d	6. b	7. b	8. c	9. d	10. a
11. c	12. a	13. d	14. d	15. a	16. b	17. a	18. b	19. c	20. a
21. c	22. c	23. a	24. d	25. c	26. a	27. a	28. b	29. b	30. a
31. a	32. a	33. c	34. d	35. a	36. a	37. b	38. c	39. d	40. d
41. c	42. b	43. c	44. d	45. c					

Unit 5

5.1 Study of Biological Source, Chemical Nature and uses of Drugs of Natural Origin Containing Following Drugs/Plant Products

5.1.1 Fibers

Fibers are hair-like materials that are continuous filaments or thread like discrete elongated pieces. Fibers are of three types: natural fiber (animal, plant and mineral fibres), manmade fibre i.e. synthetic and regenerated fibres (Example: Nylon, terylene etc). They can be spun into filaments, thread or rope. They can be used as a component of composite materials. They can also be matted into sheets to make products such as paper or felt. The earliest evidence for humans using fibers is the discovery of wool and dyed flax fibers found in a prehistoric cave in the Republic of Georgia that date back to 36,000 BP

Vegetable fibers include cotton, hemp, jute, flax, ramie, sisal and bagasse. Animal fibers consist largely of silkworm silk, spider silk, sinew, catgut, wool, sea silk and hair such as cashmere, mohair and angora, fur such as sheepskin, rabbit, mink, fox, beaver, etc. Mineral fibers include the asbestos group. Asbestos is the only naturally occurring long mineral fiber. Six minerals have been classified as "asbestos" including chrysotile of the serpentine class and those belonging to the amphibole class: amosite, crocidolite, tremolite, anthophyllite and actinolite. Short, fiber-like minerals include wollastonite and attapulgite.

Regenerated fibers are sometimes known as man-made fibers or textiles. Textile fiber produced by dissolving a natural material (such as cellulose), then regenerating it by extrusion and precipitation, as with viscose.

Type of Natural fibers	
Vegetable fibers: Vegetable fibers are generally composed mainly of cellulose: examples include cotton, jute, flax, ramie, sisal, and hemp. Cellulose fibers serve in the manufacture of paper and cloth.	**Animal fibers**: generally comprise proteins such as collagen, keratin and fibroin; examples include silk, wool, catgut, angora, mohair and alpaca.
➢ **Seed fiber:** Fibers collected from seeds or seed cases. Example: cotton and kapok ➢ **Leaf fiber :** Fibers collected from leaves. Example: fique, sisal, banana and agave. ➢ **Bast fiber:** Fibers are collected from the skin or bast surrounding the stem of their respective plant. These fibers have higher tensile strength than other fibers. Therefore, these fibers are used for durable yarn, fabric, packaging, and paper. Some examples are flax, jute, hemp ➢ **Fruit fiber:** Fibers are collected from the fruit of the plant. Example:coconut (coir) fiber. ➢ **Stalk fiber:** Fibers are actually the stalks of the plant. Example: straws of wheat, rice, barley, and other crops including bamboo and grass. Tree wood is also such a fiber.	➢ **Animal hair (wool or hairs):** Fiber or wool taken from animals or hairy mammals. Example: sheep's wool, goat hair (cashmere, mohair), alpaca hair, horse hair, etc. ➢ **Silk fiber:** Fiber secreted by glands (often located near the mouth) of insects during the preparation of cocoons. ➢ **Avian fiber:** Fibers from birds, Example: feathers and feather fiber.

Examples of Plant Fibers			
Name	**Source**	**Preparation**	**Uses**
Cotton (Purified cotton, Absorbent cotton))	Hairs of seeds of *Gossypium barbadense,* or *G. herbaceum* Malvaceae. It consists of 90% cellulose and 10 % moisture, fat etc.	Collect seeds with hair, separate hair by ginning press, (short hair useful to prepare adsorbent cotton and long hair for clothes.) removes fatty material, debris and any foreign matter by treating with soda solution for 15 hr, wash with water and bleaching agent. Dry it and use it. Following are important steps in preparation of cotton: *Ginning*: Removal of seeds and trash *Bale making*: Compression into bales *Scutching*: Mixing and blending *Lapping*: Opening and preparation of laps *Carding*: Preparation of loose strands and then thin layers *Sterilisation*	Surgical dressing, insulating material, filtering medium
Jute (Gunny)	Phloem fibres of stem of *Corchorus olitorius,* Tiliaceae. It consists of 55% cellulose, 20% hemicelluloses, 10 % lignin	Collect fibres from stem and outer skin. Extract by retting. Retting is a process of rottening of fibers due to combined effects of moisture, air, sun and microorganism so that to remove much of the cellular tissues and pectins surrounding bast-fibre bundles, and so facilitating separation of the useful fibre from the stem. There are three types of retting processes: *Water retting*: most preffered fibers are allowed to rot in optimum water conditions *Dew retting*: in limited water areas fibers spread over grass rottens due to dew formation in night *After retting*: collected fibers are allowed to dry completely and then further broken by Scutching (beating and scrapping). Scutching can be done by hand or by a machine known as a scutcher. This beaten fibers further need to sterilize and roll according to medical use.	Filtering medium, clothes, medicated sponge
Hemp	From stalks of plant *Cannabis sativa* The legality of industrial hemp varies widely between countries due to its psychoactive habitual effects. Only low psychoactive chemical containing hemp species are allowed to cultivate for fiber production.	The crop is ready for harvesting high quality fiber when the plants begin to shed pollen. Once the crop is cut, the stalks are allowed to rett (removal of the pectin by natural exposure to the environment) in the field for four to six weeks—depending on the weather—to loosen the fibers. A sequence of rollers (breakers) or a hammermill are used to separate bast fibers. The bast fiber is then cleaned and carded to the desired core content and fineness, sometimes followed by cutting to size and baling.	Rope, clothes, food, paper, textiles, plastics, insulation and biofuel

5.1.2 Plant Allergens

The substance originated from plant induces allergic reaction is called as plant allergen. The plant allergens are antigenic substances capable of sensitizing the body in such a way that unusual responses occur in hypersensitive individual. The allergy or hypersensitivity is an unwanted immunolo-gical reaction towards an antigen. Chemi-cally most of plant allergens are proteins or glycoprotein of molecular weight of 1000 - 7000 Daltons. Sometimes low molecular weight substance also causes allergy.

Process of Allergy

To very first or primary exposure to allergen, no symptoms of allergy are produced. But subsequent exposure causes release of antibodies, chemicals such as histamine, bradyklinins and other mediators into the bloodstream. These mediators then acts on a person's eyes, nose, throat, lungs, skin, or gastrointestinal tract and causes the symptoms of the allergic reaction. Future exposure to that same allergen will trigger this antibody response again. This means that every time you come into contact with that allergen, you will have an allergic reaction. When the symptoms are located to define area causes localized reaction. If it spreads throughout body causes generalized reaction which may be mild like sneezing, running nose or severe like allergic rhinitis, asthmas, articaria and dermatitis or even anaphylaxis i.e. difficulty in breathing, difficulty in swallowing, swelling of the lips, tongue, and throat or other parts of the body, dizziness or loss of consciousness.

Types of Reactions

The principal types of reactions observed in allergy are as follows:

➢ Type 1 reactions: (immediate type) (anaphylactic): The allergen causes formation of tissue sensitizing antibodies that are fixed to mast cells or leukocytes. On subsequent administration, the allergen reacts with these antibodies activating the cell and causing release of pharmacologically active substances like histamine, leukotrienes etc. and causing effects such as Urticaria, Anaphylactic shock and Asthma. Allergy develops within minutes to hours.

➢ Type II reactions: (Auto allergy): Where the allergen combines with a protein in the body, so that the body treats it as a foreign protein and forms antibodies.

➢ Type III reactions: Where antigen and antibody from complexes and activate the compliment. Leukocytes attracted to the site of reaction engulf the immune complexes and release pharmacologically active substances starting an inflammatory response.

➢ Type IV reactions: They are the delayed type allergy in which antigen-specific receptors produces the T-lymphocytes and subsequent administration will lead to local or tissue allergy like contact dermatitis.

Classification of Allergens

Inhalant	Substances distributed in atmosphere and contact nasal or buccal mucosa during respiration. Symptoms: Sinusitis, Hay fever, Sneezing, itching - Swelling of nose. Example- pollens of oak, Russian this day weed, Burmuda grass, perfumes.
Ingestant	Substances which occurs in food stuffs and cause allergies on ingestion Symptoms: Gastrointestinal disturbances, skin rash, migraine. Example-Tomato, Strawberry, Orange, Food additives.
Injectant	Substances present in the sol for parenteral administration Symptoms: Dermititis rash. Example-Antibiotics, penicillin, cepholosporins.
Contactants	Substances which on contact with epithelium produces allergy Symptoms: Dermititis, rashesh, purities Example-poison ivy, parthenium, mariogold, may apple, lobelia
Infestant	Parasitic microorganisms present in or on the body cause allergy.
Physical	Rise in temperature of body
Environmental	Climatic conditions like cool or hot
Psychosomatic	Anger and frustration

Examples Plant Allergens

Plant: Arnica, Mountain tobacco **Source** : *Arnica Montan,* Asteraceae **Allergenic compounds:** Sesquiterpene lactones, helenalin, carabron	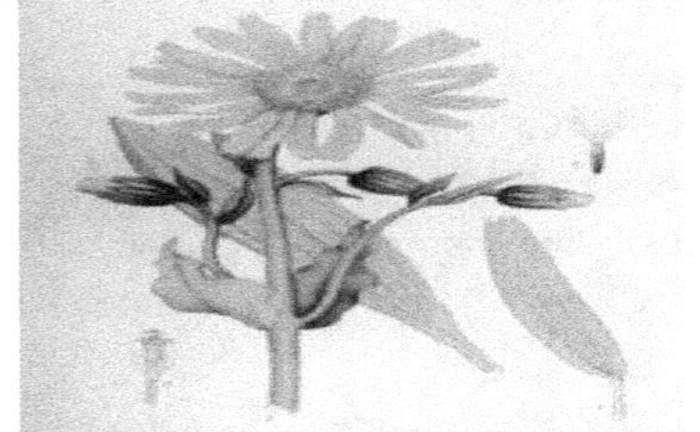
Plant: Peruvian lily **Source** : *Alstroemeria,* Amaryllidaceae **Allergenic compounds:** Pollens and sesquiterpene lactone causes tulip finger	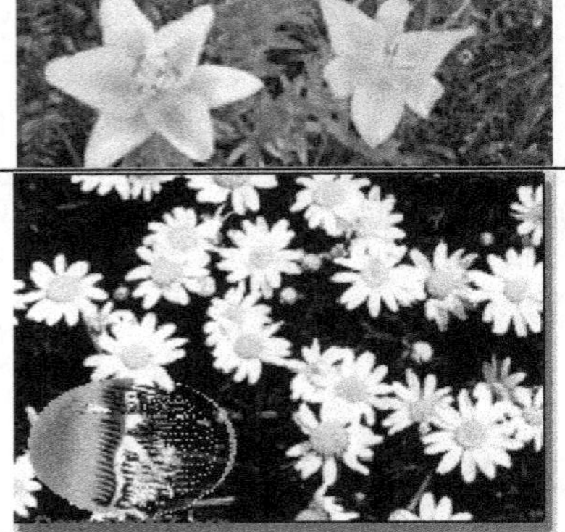
Plant: Chamomile **Source** : *Matricaria chamomilla,*Compositae **Allergenic compounds:** Pollens and oil containing Sequiterpenes causes atopic eczema	

Contd...

Plant: Horse chestnut **Source** : *Aesulus hippocastanum*Hippocastanaceae **Allergenic compounds:** Pollens	
Plant: Daffodil **Source** : *Narcissus pseudonarcissus,* Amaryllidaceae **Allergenic compounds:**Pollens and alkaloids including masonin and homolycorin	
Plant: Fig **Source** : *Ficus carica,* Moraceae **Allergenic compounds:**Furocoumarins psoralen, bergapten and the coumarins umbelliferone	
Plant: Poison oak, poison ivy **Source** : *Toxicodendron radicans* **Allergenic compounds:** Polyphenolic compounds: Urushiols	
Plant: Congress grass **Source** : *Parthenium histeroforum* **Allergenic compounds:** Parthenin	
Plant: Bermuda Grass **Source** : *Cynodondactylon,* Poaceae **Allergenic compounds:** Pollens	

Plant Allergens as Therapeutic Agents

Many times allergic plant extract are used to treat the allergic patients which is part of immunotherapy. Allergic extracts are prepared from highly pure raw material which is first defatted then extracted with sterile saline sol filter, dialyzed to remove coloring matter and irritant, concentrated and freeze dried. This immunotherapy is based on the administration of increasing amounts of the disease-eliciting allergens in order to yield allergen-specific non-responsiveness. Success of this therapy is associated with modulation of the immune response to allergenic molecules at the level of T-helper cells and the induction of blocking antibodies. The extracts used for immunotherapy are highly heterogenous preparations from natural sources and contain additional components, mostly proteins which are not well defined.

5.1.3 Hallucinogenic Plants

A hallucinogen is a psychoactive agent which can cause hallucinations, perceptual anomalies, and other substantial subjective changes in thoughts, emotion, and consciousness. The common types of hallucinogens are psychedelics, dissociatives and deliriants. Following are plants which found to be have hallucinogenic effect on central nervous system:

Common name	Plant	Active constituent
Ergot	*Cleviceps purpurea*	Ergometrine, ergotamine
Opium	*Papaver somniferum*	Morphine
Marijuana, hashish	*Cannabis sativa*	Tetrahydrocannabinol
Coca	*Erythroxylum coca*	Cocaine
Peyote	*Lophophora williamsii*	Mescaline
Coffee	*Coffea arabica*	Caffeine
Tobacco	*Nicotiana tabacum*	Nicotine
Datura	*Datura metel*	Hyoscine, Hyoscyamine
Belladonna	*Atropa belladonna*	Atropine
Nutmeg	*Myristica fragrans*	Myristicin

5.1.4 Teratogenic Plants

Teratogens are substances that may cause birth defects and developmental malformations via a toxic effect on an embryo or fetus. Following are plants which are proven with teratogenic effects.

Genus	Plant	Teratogenic effect
Lupinus	*Lupinus formosus, L. arbustus*	Cleft palate and minor front limb contractures due to piperidine alkaloid- lupines
Veratrum	*Veratrum californicum*	Cyclopamine alkaloid produces cyclopia and holoprosencephaly
Conium	*Conium maculatum*	Arthrogryposis and spinal curvature due to piperidine alkaloid coniine
Leucaena	*Leucaena leucocephala*	Skeletal defects and craniofacial malformations due to mimosin alkaloids
Astragalus	*Astragalus lentiginosus*	Delayed placentation, decreased vascularization, fetal edema and hemorrhage

Contd...

Genus	Plant	Teratogenic effect
Nicotiana	*Nicotiana tabacum, N.glauca*	Fixed excessive carpal flexure with or without lateral or medial rotation of fore or rear limbs, lordosis, irregular shaped head or cleft palate
Trachymene	*Trachymenepilosa*	Gross deformities in forelimbs, bent leg due to essential oil
Datura	*Datura metel, D. stramonium*	Malformations and reduction deformities due to scopolamine and hyoscyamine
Prunus	*Prunus serotina*	Absence of anus, plantar hind legs, rudimentary external genitalia due to isothiocyanate alkaloids
Sorghum	*Sorghum bicolor, S. controversum*	Deformities of the fetal musculoskeletal system (ankylosis or arthrogryposis) due to lathyrogenic nitriles such as β-cyanoalanine, cyanogenic glycosides, and nitrates
Senecio	*Senecio vulgaris*	Mutagenic, genotoxic, fetotoxic and teratogenic due to pyrrolizidine alkaloids due to senecionine, seneciphylline, retrorsine, riddelline, intergerrimine, spartioidine, and usaramine

5.2 Primary Metabolites: General Introduction, Detailed Study with Respect to Chemistry, Sources, Preparation, Evaluation, Preservation, Storage, Therapeutic Used and Commercial Utility as Pharmaceutical Aids and/or Medicines for the Following Primary Metabolites:

5.2.1 Carbohydrates

Primary metabolites: General introduction, detailed study with respect to chemistry, sources, preparation, evaluation, preservation, storage, therapeutic used and commercial utility as Pharmaceutical Aids and/or Medicines for the following.

Carbohydrates ('hydrates' of carbon) are the most abundant natural organic compounds defined as polyhydroxy aldehydes or ketones and their derived products.

An Aldose A Ketose Fructose Glucose Galactose

Fig. 5.1 Aldoses and ketoses

Occurrences and Distribution

They are widely distributed in plants, animals and microbes. They are synthesized in green plants and algae from water and CO_2 using solar energy in a process called photosynthesis. Included in the category of carbohydrates are the sugars, the glycogens, the starches and the celluloses. In addition, there are complex carbohydrates such as glycoproteins, glycolipids, lipopolysaccharides, etc.

Biosynthesis

Photosynthesis gives rise to various types of sugar moieties from CO_2 and light. For details see chapter 5.

Functions

➢ Chief source of energy
➢ Part of structural components
➢ Part of reserve food material
➢ Parts of very important secondary metabolites – glycosides, alkaloids and phenols
➢ Part of the backbone of genetic material i.e. Ribose in RNA, DNA
➢ Linked to proteins and lipids to form glycoproteins and glycolipids

Classification and Chemistry

Carbohydrates can be monosaccharides, oligosaccharides and polysaccharides.

Monosaccharides: Monosaccharides have two major groups : the aldoses and the ketoses. It is simplest form of carbohydrates which cannot be hydrolyzed to other sugar units under reasonably mild chemical conditions. They serve as the building-blocks for the more complex sugars. The simplest monosaccharides are the 3-carbon trioses glyceraldehyde and dihydroxyacetone. Other monosaccharides are tetroses (four carbons), pentoses (five carbons), hexoses (six carbons), heptoses (seven carbons) and octoses (eight carbons). Each exists in two series, ie., aldotetroses and ketotetroses; aldopentoses and ketopentoses; aldo-hexoses and ketohexoses, etc. Of these monosaccharides, hexoses (both aldoses and ketoses) are the most abundant. Glucose (aldohexose) is the most abundant monosaccharide. All the monosaccharides except dihydroxyacetone contain one or more asymmetric carbon atom(s) i.e., a single carbon atom having four different substituents and thus are chiral molecules. Pyrano (six membered) and furano (five membered) forms are most common in glucose and fructose repectively.

There are three important types of sugar acids: aldonic, aldaric and uronic acids. The uronic acids are components of many polysaccharides. An important sugar acid is L-ascorbic acid or vitamin C which is the lactone of hexanoic acid having an enediol structure between C-2 and C-3. Ascorbic acid is unstable and readily undergoes oxidation to dehydroascorbic acid. Ascorbic acid is present in large amounts in citrus fruits and tomatoes.

Isomeric forms explaning chemistry of crabohydrates	
Enantiomers	Aldoses and ketoses of the L-series are mirror-images of their D-counterparts. These two D- and L- forms of a sugar are known as enantiomers. Lsugars are found in nature, but they are not so abundant as D-sugars. CHO ... H—C—OH, H—C—OH, H₂C—OH = H►C◄OH, H►C◄OH, H₂C—OH ⟺ (Minor images / Not the same) HO►C◄H, HO►C◄H, HO—CH₂ = HO—C—H, HO—C—H, HO—CH₂

Contd...

Diastereoisomers	Two sugars having the same molecular formulae but not the mirror images of each other are known as diastereoisomers. Example: D-glucose and D-mannose. All these sugars are not mirror images of each other.
Epimers	Two sugars differing only in the configuration around one specific carbon atom are called epimers of each other. Thus, D-glucose and D-mannose are epimers with respect to carbon atom 2, and D. glucose and D-galactose are epimers with respect to carbon atom 4.
Anomers	From various chemical considerations it has been deduced that the **alpha and beta** isomers of D-glucose are not open-chain structures in aqueous solution but six-membered ring structures formed by the reaction of the alcoholic hydroxyl group at carbon atom 5 with the aldehydic carbon atom 1 to form a hemiacetal which renders an other chiral center at carbon atom 1, also known as carbonyl carbon atom or anomeric carbon atom. Isomeric forms of monosaccharides that differ from each other only in configuration about the carbonyl carbon atom are known as anomers. Thus, D-glucose will have two anomers designated as alpha D-glucose and beta-D-glucose.

Classification of carbohydrates		
Class	**Saccharides**	**Polysaccharides**
Properties	Low molecular weight Soluble in water Sweet taste	High molecular weight Insoluble in water Tasteless
Chemical composition	**Monosaccharides:** Simple single sugars **Examples :** Glucose, fructose, galactose	**Oligosaccharides:** 2-10 monosaccharides **Examples :**Sucrose, Maltose, Lactose	**Multiple sugar moieties** **Examples:** Starch, glycogen. Cellulose, Lignin, Chitin

Differnce between reducing and non-reducing sugars		
Reducing sugars	Reduces Fehling's solution and Tollen's reagent. These sugars have free functional groups because chemically these are hemiactals as their rings are open.	Example: All monosacharides (lactose, maltose)
Non-reducing suagrs	Do not reduces Fehling solution and Tollen's reagent because chemically these are acetals as these sugars have bonded functional groups.	Example: Sucrose
Reducing and non-reducing sugars		

Sucrose
Sucrose- Non-reducing sugar
Sucrose=glucose+fructose

Galactose   Glucose
Lactose
Lactose-reducing sugar
Lactose=glucose+galactose

Maltose
Maltose-reducing sugar
Maltose=glucose+glucose

Oligosaccharides: Oligosaccharides (Greek Oligo 'few') contain from two to ten monosaccharide units joined through glycosidic linkage or bond. They are hydrolyzable into constituent monosaccharide units. Depending on the number of monosaccharide units that are linked, the oligosaccharides are further classified as disaccharides (two sugar units), trisaccharides (three sugar units), tetrasaccharides (four sugar units), etc. Amongst these, disaccharides are the most important class because of their biological role and relative abundance in natural products. The most abundant disaccharides in nature are maltose, sucrose and lactose. Those with potentially a free aldehyde or a ketone group can reduce Fehling's solution, hence are called reducing disaccharides. The reducing disaccharides have most of the properties of monosaccharides i.e. they can form osazones and show mutarotation, etc.

Polysaccharides: Polysaccharides are polymers of monosaccharide units joined in long linear or branched chains through glycosidic bonds. Hydrolysis of polysaccharides yields many units of constituent monosaccharides.

Polysaccharides have two major biological functions: a) as a storage form of fuels and b) as structural elements in living organisms. The bulk of carbon found in nature exists in the form of polysaccharides. Complex sugars of high molecular weight; polymers of several units of monosaccharides or either derivatives with linear or branched chains. Upon hydrolysis by acids or enzymes, they are broken down into various intermediate products and finally into their consituent monosaccharides or their derivatives. They are tasteless, apparently amorphous, some are crystalline. Mostly insoluble in cold water but form a sticky or gelatinous solutions They differ in the nature of their recurring monosaccharides units, in the length of their chains and in the degree of branching. Polysaccharides are often called as glycans. Those containing glucose are called as glycans (starch and glycogen); those containing mannose are called mannans and those containing galactose units are called galactans. The most common homopolymer in animal cells is glycogen, the storage form of glucose. Glycogen is a very large, branched polymer of glucose residues. Most of the glucose units in glycogen are linked by α-1,4-glycosidic bonds. The branches are formed by α-1,6-glycosidic bonds, present about once in 10 units. Amylopectin, the branched form, has about 1 α-1,6 linkage per 30 α-1,4 linkages, in similar fashion to glycogen except for its lower degree of branching.

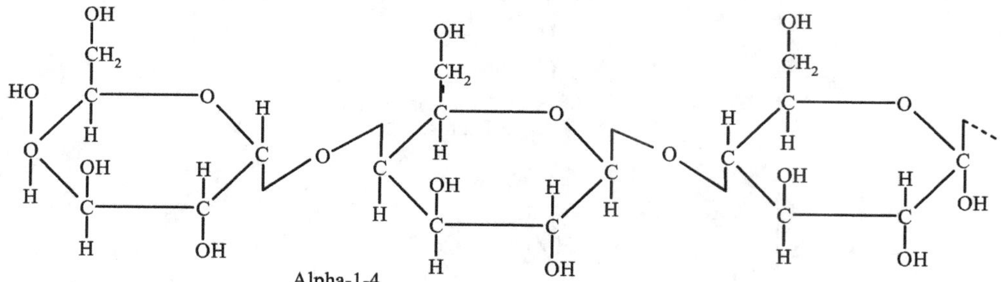

Fig. 5.2 Linkages present in sugars

Classification of Carbohydrates	
Based on function	
1. **Structural polysaccharides**: These polysaccharides serve as structural components of living organisms. Example: cellulose (plant cell wall), chitin (exoskeleton of some insects), etc.	2. **Storage/ reserve / nutrient polysaccharides**: These polysaccharides function as reserve or storage form of fuel in living organisms Example: starch (plants), glycogen (animal cells) etc.
Based on composition	
1. **Homopolysaccharides**: These are made up of single kind of monosaccharide residues or their derivatives. Example: Starch, glycogen, cellulose, chitin, inulin, etc.	2. **Heteropolysaccharides**: These are made up of two or more different kinds of monosaccharide units or their derivatives. Example: Hyaluronic acid, heparin, pectins, gums, mucilages, chondroitins, etc.

Method of Analysis

Qualitative Chemical Tests

Test	Procedure	Inference
Molisch's test [Dissolve 3.75 g of 1-naphthol in 25 ml of Ethanol 99%.]	Mix 1 ml reagent in 2 ml of test solution. Add 1 ml of concentrated sulfuric acid.	Red to violet ring depending on the amount of sugar appears at the junction of the two liquids.
Iodine test for starch	Mix 0.5 ml of iodine solution with 1 ml of the test solution.	Starch gives deep blue color.
Fehling's test [Fehling's "A" is 7 g copper(II) sulfate pentahydrate dissolved in distilled water containing 2 drops of dilute sulfuric acid. Fehling's "B" is 35g of potassium tartrate and 12g of NaOH in 100 ml of distilled water. These two solutions should be stoppered and stored until needed.]	Mix 1 ml of Fehling's solution 'A' with 1 ml of Fehling's solution 'B' and 1 ml of test solution. Then, boil it.	Yellow to red precipitate indicates presence of reducing sugars
Benedict's test [Benedict's reagent is prepared by mixing 17.3 grams of copper sulfate pentahydrate, 100 grams of sodium carbonate, and 173 grams of sodium citrate in distilled water (required quantity).]	Mix 2 ml of Benedict's reagent with 2 ml test solution. Boil it in a water bath.	Formation of red, yellow or green colored precipitate depending on the sugar concentration indicates presence of reducing sugars
Barfoed's test [Barfoed's reagent is 0.33 molar solution of copper (II) acetate in 1% acetic acid solution.]	Mix 2 ml of Barfoed's reagent with 1 ml of the test solution. Boil it and wait.	Brick-red precipitate of monosaccharides.
Seliwanoff's test for ketohexoses [Seliwanoff's Reagent is 110 mg of Resorcinol in 220 ml of 3N HCl.]	Mix 2 ml of Seliwanoff's reagent with 1 ml of test solution. Boil.	Deep red color due to ketohexoses.
Bial's test for pentoses [Bial's reagent is 0.4 g orcinol, 200 ml of concentrated hydrochloric acid and 0.5 ml of a 10% solution of ferric chloride.]	Mix 5 ml of Bial's reagent with 1 ml of test solution. Warm slowly.	Green color precipitate due to pentoses.

Extraction

Extraction of carbohydrates is a very simple process. Being polar in nature, sugars can be extracted in water, acetone or alcohols. The mucilage or gum containing polysaccharide extracts can be precipitated by slow addition of ethanol or acetone. Sometimes solution of sodium chloride or ammonium oxalate is also useful for fractionation of sugars. Extraction with enzyme, dilute acid or water are the preferred methods for carbohydrate isolation. Here, one general method of carbohydrate extraction is mentioned.

Extraction of Frre sugars: Take accurately weighed quantity of sample. Add sufficient quantity of 50% ethanol or methanol. Extract by reflux or ultrasonication method for 1 hour at 50°C. Then centrifuge at 600 rpm for 20 min. Remove and store supernatant and re-extract marc by same procedure until Molisch test is negative. Combine the supernatants and heat at 80°C for 20 min to inactivate endogenous enzymes. Then centrifuge at 6000 rpm for 20 min. Collect the supernatants and evaporate to dryness in a rotary vacuum evaporator at 40°C to give dry massof total carbohydrates.

Extraction of polysachharides: Extract the powder with hot water. Fractionate it with ether-benzene (1:1) to remove lipids. Now precipitate water extract into alcohol or acetone. Collect and dry precipiate.

Estimation

To estimate total carbohydrates, phenol-sulfuric acid or anthrone method is most useful.

Agar	
Synonyms	Agar-Agar, Isinglass, Vegetable gelatin
Biological Source	Agar is the dried hydrophilic colloidal polysaccharide complex extracted from the red algae belonging *Gelidium amansii* belonging to the family Gelidaceae. The most common agar-producing genera are Gelidium; Gracilaria; Acanthopeltis; Ceramium and Pterocladia.
Geographical Source	Japan, Australia, India, New Zealand, Korea, Spain, South Africa, USA
Description	Colour : Yellowish white Odour : Odourless Taste : Bland, mucilaginous Shape : various shapes like: bands, strips, flakes, sheets and coarse powder
Chemical Constituents	It is complex range of polysaccharide chains having alternating α–(1→3) and β–(1-4) linkages. It contains two major fractions i.e. Agarose (neutral gelling fraction consisting (+) –galactose and 3,6-anhydro-(–)-galactose moieties;) responsible for the gel-strength of agar and agar pectin (sulphated non-gelling fraction consisting sulphonated polysaccharide wherein both uronic acid and galactose moieties are partially esterified with sulphuric acid)
Substituents/Adulterants	Gelatin
Uses	It is used in making photographic emulsions, sizing silks and paper, preparation of bacteriological culture media, gels in cosmetics, ointments and in the dyeing and printing of fabrics and textiles. It is most famous as thickening agent in confectionaries and extensively used as a bulk laxative. 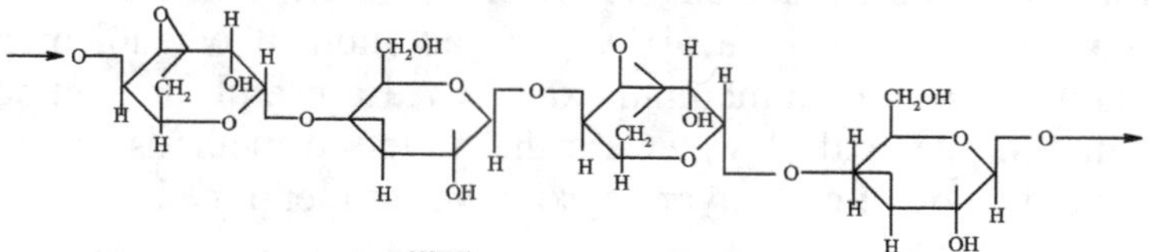 agarose

Contd...

Acacia	
Synonyms	Indian gum; Gum Acacia; Gum Arabic.
Biological Source:	It is the dried gummy exudation from the stems and branches of *Acacia Senegal* and *Acacia arabica*, family; Leguminoseae.
Geographical Source:	India, Arabia, Sudan and Kordofan (North-East Africa), Sri Lanka, Morocco, and Senegal (West Africa).
Cultivation and Collection	Acacia is recovered from wild as well as duly cultivated plants in the following manner, such as: **(a)** *From wild plants:* The Gum after collection is freed from small bits of bark and other foreign organic matter, dried in the sun directly that helps in the bleaching of the natural gum to a certain extent, and *From cultivated plants:* Usually, transverse incisions are inflicted on the bark which is subsequently peeled both above and below the incision to a distance 2-3 feet in length and 2-3 inches in breadth. Upon oxidation, the gum gets solidified in the form small translucent beads, sometimes referred to as 'tears'. Tears of gum normally become apparent in 2-3 weeks, which is subsequently hand picked, bleached in the sun, garbled, graded and packed.
Description	Colour : White, pale-yellow Odour : Odourless Taste : Bland, mucillagenous. Shape and Size : Spheroidal or ovoid in shape Appearance : Opaque, fracture is brittle and glossy.
Chemical Constituents:	It contains mainly four chemical constituents, namely: (–) arabinose; (+) – galactose; (–)–rhamnose and (+) glucuronic acid. It also contains a peroxidase enzyme.

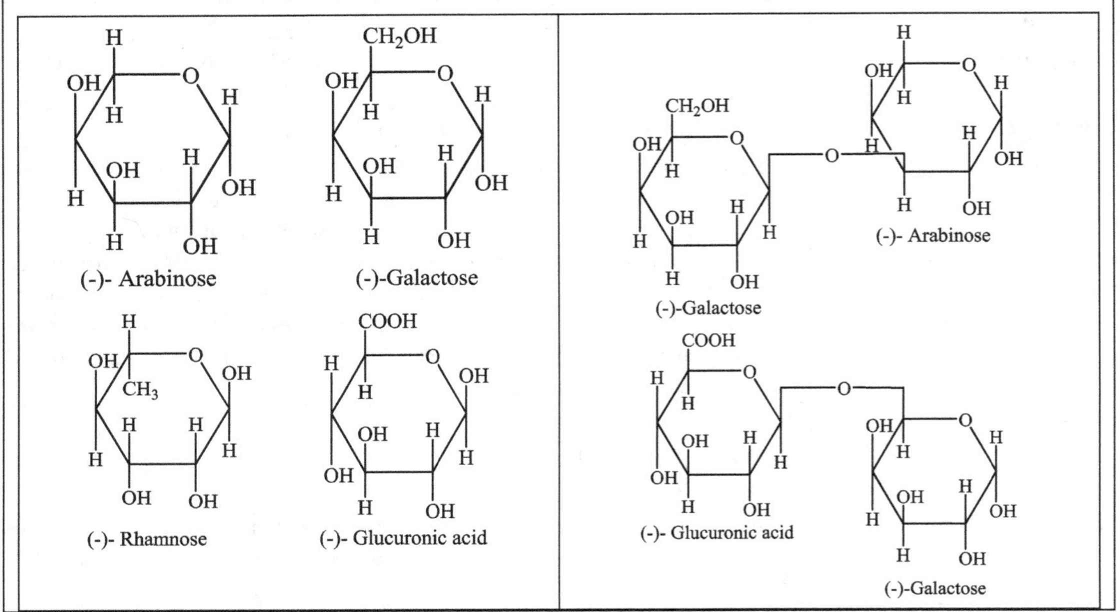

Chemical Tests

Lead Acetate Test	Treat aqueous solution with lead-acetate solution	Heavy white precipitate
Borax Test	Treat aqueous solution with borax	Stiff translucent mass
Enzyme test	Treat aqueous solution with benzidine in alcohol together with a few drops of hydrogen peroxide (H_2O_2),	Distinct–blue colour due to peroxidase enzyme
Reducing Sugars Test	Treat aqueous solution with dilute HCl and Fehling's solution	Brick-red precipitate
Tragacanth distinguishing test	Treat aqueous solution with lead acetate	No precipitate (a clear distinction from Agar and Traga-canth)
Starch and dextrin distin-guishing test	Treat aqueous solution with Iodine solution	No colour change (a marked distinction from starch and dextrin)
Tannins distin-guishing test	Treat aqueous solution with $FeCl_3$ solution	No bluish-black colour (an apparent distinction from tannins).

Uses: It is used as mainly demulscent, thickening agent, binding agent and colloidal stabilizer.

Tragacanth	
Synonym	Gum Tragacanth, White Gavan
Biological Source	It is dried gummy exudation from *Astragalus gummifer* Labill. belonging to the family of *Leguminoseae*.
Geographical Source	Iran, Iraq, India, Armenia, Syria, Greece and Turkey.
Collection:	The thorny shrubs of **tragacanth** normally grow at an altitude of 1000-3000 meters. As an usual practice transverse incisions are inflicted just at the base of the stem, whereby the gum is given out both in the pith and medullary rays. Thus, the absorption of water helps the gum to swell-up and subsequently exude through the incisions. The gummy exudates are duly collected and dried rapidly to yield the best quality white product. It usually takes about a week to collect the gum exudates right from the day the incisions are made; and this process continues thereafter periodically.
Description	**Colour** : Pale white **Odour** : Odourless **Taste** : Tasteless **Shape:** Curved or twisted ribbon shape flakes with markings of concentric ridges which indicates successive exudation and solidification. Fracture is normally short and horny.

Contd...

	Size: $25 \times 12 \times 12$ mm. **Appearance:** Translucent
Chemical Constituents	It consists of two major fractions i.e. water soluble **'traga-canthin'** and water-insoluble **'bassorin'.** Tragacanthin do not contain methoxyl groups whereas bassorin contains methoxyl moieties and hence yields the most viscous mucilages.

Chemical Test			
	Acid test	Treat aqueous solution with conc. HCl	Red colour
	Ruthenium Red test	Treat aqueous solution with 0.1% aqueous Ruthenium Red solution	Pink colour
	FeCl₃ test	Boil aqueous solution with 10% aqueous $FeCl_3$	Deep-yellow precipitate.
	Lead acetate test	Treat aqueous solution with lead acetate.	Heavy precipitate

Substituents/ Adulterants	Karaya gum
Uses	It is used as a demulcent and employed as an emollient, suspending agent, binding agent, emulsifying agent and stabilizing agent in pharmaceutical and food industry, oils and waxes.

Honey	
Synonyms	Madhu, Madh, Mel, Honey
Biological Source	It is sweet secretion found in the honey comb secreted by various species of bees, such as: *Apis dorsata, Apis florea, Apis indica, Apis mellifica,* belonging the natural order *Hymenotera* (Family: *Apideae*).
Geographical Source	Africa, India, Jamaica, Australia, California, Chili, Great Britain and New Zealand
Preparation	Honey is produced by bees as a food source. Generally, honey bees reside in colonies and produces honey and beeswax. Every colony has one *'queen'* or *'mother bee'*, and number of worker bees. The worker bees raise larvae and collect the nectar that will become honey in the hive. Invertase, is one of the enzymes synthesized by the body of bees and present in the saliva, converts the nector into the invert sugar. It means invertases and digestive acids hydrolyze sucrose to give the monosac-charides glucose and fructose and finally a product honey, containing approximately 80% invert sugar and 20% water is ready. As soon as the cell is filled up completely, the bees seal it with wax to preserve it for off-season utility. This seal can be broken by sterilized sharp knife and honey is extracted from that, often using a honey extractor. Honey is then filtered and warmed the separated combs to recover the beeswax.
Description	Appearances: Pale yellow to reddish brown viscid fluid Odour: Pleasant and characteri-stic, depends upon the surrounding flowers Taste: Sweet, Slightly acrid, depends upon the sur-rounding flowers Specific gravity : 1.35-1.36 Specific rotation : +3o to –15o Total Ash : 0.1-0.8%

Contd...

Chemical Constituents	The average composition of honey rangles as follows: Moisture 14-24%, Dextrose 23-36%, Levulose (Fructose) 30-47%, Sucrose 0.4-6%, Dextrin and Gums 0-7% and Ash 0.1-0.8%. Besides, it is found to contain small amounts of essential oil, beeswax, pollen grains, formic acid, acetic acid, succinic acid, maltose, dextrin, colouring pigments, vitamins and an admixture of enzymes Example- diastase, invertase and inulase. Interestingly, the sugar contents in honey varies widely from one country to another as it is exclusively governed by the source of the nector (availability of fragment flowers in the region) and also the enzymatic activity solely controlling the conversion of nector into honey.
Uses:	It is used as a sweetening agent in confectionaries, demulcent for coughs, colds, sore-throats and constipation and as a good nutrient source
Substituents / Adulterants:	Artificial invert sugar or cane-sugar syrup.

5.2.2 Proteins

Proteins (Greek, proteios – primary or first), also known as polypeptides, are the high-molecular-weight polymers of large chains of amino acids. The amino acids in a polymer are joined together by peptide bonds between the carboxyl and amino groups of adjacent amino acid residues. Generally the proteins are three dimensional in nature due to the fact that the each amino acid which forms protein has its own enantiomeric structure.

Properties

➤ A protein in solution shows changes in solubility as a function of pH, ionic strength, temperature and the dielectric properties of the solvent.

➤ Excepting the chromo-proteins, they do not have any characteristic color, odour, or taste.

➤ Proteins are precipitated from solution by heavy metal ions ($AgNO_3$, $CuSO_4$, lead acetate, mercuric chloride), alkaloidal reagents (trichloroacetic acid, picric acid, metaphosphoric acid), and concentrated salt solution [$(NH_4)_2SO_4$, Na_2SO_4, $NaCl$)]. The precipitation is the result of the destabilization of protein-solvent interaction.

➤ Most proteins have distinct light absorption maxima at 280 nm due primarily to the presence of tyrosine, tryptophan and phenylalnine.

➤ Due to denaturation protein usually losses its three dimensional structure and biological activity

➤ Proteins can be hydrolyzed completely to yield a mixture of constituent amino acids as end-products by an acid (6M HCl for 12-36 hours at 100-110°C), a base (2M NaOH) or by enzymes (proteases).

Functions

Proteins from plants are an important source in food and feed. Proteins are actually the genetic information storing components of plants. These are involved in storage, transport, form structural components and carry out the reactions in the form of enzymes. The two steps (transcription and translation) in the biosynthesis of proteins depends on information encoded by genes. Each protein has its own unique amino acid sequence that is specified by the nucleotide sequence of the gene encoding this protein. The genetic code is combination of three-nucleotide sets i.e. codons and each three-nucleotide combination designates an amino acid, for example : AUG (adenine-uracil-guanine) is the code for methionine.

Classification

Classification of proteins based on composition
1. *Simple proteins*: These proteins yield only -amino acids on complete hydrolysis
2. *Complex or conjugated proteins*: These proteins give in addition to amino acids an organic or inorganic non-protein moiety called prosthetic group on hydrolysis. Following are examples of complex or conjugated proteins

Conjugated protein	Prosthetic group	Example
Lipoproteins	Lipid	Plasma 1 -lipoproteins
Glycoproteins	Carbohydrate	Immunoglobulins
Nucleoproteins	Nucleic acid	Ribosomes
Flavoproteins	FAD	Succinate dehydrogenase
Phosphoproteins	Phosphoric acid	Casein (milk)
Chromoproteins	Colored substance	Hemoglobin (contains heme)
Metalloproteins	Metal ion	Ferrition (contains ferric hydroxide)

Classification of proteins according to their functions		
Functional class	**Example**	**Occurrence or biochemical function**
Catalytic	Enzymes	Hydrolysis, oxidation, reduction synthesis and degradation of macromolecules etc.
Structural	Collagen Glycoproteins a-Kration sclerotin Fibroin Viral-coat	Framework of bone, tendons and connective tissue Cell coats and wall Component of hair, wool, skin. Nails, feathers and hoofs Exoskeletons of insects Component of silk of cocoons, spider webs Sheath around nucleic acid protein
Contractile	Actin and mysin Dynein	Contraction of muscle fibers Cilia and flagella
Protective	Antibodies Fibrinogen	Natural defense in vertebrates Precursor of fibrin in blood clotting
Transport	Hemoglobin Serum albumin	Transport of O2 in vertebrate blood Transport of fatty acids in blood
Respiratory	Cytochrome	Mitochondrial electron transport chain
Hormonal	Insulin Growth hormone	Regulates blood glucose level Stimulates growth of bones

Contd...

Storage	Gliadin	Wheate seed protein
	Zein	Corn seed protein
	Casein	A milk protein
	Ferrition	Iron storage in spleen
	Ovalbumin	Egg-white protein
Toxins	Ricin	Toxic protein in castor bean
	Diphtheria toxin	Bacterial toxin
	Gossypin	Toxic protein in cotton seed
Vision	Rhodopsin	Visual cycle in eye
Membrane	Na+ − K + ATPase	Active transport

Chemistry

Amino Acids are the Basic Structural Units of Proteins. The twenty naturally occurring amino acids that make up proteins can be grouped according to many criteria, including hydrophobicity, size, aromaticity, or charge. Amino acids are linked by amide bonds to form peptide chains. The peptide bond has two resonance forms that contribute some double-bond character and inhibit rotation around its axis, so that the alpha carbons are roughly coplanar. The other two dihedral angles in the peptide bond determine the local shape assumed by the protein backbone. The end of the protein with a free carboxyl group is known as the C-terminus or carboxy terminus, whereas the end with a free amino group is known as the N-terminus or amino terminus. The words protein, polypeptide, and peptide are a little ambiguous and can overlap in meaning. Protein is generally used to refer to the complete biological molecule in a stable conformation, whereas peptide is generally reserved for short amino acid oligomers often lacking a stable three-dimensional structure.

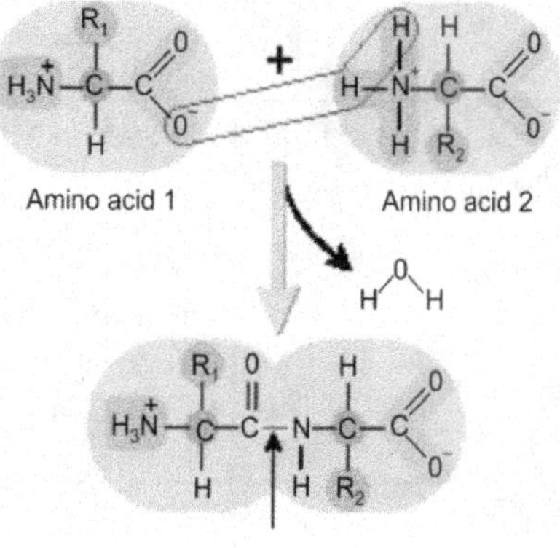

Fig. 5.3 Peptide bond fromation

Biochemists often refer to four distinct aspects of a protein's structure:

➢ Primary structure: It is just the amino acid sequence.

- Secondary structure: It is regularly repeating local structures stabilized by hydrogen bonds. The most common examples are the alpha helix, beta sheet and turns.
- Tertiary structure: Tertiary means folded structure which is generally stabilized by formation of a hydrophobic core and or salt bridges, hydrogen bonds, disulfide bonds, and even posttranslational modifications.
- Quaternary structure: The structure formed by several protein molecules (polypeptide chains), usually called protein subunits in this context, which function as a single protein complex.

Extraction

Proteins can be present in the from of enzymes as well as antibodies but in extraction and isolation of proteins from plant tissues it is necessary to follow following general steps:

- Defatting with ether to remove excess lipids
- Treatment with buffer of p^H 6-8 to neutralize acidic environment in cell sap
- Addition of reducing substances like ascorbic acid to deactivate enzyme phenolase
- addition of Polyvinyl pyrrolidone (PVP) to remove tannins
- Processing as early as fast to avoid action of proteolytic enzymes preferably at low temperature range
- Now add ammonium sulphate to obtain precipitate of proteins
- Collect precipitate and analyse for molecular weight by gel chromatography and for composition by gel electrophoresis

Method of Analysis

Chemical Tests

Test	Procedure	Inference
Biuret test [Biuret reagent is prepared by mixing 1.5 gram of pentavalent copper sulphate (CuSO4), 6 gram of Sodium potassium tartarate (chelating agent) in 500 ml of distilled water and 375 ml of 2 molar Sodium hydroxide. Mix and make final volume to 1000 ml by adding distilled water.	Mix 2 ml test solution with 2 ml Biuret reagent.	Violet to pink color
Millon's test [Millon's reagent is Mercuric Nitrate-160 g, Mercurous Nitrate-160 g, Conc. Nitric acid-400 ml and Distilled water-600 ml	Mix 2 ml test solution with 2 ml Millon's reagent. Boil it.	Red color
Xantho-protein test	Mix 2 ml test solution with 2 ml Conc. H2SO4	White precipitate
Precipitation test	Mix 2 ml test solution with 2 ml 5% HgCl2 or 5% ammonium sulphate	White precipitate
Lead acetate test	Mix 2 ml test solution with 2 ml 40 % NaOH, 0.5 ml lead acetate solution. Boil.	Black to brown colour

Estimation

Kjeldahl, Lowery and Biuret method are commonly used to estimate proteins.

Gelatin

Gelatin is a mixture of peptides and proteins produced by partial hydrolysis of collagen extracted from the skin, bones, and connective tissues of animals such as domesticated cattle, chicken, pigs, and fish. Amino acids present in geleatin are Glycine 21%, Proline 12%, Hydroxyproline 12%, Glutamic acid 10%, Alanine 9%, Arginine 8%, Aspartic acid 6% and Other 22%.

Gelatin preparation involves following steps:

- *Pretreatment*: acid, alkali, and enzymatic hydrolysis to remove excess calcium, fat and salt. Gelatin obtained from acid-treated raw material has been called type-A gelatin and the gelatin obtained from alkali-treated raw material is referred to as type-B gelatin
- *Extraction*: neutral or acidic water used to extract pure gelatin at appropriate temperatures by multiple steps
- *Recovery*: This step involves filtration, evaporation, drying, grinding, and sifting

It is widely used as gelling agent, stabiliser, thickening agent, binding agent, capsule shell ingredients in food and pharmaceutical industry.

Casein

Casein is, a phosphoprotein, commonly found in mammalian milk. It constitutes to 80% of the proteins in cow's milk 20-45% of the proteins in human milk. The most common form of casein is sodium caseinate Casein contains amino acids, carbohydrates, and two essential elements, calcium and phosphorus. It contains high number of proline residues without disulfide bridges. It is water insoluble.

Casein breaks down in the human stomach to produce the opioid peptide casomorphin. Casomorphin is an exogenous opioid peptide pertaining to the class of exorphins which include opioid food peptides like Gluten exorphin and opioid food peptides. Exorphins mimic the actions of endorphines because they bind to the same opioid receptors in the brain. It is major component of cheese, used as a food additive, protein supplement, tooth remineralization product etc. It is also used in glue, paint, plastics etc.

5.2.3 Proteolytic Enzymes

One of the most important proteins in nature are enzymes which can be defined as an organic catalysts produced by the living cells but capable of acting outside cells or even in-vitro. Enzymes are also called as biological catalysts. There are additional non-protein moieties usually present which may or may not participate in the catalytic activity of the enzyme. Example: minerals: Cu, Fe, Zn. Other factors often found are metal ions (cofactors) and low molecular weight organic molecules like vitamins (coenzymes).

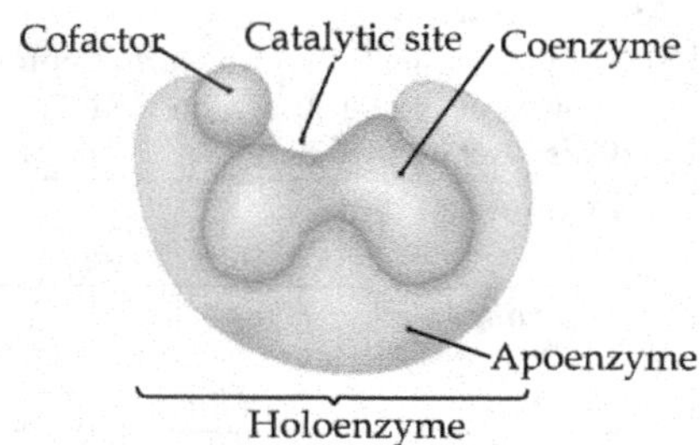

Fig. 5.4 Typical parts of enzymes

➢ **Terminology:** An inactive enzyme, without the cofactor is called an apoenzyme, while the complete enzyme with cofactor is the holoenzyme. Apoenzyme is the protein component of the enzyme.

➢ **Cofactor:** The non-protein component of the enzyme molecule required for complete activity. Cofactors can be divided into two broad groups: organic cofactors, such as flavin or heme, and inorganic cofactors, such as the metal ions Mg_2^+, Cu^+, Mn_2^+. They can also be classified depending on how tightly they bind to an enzyme, with loosely-bound cofactors termed coenzymes and tightly-bound cofactors termed prosthetic groups.

Properties

➢ Chemically all enzymes are proteins.

➢ They are highly selective and specific (regiospecificity as well as stereo specificity).

➢ Reaction can be catalyzed to the exclusion of side-reactions, eliminating undesirable by-products. Thus, higher productivities plus reduced material costs can be obtained.

➢ Product is generated in an uncontaminated state thereby reducing purification costs.

➢ Often a smaller number of steps may be required to produce the desired end-product. They catalyze only the reactions of very narrow ranges of reactants (substrates).

➢ These can be regenerated during the course the reaction

Sources of Enzymes

Biologically active enzymes may be extracted from any living organism, over 50% are from fungi and yeast and over 30% are from bacteria with the remainder divided between animal (8%) and plant (4%) sources.

	IUPAC classification of enzymes is as follows:	
Oxidoreductases	These enzymes catalyze oxidation or reduction reactions by transfer of hydrogen or electrons.	succinic dehydrogenase, oxidases
Transferases	These enzymes are involved in transferring functional groups between donors and acceptors. The amino, acyl, phosphate, one-carbon and glycosyl groups are the major moieties that are transferred.	Transminase, kinase
Hydrolases	This group of enzymes can be considered as special class of transferases in which the donor group is transferred to water. The generalized reaction involves the hydrolytic cleavage of C-O, C-N, O-P and C-S bonds. The cleavage of the peptide bond by peptidases is good example of this reaction.	Peptidases, esterase
Layses	These enzymes remove the groups of water, ammonia or CO_2 from the substrate to cleave double bond or conversely, add these groups to double bonds	Aldolase
Isomerases	These are a very heterogeneous group of enzymes that catalyze isomerizations (i.e., structural rearrangements within a molecule) of several types. These include cis-trans, keto-enol, and adose-ketose interconversion	Mutases involve the intramolecular transfer of a group such as phosphoryl group. Furmarase,
Liagases (synthetases)	Two molecules are joined together at the expense of breakdown of nucleosidetri-phosphates.	pyruvic carboxylase, citric acid synthtase

<table>
<tr><td colspan="5" align="center">Examples of Proteolytic enzymes</td></tr>
<tr><td>Sr. No.</td><td>Name of drug and synonym</td><td>Biological source</td><td>Type of Enzyme</td><td>Uses</td></tr>
<tr><td>1</td><td>Bromelian (plant protease Concentrate)</td><td>Stem of pineapple plant Ananascomosus (Bromeliaceae)</td><td>Mixture of proteolytic enzyme</td><td>Anti inflammatory for soft tissues</td></tr>
<tr><td>2</td><td>Papaine</td><td>Latex of unripe fruit of tropical melon tree Carica papaya (Caricaceae)</td><td>Proteolytic enzyme</td><td>Meat tenderiser, clarification of beverages</td></tr>
<tr><td>3</td><td>Pepsin</td><td>Glandular layer of fresh stomsch of hog, Sus scrofa (Suidae)</td><td>Proteolytic enzyme</td><td>Conversion of protein into peptone and proteose</td></tr>
<tr><td>4</td><td>Streptokinase</td><td>Culture filtrates of beta-hymolyticStreptococci group c.</td><td>Plasminogen activator enzyme</td><td>Treatment of thromboembolic disorder</td></tr>
<tr><td>5</td><td>Seratio-peptidase</td><td>Bacteria belonging to genus Serratia</td><td>Proteolytic enzyme</td><td>Anti-inflammatory especially to enhance antibiotic effects</td></tr>
<tr><td>6</td><td>Urokinase</td><td>Human urine or kidney tissue cultures</td><td>Fibronolysis activating enzyme</td><td>Lysis of blood clots or fibrin in pulmonaryembolism and inferior chamber of eye</td></tr>
</table>

5.2.4   Lipids (Waxes, Fats, Fixed Oils)

Lipids (Greek, 'lipos'-fat) are the hydrophobic compounds used to supply energy. Lipids includes fixed oils, fats, fatty acids, glycerols, waxes, monoglycerides, diglycerides, triglycerides, phospholipids, sphingolipids, sterols (chlolesterol), prenols (retinol) and polyketides.

Occurrence and Distribution

Fats and oils are widely distributed in nature in both plant and animal tissues. They occur in relatively high concentration in seeds of certain plants (oilseeds) where they function to supply food for use of the growing seedlings. Animals store deposits of fats in their adipose tissues; these stored fats constitute a reserve which can be used as the source of energy.

Biosynthesis

Acetate pathway builds various types of lipids and oil moieties from acetyl-coA condensation.

Functions

- Sources of metabolic energy
- Structural components of the brain and cell membranes
- They carry fat-soluble vitamins (A, D, E, K) and are vital parts of the cell signaling.
- They also found to have potential source of antioxidant compounds.
- As a protective water proof coating on the surface of cuticle of leaves or fruits of plants, feathers of birds and as insect secretions
- Intense biological activity – some have profound biological activity; they include some of the vitamins and hormones.

- Fats stored subcutaneously in warm blooded animals serve as insulation against an unfavorable environment and also fatty tissues around vital organs give protection against mechanical injuries.

Properties

- Soluble in nonpolar solvents but only sparingly soluble in water
- Greasy or fat-like in nature and show transluecent properties
- The glyceride esters of saturated fatty acids are usually liquids at room temperature

Classification

Simple lipids	These are esters of fatty acids with alcohols; saponifiable; include the most abundant of all lipids such as fats and oils or triglycerides and the less abundant waxes.
Compound or complex lipids	These are esters of fatty acids containing other groups in addition to alcohol and fatty acids; saponifiable; include phosphoglycerides and sphin-golipids.
Derived lipids	These are derived from the hydrolysis of above two classes of lipids; nonsaponifable (except fatty acids); include fatty acids, sterols, terpenes and fats soluble vitamins.

Chemistry

Glycerol is a trihydric alcohol and is a constituent of all fats and oils. It has the ability to react with three molecules of fatty acids to form a triple ester called a triglyceride. Glycerol and fatty acids are the backbone structures of all fats and oils.

Fatty acid is a carboxylic acid with long aliphatic chain which is either saturated or unsaturated.

Fats may be either solids or liquids at room temperature. Chemically, these are triesters of glycerol and fatty acids. Fatty acids consist of the carboxyl group (-COOH) at one end of the aliphatic side chain. Hydrolytic removal of glycerol from fats or oils produces fatty acids. Saturated fatty acids do not contain double bonds in the carbon chain. Monounsaturated fatty acids usually contain a cis-olefinic bond in a limited number of preferred positions in the chain. Polyunsaturated fatty acids have two to six cis double bonds. Most of these double bonds have a cis-configuration. The positions of the double bonds of unsaturated fatty acids are indicated by the symbol n where the subscript indicates the position of the first cabon in the double bond, numbering from the carboxyl carbon as C-1. Thus the C18 fatty acid has one cis double bond between carbons 9 and 10 is called cis 9 octadecenoic acid.

Waxes (Example: bees wax, carnauba wax, paraffin) are types of lipids that contain a long-chain of alkanes, alkyls, alkane esters, fatty acids, fatty alcohols or even terpenes. These are water-insoluble, solid esters of higher fatty acids with long chain mono hydroxylic fatty alcohols or sterols. They differ from fats and oils in that glycerol is replaced by high molecular weight alcohols or sterols. They are the less abundant class of lipids; saponifiable in nature and very resistant to atmospheric oxidation. Because of these properties, they are used in furniture and automobile polishes.

Examples of true waxes are beeswax, carnauba wax (from the carnauba plant) and spermaceti (spem whale wax). Beeswax and spermaceti are composed mainly of palmitic acid esterified with either hexacosonol ($C_{26}H_{53}OH$) or triacontanol ($C_{30}H_{61}OH$). Carnauba wax, the hardest known wax consists of fatty acids esterified with tetracosanol ($C_{24}H_{49}OH$) and tetratriacontanol ($C_{34}H_{69}OH$).

Waxes are found as protective coatings on skin, fur and feathers of animals and birds and on leaves and fruits of higher plants and on exoskeleton of many insects.

Phospholipids (Example: lecithin, cephalin, phosphatidate) are made of only two fatty acids, glycerol, phosphoric acid and simple organic molecules such as choline, serine or ethanolamine.

Similarly sphingomyelin is derived from sphingosine instead of glycerol. Sphingosine (4-sphingenine) is a C18 amono alcohol containing a long unsaturated hydrocarbon tail.

Method of Analysis

Qualitative Chemical Tests

Test	Procedure	Inference
Filter paper test	Press the powder between filter paper.	Permanent oily spot
Solubility test	Mix oil in alcohol	Insoluble
Sudan red III test	Treat the test solution with Sudan red III	Red colour
Tincture alkana test	Treat the test solution with tincture alkana	Red colour

Quantitative Chemical Tests

1. *Saponification number or value:* It is the number of milligrams of KOH required to completely saponify one gram of fat or oil. The higher the   saponification number, the shorter the average carbon chain length of the fatty acids in a fat or an oil.

2. *Iodine number or value:* It is the number of grams of iodine absorbed by 100 grams of a fat or oil. It is a measure of degree of unsaturation of the fatty acids in a fat or oil.

3. *Acid value:* It is the number of milligrams of KOH required to neutralize the free fatty acids in one gram of a fat or oil. It is a measure of free fatty acid content in a fat or oil

4. *Solid fat content (SFC):* The solid fat content is defined as the percentage of the total lipid that is solid at a particular temperature, i.e. SFC = 100 M solid /Mtotal, where Msolid is the mass of the lipid that is solid and Mtotal is the total mass of the lipid in the food.

5. *Cloud point:* This gives a measure of the temperature at which crystallization begins in liquid oil. A fat sample is heated to a temperature where all the crystals are known to have melted (Example: $130^{\circ}C$). The sample is then cooled at a controlled rate and the temperature at which the liquid just goes cloudy is determined. This temperature is known as the cloud point, and is the temperature where crystals begin to form and scatter light. It is often of practical importance to have an oil which does not crystallize when stored at $0^{\circ}C$ for prolonged periods. A simple test to determine the ability of lipids to withstand cold temperatures without forming crystals is to ascertain whether or not a sample goes cloudy when stored for 5 hours at $0^{\circ}C$.

6. *Smoke point:* The smoke point is the temperature at which the sample begins to smoke when tested under specified conditions. A fat is poured into a metal container and heated at a controlled rate in an oven. The smoke point is the temperature at which a thin continuous stream of bluish smoke is first observed.

7. *Flash point:* The flash point is the temperature at which a flash appears at any point on the surface of the sample due to the ignition of volatile gaseous products. The fat is poured into a metal container and heated at a controlled rate, with a flame being passed over the surface of the sample at regular intervals.

8. *Fire point*: The fire point is the temperature at which evolution of volatiles due to the thermal decomposition of the lipids proceeds so quickly that continuous combustion occurs (a fire).

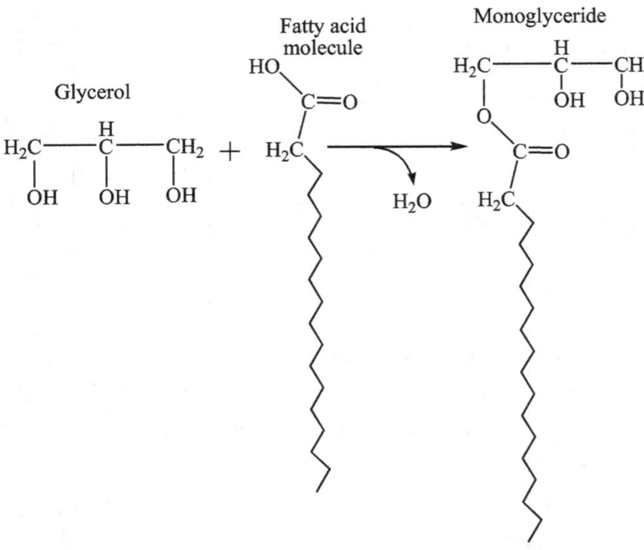

Fig. 5.5 Formation of glycerides

Table 5.9 Analytical standards for few fatty oils.

Analytical standards for few fatty oils				
Sr. No.	Drugs	Acid Value	Saponification value	Iodine value	Refractive index
1	Arachis oil	≤ 0.5	185 - 195	85 - 105	1.467 - 1.470
2	Black mustard oil	61%	173-184	96-194	1.472-1.4733
3	Carnauba wax	04-07	78-89	13-15	1.459
4	Castor oil	≤ 2	176 - 187	82 - 90	1.4758 -1.4798
5	Chaulmoogra oil	≤ 10	195-213	93-104	1.472-1.476
6	Cocoa butter	1.68	188-195	35-40	1.4637-1.4578
7	Cod liver oil	≤ 2	180-190	145-180	1.4705-1.4745
8	Corn oil	2-6	187-196	109-133	1.0464-1.468
9	Hydrous wool fat	≤ 1	90-105	18-36	1.431-1.439
10	Jojoba oil	0.30-0.50	90-92	80-81	1.4648
11	Karanja oil	6-7	181-182	89-90	1.4736-1.4739
12	Kokum butter	≤ 3	185-190	35-37	1.4565-1.4575

Contd...

Sr. No.	Drugs	Acid Value	Saponification value	Iodine value	Refractive index
13	Lard	01-02	192-198	52-56	1.4520-1.4550
14	Linseed oil	≤ 4	188-195	160-200	1.4786-1.4815
15	Neem oil	≤ 2	195-205	68-75	1.417-1.4627
16	Olive oil	≤ 6.6	190-195	79-88	1.4677–1.4705
17	Poppy seed oil	3-13	188-196	132-158	1.467-1.470
18	Rice bran oil	04-05	181-189	99-108	1.470-1.473
19	Safflower oil	01-9	188-194	140-150	1.472-1.475
20	Sesame oil	≤ 2	188-195	103-116	1.472-1.4776
21	Shark liver oil	≤ 2	> 170	> 90	1.459-1.477 at 40^0
22	Spermaceti	10–18	125-136	03-05	1.433 at 80^0C
23	Suet	≤ 2	192-195	33-45	1.449-1.451
24	Wheat germ oil	06-20	179-190	115-130	1.469-1.478
25	Yellow bees wax	05-10	90-103	6-13	1.4410-1.4430

Extraction

Fatty acid extraction involves three step processes. The first step is to extract total fatty acids in samples and second step is to convert all fatty acid such as triacyl-glycerols, phospholipids, and sphin-golipids, to methyl esters using esteri-fication procedure. The last step is to quantify fatty acid methyl esters by gas chromatography.

To extract and analyze total lipids from plant tissues is a difficult task. Ether extraction is the classical method for lipid determination. Hexanes can be an acceptable alternative to diethyl ether as a solvent. But isopropanol is the most preferred solvent to deactivate lipases which rapidly hydrolyze phospholipids and glycolipids and increases the amount of free fatty acids in the extract. Recent trend is the use of solvents in combination for extraction of total lipids from plant tissues. Hexane: isopropanol (3:2, vol/vol) or chloroform: methanol (2:1) can be selected. Extracted lipid fraction must be stored with addition of 0.005 % butylated hydroxytoluene until next use to avoid degradation.

Soxhlet extraction is one of the most commonly used methods for deter-mination of total lipids in dried foods. This is mainly because it is fairly simple to use and is the officially recognized method for a wide range of fat content determinations. The main disadvantages of the technique are that a relatively dry sample is needed (to allow the solvent to penetrate), it is destructive, and it is time consuming. For high moisture content foods it is often better to use batch solvent or nonsolvent extraction techniques. Many instrumental methods are simple to operate, rapid, reproducible, require little sample preparation and are nondestructive. Instrumental methods are most useful for rapid measurements of fat content on-line or in quality assurance laboratories of food factories where many samples must be measured rapidly.

Estimation

Estimation of total lipid amount in a biological sample may be done by gravimetry or by colorimetry.

Chaulmoogra oil	
Common name:	Hydnocarpus oil, Gyno-cardia oil.
Biological source:	It is obtained from seeds of the plant *Taraketogenos kurzil* king belonging to family Flacourtriaceae.
Geographical source:	Native to Myanmar, Thailand, East India, and Sri Lanka.
Morphology-	**Colour:** Yellow to yellowish brown, Odour: Characteristic, Taste: Acrid
Chemical constituents:	Oil contains esters of unsaturated fatty acids, Chaulmogric acid, hydrocarpic acid and palmitic acid.
Uses:	It is used externally in treatment of Leprosy, Psoriasis, Rheumatism Chaulmoogric acid
Castor oil	
Common name:	Ricinus oil
Biological source:	oil is obtained from plant *Ricinus comunis* family Euphorbeaceae
Geographical source	India.
Morphology	Colour: Pale yellow, Odour: Slight and characteristic, Taste: Bland followed by acrid
Chemical constituents	Oil contains triagycerides of recinolic acid (80%) and also iso ricinolic acid, linoleic acid, staric acid and isostaric acid.
Uses	Cathartic, Laxative, Lubricant, Preparation of soaps
Bees wax	
Common name	Yellow beeswax
Biological source	It is btained from the honey comb of the bees Apis mellifica, A.indica (Apidae)
Chemical constituents	Myricyl palmitate, cerotic acid, Cerolein
Use	Hardening agent, ointment base
Wool Fat	
Synonym	Hydrous lanoline; Lanoline; Purified lanolin; AdepsLanae.
Biological Source	It is secreted by the hairs constituting the fleece of the sheep Ovis aries, family Bovidae.
Geographical Source	Australia, U.S.A., India.
Method of preparation	Wool fat may also be extracted by scouring the fleeces with hot water, and allowing the emulsion thus produced to stand, when impure wool fat rises as a cream. This can be cleansed by repeatedly mixing with water and separating by centrifugation, the resulting wool fat being subjected to a final process of purification

Contd...

Description	Colour – Whitish yellow; Odour – Faint and characteristic; Taste – Bland; Extra features – It is found in the form of ointment like mass and on heating in water bath, it separates into two layers.
Chemical constituents	Wool fat consists chiefly of cholesteryl and iso-cholesteryl alcohols combined with lanoceric, lanopalmitic, carnaubic, myristic, a little oleic, and possibly also palmitic and cerotic acids. Lanolin is also frequently, but incorrectly, referred to as wool fat (adeps lanae) by many of the world's pharma-copoeias even though it has been known for more than 150 years that lanolin is devoid of glycerides and is in fact a wax, not a fat.
Uses:	Wool fat is largely used as an emollient and for promoting the absorption of drugs by the skin.

5.2.5 Marine Drugs

Approximately 70% earth surface is covered by water and enclosed nearly 3 lakh known species of plants and animals. Human tries to understand oceanic resources since ancient time. Chinese and Japanese are very famous to use these resources to treat goiter or cancer like disease. Most of the marine organisms are soft and sessile then how they protect from their predators as well as large bacterial growth in sea water. That's possible due to secondary metabolites. India is blessed with more then 8000 km coastline but very few institutes and industries are involved in marine research.   Why sponges are anticancer? The reason is that to occupy maximum space they kill nearside sponge's growing cell and protects own normal cell. Several molecules (like sterols, steroidal alkaloids, terpenoids, isoprenyl quinols, furanoids, sesquiterpenoids, triprenyl phenols, guanino and sulphone units) isolated from these marine organisms (micro-organisms, algae, fungi, invertebrates, and vertebrates like sponges, jelly fishes, sea anemones, gorgonians, corals, bryozoans, molluscs, echinoderms, tunicates, and crystaceans) are currently under study.

➤ All sponges are sessile aquatic animals. They are multicellular organisms which have bodies full of pores and channels allowing water to circulate through them, consisting of jelly-like mesohyl sandwiched between two thin layers of cells. Sponges do not have nervous, digestive or circulatory systems. Instead, most rely on maintaining a constant water flow through their bodies to obtain food, oxygen and remove wastes

➤ Corals are marine animals typically living in compact colonies of many identical individual "polyps". Polyps are approximately cylindrical in shape and elongated at the axis of the body. Cephalopods are mollusks. These exclusively marine animals are chara-cterized by bilateral body symmetry, a prominent head, and a set of arms or tentacles (muscular hydrostats) modi-fied from the primitive molluscan foot.

➤ Clam is one of the many interesting species of mollusks.

➤ Sea cucumbers are marine animals with a leathery skin and an elongated body containing a single, branched gonad.

➤ Sea anemones (flower like) are a group of water-dwelling, predatory animals.

➤ Coelenterata is an obsolete term hollow body cavity surrounded by sensory tentacles. These animals generally reproduce asexually by budding.

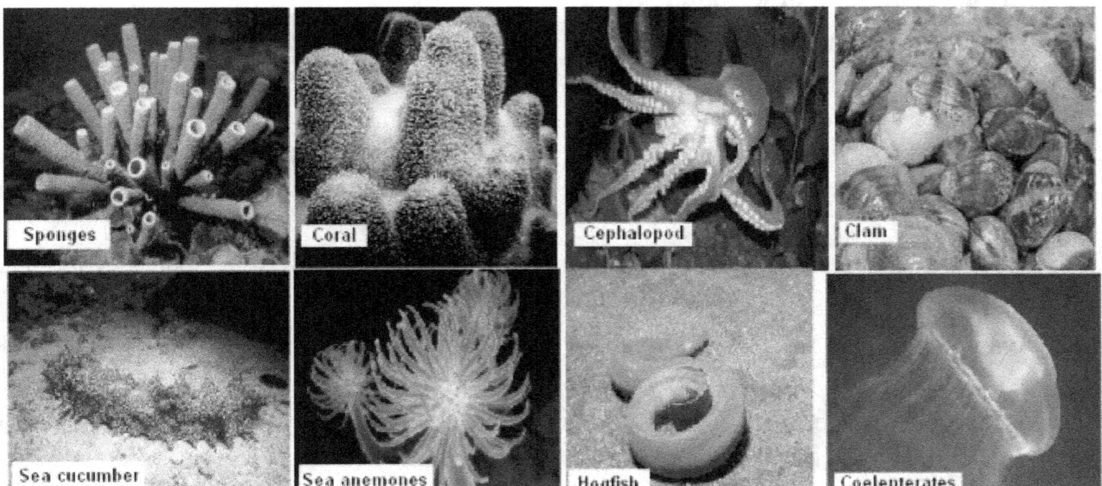

Common Marine bioactive molecules

Protein and Peptides

➤ *Collagen*: obtained from various fishes used as edible coating in meat industry (e.g. sausages), Anti-oxidant, anti-hypertensive and anti-skin-aging activities.

➤ *Gelatin*: obtained from Cold-water fishes used as stabilizer, texturizer, or thickener in ice cream, jam, yogurt, cream cheese, margarine, confectionaries, utilized in low fat foods and clarifiers, prevents and treat chronic atrophic gastritis

➤ *Albumin*: obtained from mollusks, crustaceans, low-fat fish used as whipping, suspending, or stabilizing agent, anticoagulant and antioxidant properties

Poly-Saccharides

➤ *Carrageenan:* obtained from macroalgaes used in gel formation and coatings in the meat and dairy industry, anti-HIV activity and anticoagulant properties

➤ *Agar agar:* obtained from Red Alga like Gelidium, Gracilaria, Hypnea and Gigartina used in gel formation and food gums

➤ *Fucans and fucanoids:* obtained from Cell walls of brown algae, sea urchin eggs, sea cucumbers used as nutraceutical supplements, anticoagulant, antiviral, antithrombotic, proliferative and anti-inflammatory

➤ *Chitin, chitosan, and derivatives*: obtained from shrimp, crab, lobster, prawn and krill used as gelling agents, edible protective films, clarification and de-acidification of fruits, increase dietary fiber, reduce lipid absorption, antitumor, bactericidal and fungicidal activities

Fatty acids

➤ *Omega-3 fatty acids*: obtained from almost all marine sources used as nutraceuticals (fish oil and capsules), fortification of livestock, feed and infant formula, found to have numerous health benefits (e.g. visual and neurodevelopment, reduce risk of cardiovascular problems, ameliorate diseases such as arthritis and hypertension)

Phenolic compounds and other pigments

➤ *Phlorotannins*: obtained from brown algae used as active ingredients in the nutraceuticals, antioxidant activity

➤ *Carotenoids*: β-carotene, and lutein: obtained from *Dunaliella salina, Sarcina maxima, Chlorella protothecoides, Chlorella vulgaris* and*Haematococcuspluvialis* used as natural food colorant, nutraceutical agents, vitamin A precursors, antioxidants, anti-carcinogenic and anti-inflammatory

➤ *Chlorophylls*: obtained from *S. platensis* and *A. flos-aquae* used as natural food and beverage colorants, anticancer activity, natural pigment

Marine enzymes

➤ *Gastric proteases (pepsins, gastricsins and chymosins):* obtained from various fish body viscera like atlantic cod, carp, harp seals, and tuna etc. used as cCold renneting milk, fish feed digestion aid and helps in digestion

➤ *Serine and cysteine proteases*: obtained from Crustaceans, mollusks and short-finned squid used in preventing unwanted color changes in food products, meat tenderizing, curing of Herring, squid fermentation and helps in digestion

➤ *Lipases*: obtained from Atlantic cod, seal, salmon, sardine, Indian mackerel and red sea bream used in fats and oils industry and helps in digestion

➤ *Transglutaminase*: obtained from Red sea bream, rainbow trout, atka mackerel, walleye, Pollock liver and scallop used to create protein cross-links to improve rheological properties of gels, i.e., surimi, gelatin and resistance to proteolytic degradation

Vitamins and Minerals

➤ *Fat and water soluble vitamins, iron, iodine, manganese and zinc*: obtained from almost all marine sources used in food, pharma and nutraceutical industries, health benefits as they provide transport inside cells and also serve as cofactors during metabolic processes

Examples of Marine Pharmaceuticals

Compound Name (Trademark)	Source	Company/Institution (City, State, Country)	Use
Cytarabine (Cytosar-U®; Depocyt®)	Spongothymidine/sponge *Cryptotethya crypta*	Bedford, USA; Enzon, USA	Cancer
Trabectedin (Yondelis®)	Ecteinascidin 743/ tunicate *Ecteinascidiaturbinata*	PharmaMar, Spain	Cancer
Eribulin mesylate (Halaven®)	Halichondrin B/sponge *Halichodriaokadai*	Eisai, Japan	Cancer
Brentuximab vedotin (SGN-35) (Adcetris®)	Dolastatin 10/sea hare *Dolabellaauricularia*	Seattle Genetics, USA; Takeda GRDC, Japan	Cancer

Contd...

Compound Name (Trademark)	Source	Company/Institution (City, State, Country)	Use
Pliditepsin (Aplidin®)	Ascidian *Aplidium albicans*	PharmaMar, Spain	Cancer
PM00104 (Zalypsis®)	Jorumycin/sea slug *Jorunafunebris*	PharmaMar, Spain	Cancer
Lurbinectedin (PM01183)	Ecteinascidins/tunicate *Ecteinascidiaturbinata*	PharmaMar, Spain	Cancer
CDX-011	Dolastatin 10/sea hare *Dolabellaauricularia*	Seatle Genetics, USA	Cancer
SGN-75	Dolastatin 10/sea hare *Dolabellaauricularia*	Seatle Genetics, USA	Cancer
PM060184	Sponge *Lithoplocamialithistoides*	PharmaMar, Spain	Cancer
Marizomib	Salinosporamide A/Marine actinomycete *Salinisporatropica*	Nereus Pharmaceutical, USA	Cancer
ASG-5ME	Dolastatin 10/sea hare *Dolabellaauricularia*	Astellas, USA	Cancer
Soblidotin	Dolastatin 10/sea hare *Dolabellaauricularia*	Aska Pharmaceuticals, Japan	Cancer
Synthadotin	Dolastatin 15/Sea hare *Dolabellaauricularia*	Genzyme Coporation, USA	Cancer
Elisidepsin (Irvalec®)	Kahalides/ *Sea slug Elysia rufescens*	PharmaMar, Spain	Cancer
Plinabulin (NPI-2358)	Halimide (NPI-2350)/marine fungus *Aspergillus sp.*	Nereus Pharmaceutical, USA	Cancer
Tasidotin (ILX-651)	Dolastatin 15/sea hare *Dolabellaauricularia*	Genzyme Corporation, USA	Cancer
Hemiasterlin	Sponge *Hemiastrella minor*	Eisai, Japan	Cancer
Kahalalide F	Sea slug *Elysia rufescens*.	PharmaMar Spain; Hawai University, USA	Cancer
Squalamine	Dogphish shark *Squalus acanthias*	Genaera, USA	Cancer
HTI-286	Hemiasterlin/sponge *Hemiastrella minor*	Wyeth, USA	Cancer
Discodermolide	Sponge *Discodermiadissouta*	Novartis, Switzerland; Harbor Branch, USA	Cancer
E7389	Halichondria B/sponge *Halichondriaokadai*	Eisai, Japan	Cancer
Spisulosine (ES-285)	Marine clam *Spisulapolynyma*	PharmaMar, Spain	Cancer
KRN-7000	Agelasphins/sponge *Agelasmauritianus*	Vrije Universiteit Medical Center, Netherlands	Cancer
Æ-941 (Neovastat®)	Shark cartilage	Æterna, Canada)	Cancer

Contd...

Compound Name (Trademark)	Source	Company/Institution (City, State, Country)	Use
NVP-LAQ824	Psammaplin A/sponge *Aplysinellarhax*	Dana-Farber Cancer Institute, USA	Cancer
Conotoxin G (CGX-1160)	Marine snail *Conus geographus*	Cognetix, USA	Pain
IPL-576092 and derivatives	Contignasterol/Sponge *Petrosiacontignata*	Aventis, France	Anti-asthmatic
Vidarabine (Vira-A®)	Spongouridine/sponge *Cryptotethya crypta*	King Pharma, USA	Anti-viral
Ziconotide (Prial®)	ω-Conotoxin/marine snail *Conus magus*	Elan Corporation, Ireland	Neuropahtic Pain
Omega-3-acid ethyl esters (Lovaza®)	Omega-3-fatty acids/fish	GlaxoSmithKline, UK	Hyper-triglyceridemia
Iota-carrageenan (Carragelose®)	Iota-carrageenan/red Algee *Eucheuma/Cnondus*	Marinomed, Austria; Boehringer Ingelheim, Germany	Antiviral Viral
DMXBA (GTS-21)	Anabeseine/worm *Paranemertes peregrina*	Comentis, USA	Alzhemier's
Bryostatin I	Bryozoan *Bugula neritina*	NCI, USA	Cancer and Alzheimer's
Pseudopterosins	Pseudopterosins /Soft coral *Pseudoptergorgiaelisabethae*	VimRx Pharmaceuticals, USA	Wound healing

Anti-malarial Marine drugs

Chemical compound	Source	Chemistry
Bromotyrosine derivative araplysillin I	From South Pacific Solomon Islands sponge Suberea ianthelliformis	Araplysillin I
Glycosphingolipids axidjiferoside A–C	From Senegal marine sponge Axinyssa djiferi with potent antimalarial activity against chloroquine-resistant FcB1/Colombia P. falciparum strain	axidjiferoside A n = 18 axidjiferoside B n = 17 axidjiferoside C n = 19

Contd...

Pentacyclic ingamine alkaloid dihydroingenamine D	From sponge Petrosid which showed strong antiplasmodial activity against P. falciparum	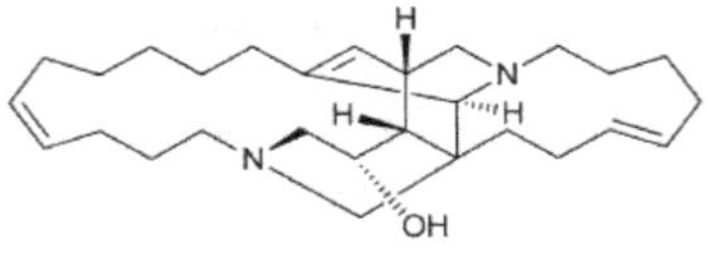 dihydroingenamine D
Alkaloid 19-hydroxypsammaplysin E	From Indonesian marine sponge Aplysinella strongylata showed notable antimalarial activity against the P. falciparum chloroquine-sensitive strain	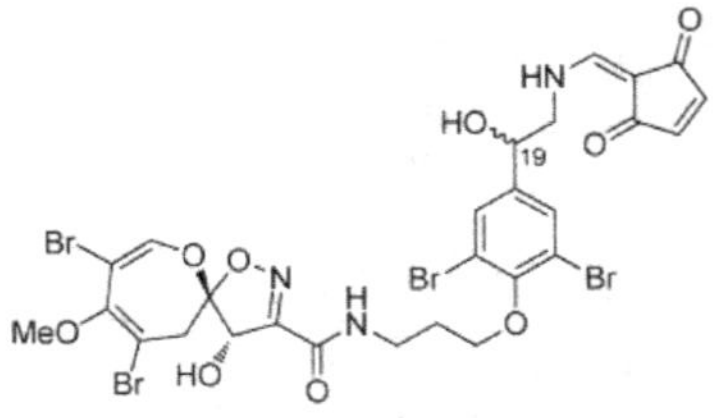 19-hydroxypsammaplysin E
Thiazine alkaloids-Thiaplakortone A	From the Australian marine sponge Plakortis lita which showed potent activity against the human malaria parasite Plasmodium falciparum strains	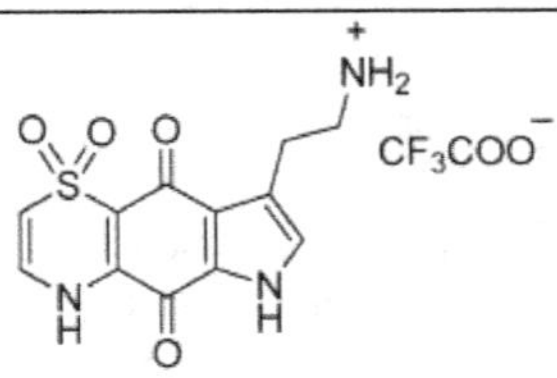 thiaplakortone A
Anti-diabetic Marine Drugs		
Phenolic compound Octaphlorethol A	From the marine brown alga Ishige foliacea	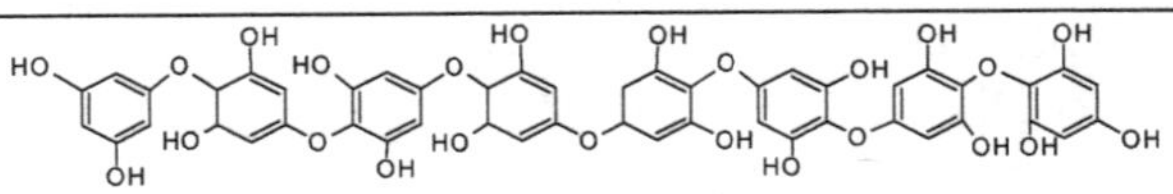 Octaphlorethol A
Immunomodulatory Marine Drugs		
Cembrane-type diterpenoid lobocrassin B	From marine soft coral Lobophytum crissum, demonstrated immunomodulatory effects	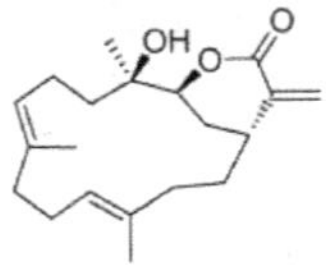 lobocrassin B
Mycophenolic acid derivative, penicacid B	From South China sea fungus Penicillium sp. SOF07, inhibited splenocyte lymphocyte proliferation by a mechanism that	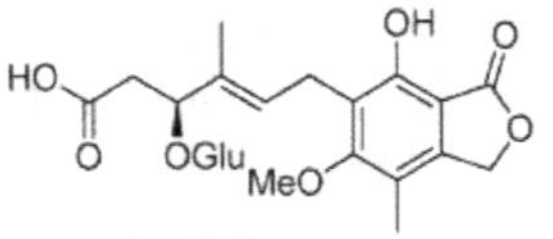 penicacid B

Contd...

	involved inhibition of inosine 5′-monophosphate dehydrogenase, an essential rate-limiting enzyme in purine metabolic pathway and an "important drug target for immunosuppressive" activity	
Anti-nociceptive, anti-inflammatory and analgesic Marine Drugs		
Convolutamydine-A	From Floridian marine bryozoan Amantia convoluta, demonstrating that it caused peripheral anti-nociceptive and anti-inflammatory effects	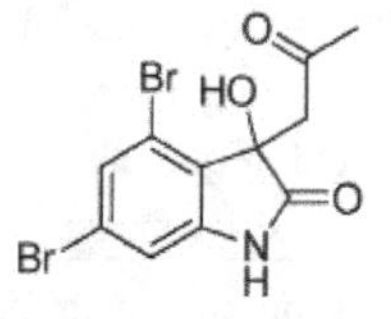 convolutamydine A
Polypeptides APHC1 and PAHC3	From sea anemone Heteractis crispa, shown to have significant anti-nociceptive and analgesic activity	-
Neuro-protective Marine Drugs		
Octopamine derivative ianthellamide A	From Australian marine sponge Ianthella quadrangulate, increased endogenous kynurenic acid in rat brain, as well as selectively inhibited the kynurenine 3-hydroxylase in vitro, thus revealing that modulation of the kynurenine pathway of tryptophan metabolism by this compound suggested "potential as a neuroprotective agent"	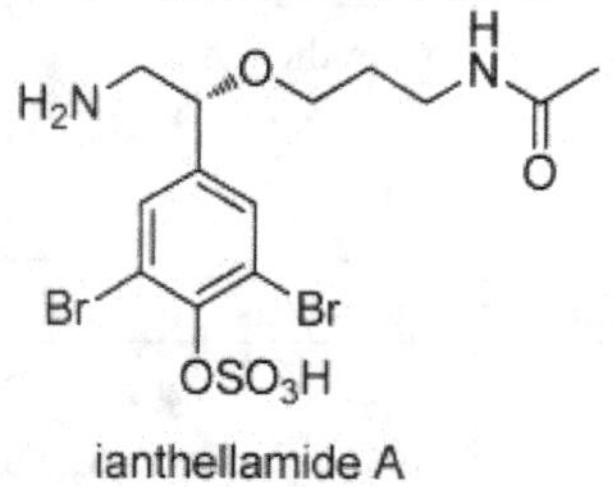 ianthellamide A

Marine drugs acting on Cardiovascular system

Compound	Source	Chemistry	Use	Structure
Saxitoxin	Butter clam (type of clam-closed shell) *Saxidomus giganteus*	Toxin	Hypotensive	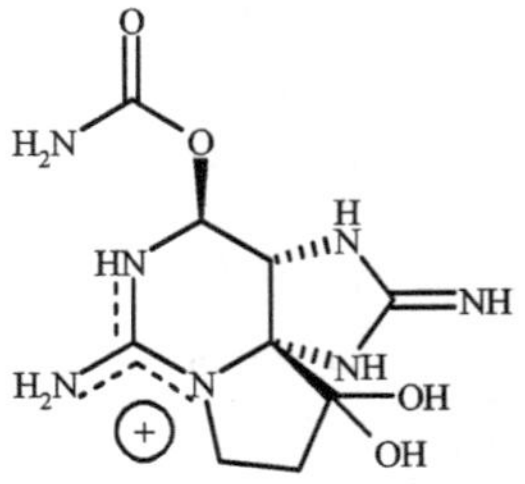
Spongosine	Carribean sponge *Cryptotethi a crypta*	Nucleoside	Hypotensive	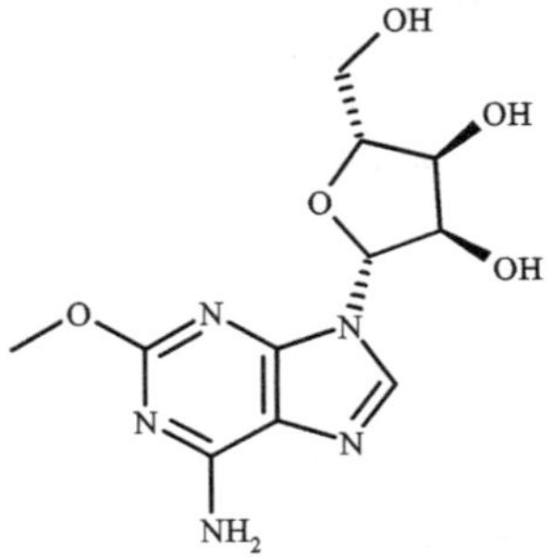
Eptatretin	Hogfish (pig like mouth) *Eptatretus stoutii*	Amide	Cardiac stimulant	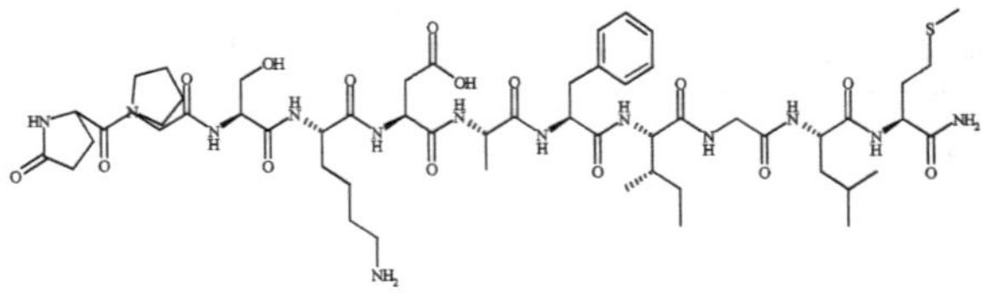

Marine drugs acting on Cardiovascular system

Compound	Source	Chemistry	Use	Structure
Eledosin	Cephalopod (pleural head) *Eledone moschata*	Peptide belonging to the tachykinin family of neuro-peptides.	Hypotensive	Polypeptide
Laminine	Algae *Laminaria angustata*	Phyto proteins	Hypotensive	Amino acid sequence
Antho-pleurins	Coelenterate s (sac like) *Anthoplerur a xantho-grammica*	Peptides	Cardio tonic	Anthopleurins are water-soluble proteins., and contain three disulfide bridges

Contd...

| Autono-mium | *Verongia fistularis Yellow Tube Sponge* | Like adrenaline and acetylcholine | Cardio tonic | 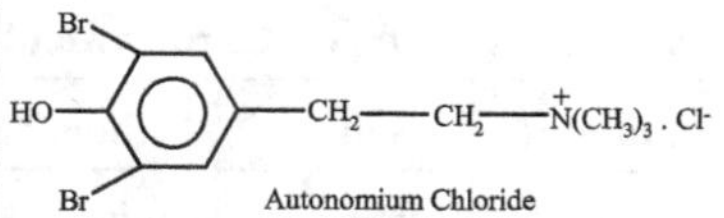 Autonomium Chloride |
| ATX-II | Sea anemones (flower type predators) | Polypeptide | | Polypeptide |

Marine drugs acting on Cardiovascular system

Compound	Source	Chemistry	Use	Structure
Holothu-rians	Sea cucumber *Phyllum echino-dermata*	Triterpenoid saponins	Cardiotonic	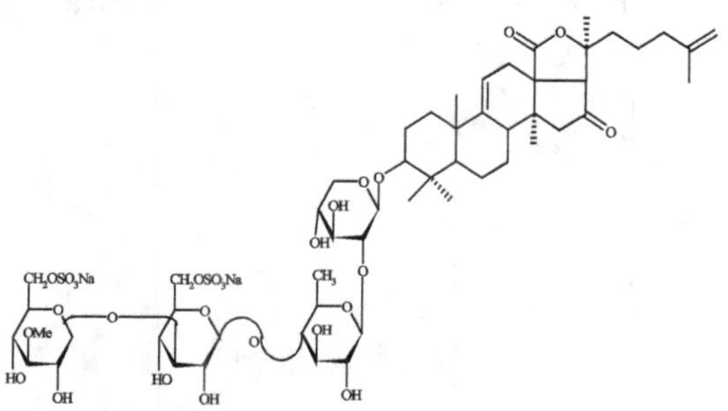

Anticancer marine drugs

Compound	Source	Chemistry	Use	Structure
Ecteinascidin	Caribbean tunicate *Ecteinascidia turbinata*	Alkaloid	Anticancer	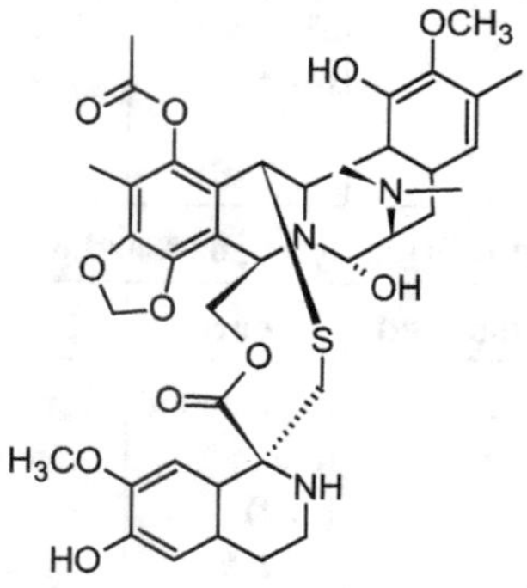 Ecteinascidin-743 (Eribulin, Yondelis)
Dolastatin 10	Sea hare *Dolabella auricularia*	Amine	Anaplastic large cell lymphoma (ALCL) and Hodgkin's lymphoma	Dolastatin 10 and related analogs found to be too toxic, cause peripheral neuropathy, and lack efficacy in the treatment of cancer. Hence, monoclonal antibody conjugated drug, brentuximab vendotin, is marketed as Ascentris®, and has been approved for treating anaplastic large cell lymphoma (ALCL) and Hodgkin's lymphoma.

Contd...

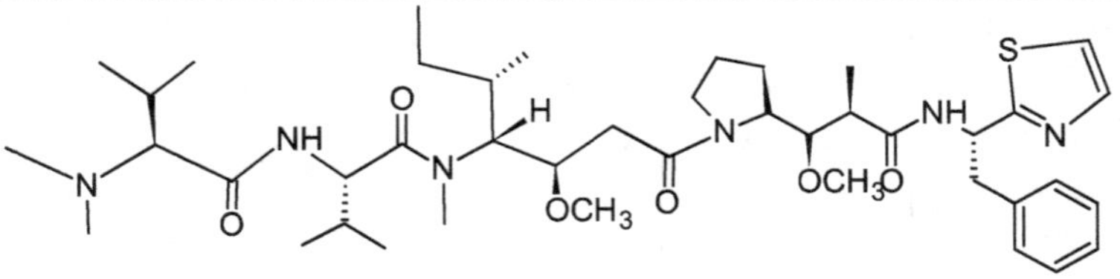 Dolastatin 10 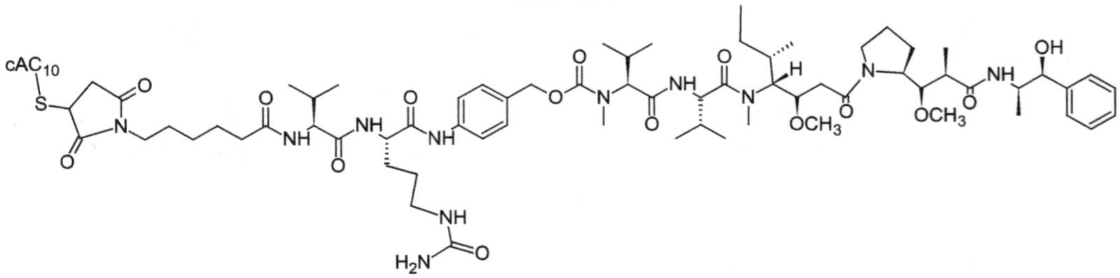 Brentuximab vedotin (Ascentris)				
Halichondrin B	Sea sponge *Halichondria okadai*	Lactones	Breast carcinoma 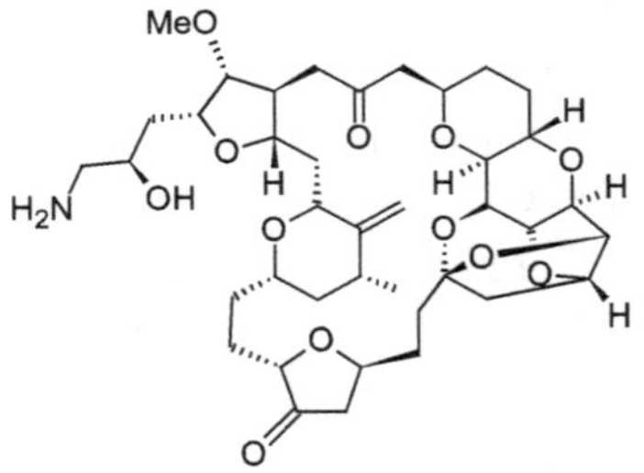 E789(Halaven) 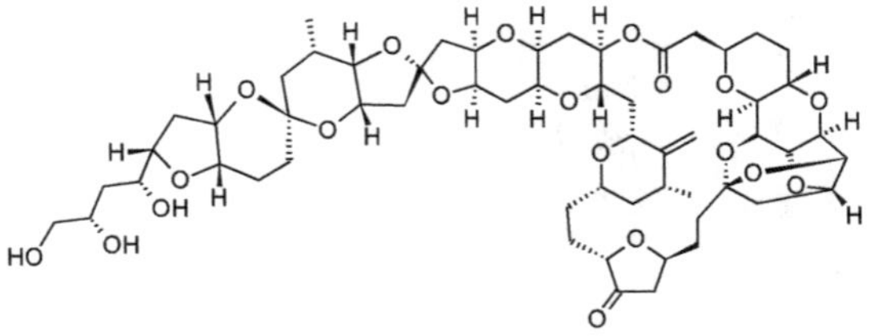 Halichondrin B	
Salinosporamide A	Marine genus of streptomycete bacteria known as *Salinispora*	Alkaloid	Multiple myeloma	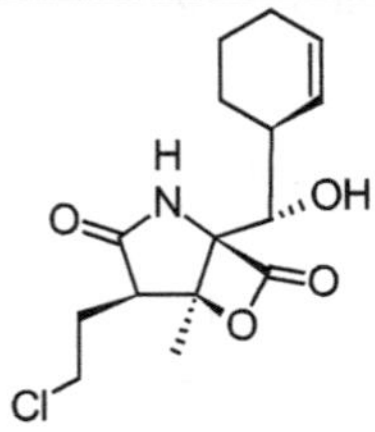 Salinosporamide A

Contd...

Crassin acetate	Cembranoids (Invertebrates like thick welvet type) *Pseudoplexaura porosa*	Cyclic diterpenes	In vitro human leukemia and Hela Cells	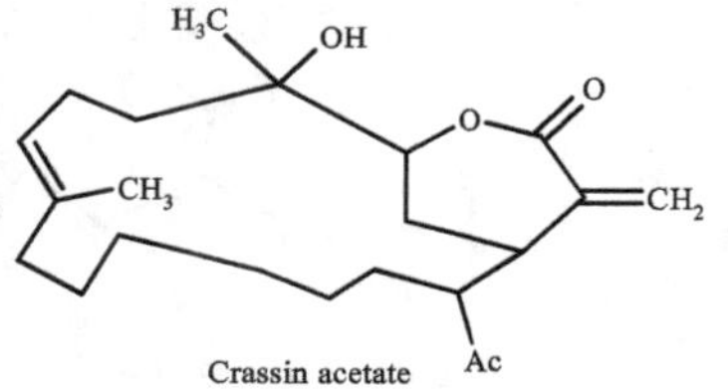 Crassin acetate
Ara-C (cytosine arabinoside)	Carribbean sponges	Synthetic compound based on knowledge of spongosine	Carcinaoma, sarcoma	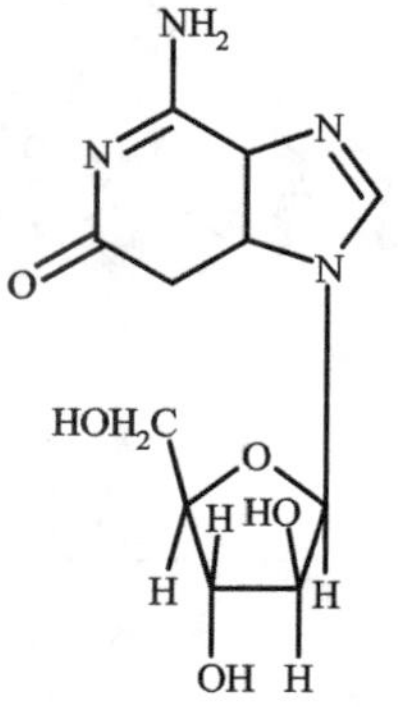 Ara-C
Simularin	Soft coral *Sinularia flexibilis*	Cembranoids (14-C cyclic diterpenoid with exocyclic lactone)	Anticancer	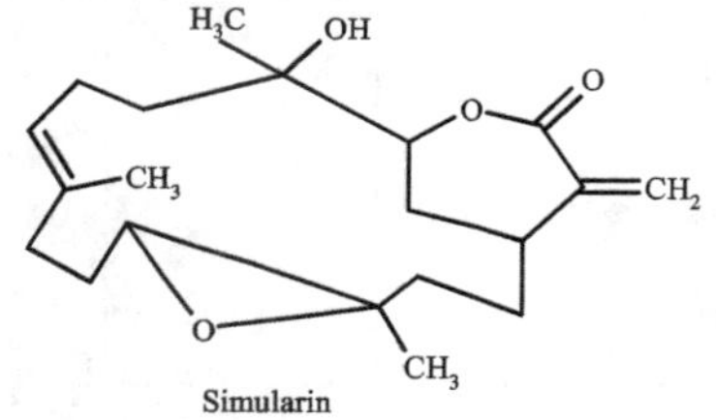 Simularin
Asperdiol	from gorgonian coral *Euniceaknighti*	Non lactone cembranoid	leukemia	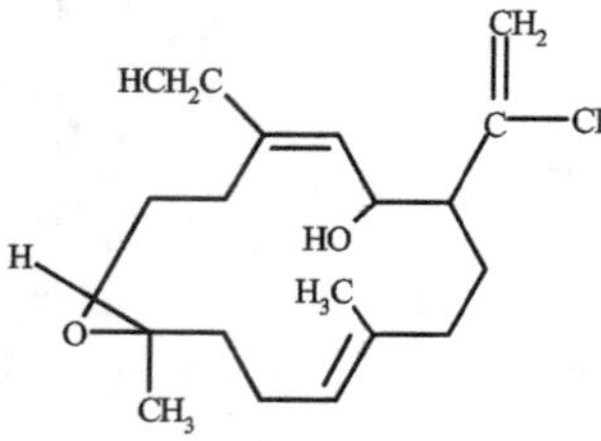 Asperdiol
Geranyl Hydroquinone	*Aplidium* species	Quinone	Anticancer	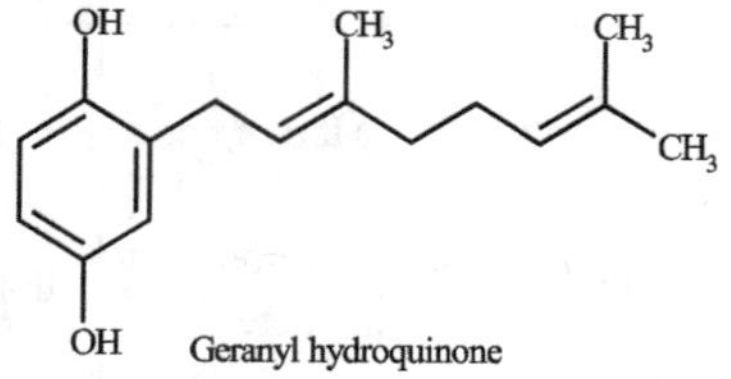 Geranyl hydroquinone

Contd...

Anti-inflammatory marine drugs

Compound	Source	Chemistry	Use	Structure
Manolide	*Songe Luffariella variabilis*	Phospholipase A2 inhibitor sester terpene	Analgesic and anti-inflam-matory	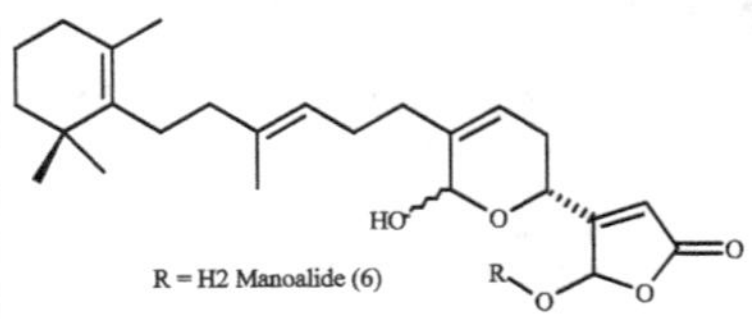 R = H2 Manoalide (6)
Dendalone 3 hydroxy butyrate	*Songe Phyllospongia dendyi*	Terpenoid	Anti-inflam-matory	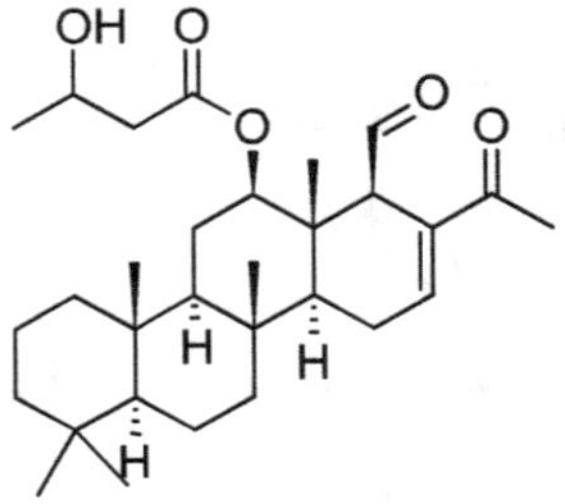 Dendalone 3 hydroxy butyrate
Flexibilide	*Soft coral Sinularia flexibilis*	Diterpenoid cembrane	Anti-inflam-matory	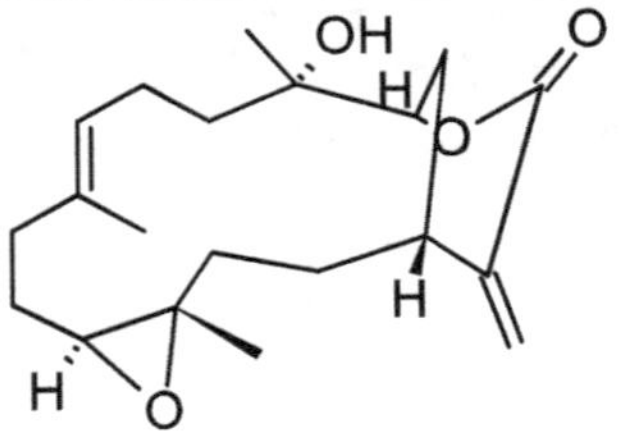 Flexibilide

Antimicrobial marine drugs

Compound	Source	Chemistry	Use	Structure
Zoranol and iso-zoranol	Dctyopteris zonaroides (Brown Algae)	Flavonoid	Antimicrobial	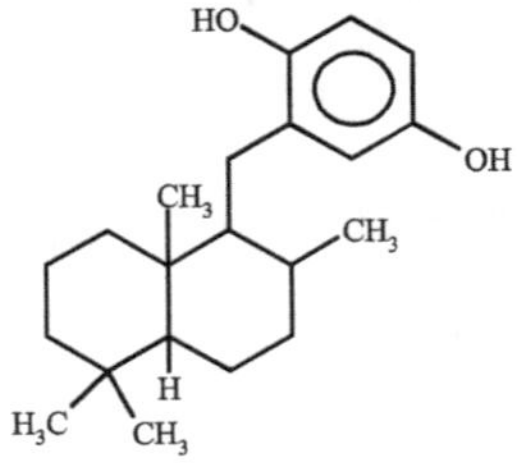 Zonarol
Thelpin	Annelida, *Thelepus setosus*	Bromophenol compound	Antimicrobial	
Eunicin	Gorgonian corals, *Eunicia mammosa*	Diterpene	Antimicrobial	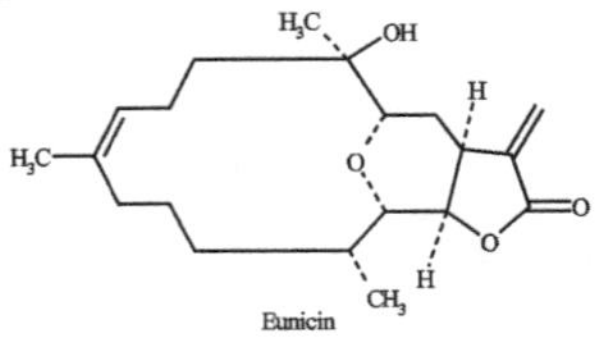 Eunicin

Antibiotic marine drugs				
Compound	**Source**	**Chemistry**	**Use**	**Structure**
Cycloeudesmol	Red algae Chondria oppositiclada	Eudesmol (sesquiterpenoid)	Antibiotic	Cycloendesmol
variabilin	Sponge, Ircinia oros	Furanos ester terpene	Antibiotic	Variabilin

Anthelmintic marine drugs				
Compound	**Source**	**Chemistry**	**Use**	**Structure**
Kainic acid	Red algae Digenia simplex	Pyrrolidine-2-carboxylic acid	Antiascaria tic activity	Kainic acid
Domoic acid	Red algae Chondria armata	Heterocyclic amino acid	Antiascaria tic activity	Domoic acid

Marine toxins

Compound	Source	Chemistry	Use
Palytoxin	Zoanthids like *Palythoa toxica*	Non-peptide substances	Intense vasoconstrictor
Didemnins A-E, G, X and Y	Caribbean tunicate (sea squirt) of the genus *Trididemnum solidum*	Depsipeptides	Antiviral agent
Anatoxins	Blue-green alga *Anabaena flosaquae*	Alkaloid	Agonist for the nicotinic acetyl-choline receptor
Ciguatoxin	*Gambierdiscus toxicus*, a type of dinoflagellate	lipid-soluble polyether compounds	Lowers the threshold for opening voltage-gated sodium channels in synapses of the nervous system. The condition is known as ciguatera.

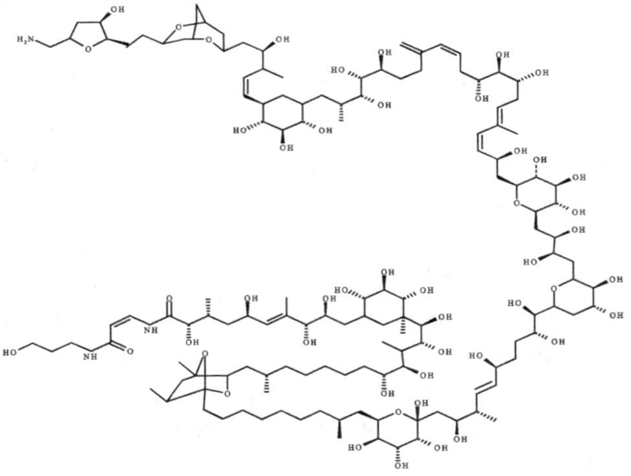

Palytoxin

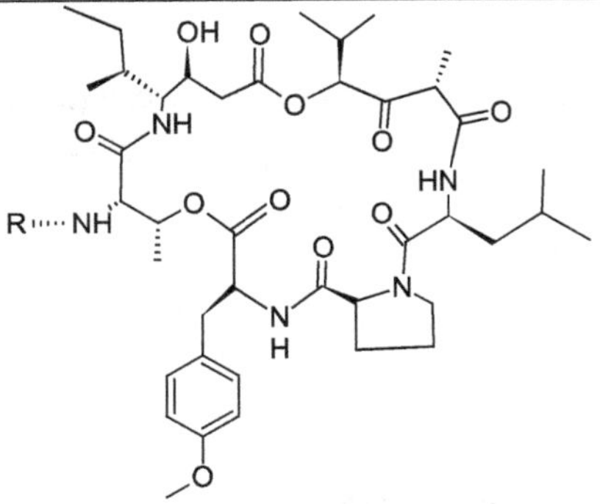

Didemnin A   R = N-Me-L-Leu
Didemnin B   R = Lac-Pro-N-Me-L-Leu
Didemnin C   R = Lac N-Me-L-Leu

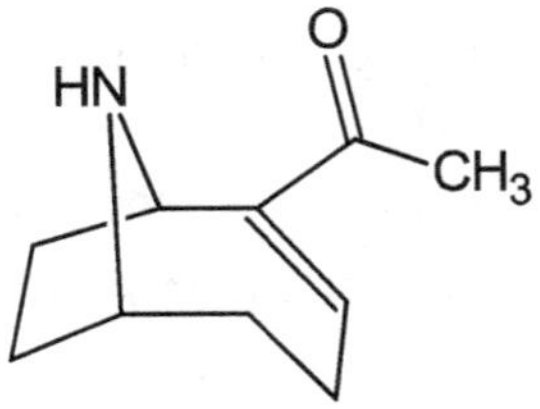

Anatoxin

Ciguatoxin

Subjective Questions

1. Give account on biological source, chemical nature and uses of fibers?

2. Give account on biological source, chemical nature and uses of Hallucinogens?

3. Give account on biological source, chemical nature and uses of Teratogens?

4. Give account on biological source, chemical nature and uses of Natural allergens?

5. Give account on sources, chemistry, preparation, evaluation, preservation, and storage, therapeutic used and commercial utility of Agar/Tragacanth / Honey.

6. Give account on sources, chemistry, preparation, evaluation, preservation, storage, therapeutic used and commercial utility of Proteins: Gelatin or casein

7. Give account on sources, chemistry, preparation, evaluation, preservation, storage, therapeutic used and commercial utility of Proteolytic enzymes: Papain, bromelain, serratiopeptidase, urokinase, streptokinase, pepsin

8. Give account on sources, chemistry, preparation, evaluation, preservation, storage, therapeutic used and commercial utility of Lipids(Waxes, fats, fixed oils) : Castor oil, Chaulmoogra oil, Wool Fat, Bees Wax

9. Give account on sources, chemistry, preparation, evaluation, preservation, storage, therapeutic used and commercial utility of Marine Drugs: Novel medicinal agents from marine sources

10. What is chemical difference between fats and waxes?

11. Differentiate agar and tragacanth based on chemical testing?

12. Differentiate between reducing and non reducing sugar.

13. Explain saturated and non non-saturated lipid.

14. Differentiate between essential and non-essential Amino acids.

15. Write a note on essential fatty acids.

Multiple Choice Questions (MCQs)

1. How much amount of cellulose is present in raw cotton?
   a. 90 -94%
   b. 95 – 99%
   c. 80 -85%
   d. 95 -100%

2. Absorbent cotton wool I.P has standard water soluble extractive value
   a. Not more than 0.5%
   b. Not more than 0.1%
   c. Not more than 1%
   d. Not more than 1.5%

3. Which of the following reagent is used to differentiate between raw cotton and absorbant cotton?
   a. Cuoxam reagent
   b. Dragendroff's reagent
   c. Hagger's reagent
   d. Wagner's reagent

4. Cotton is soluble in
   a. 60% sulphuric acid
   b. 60% hydrochloric acid
   c. 66% sulphuric acid
   d. 66% hydrochloric acid

5. Biological source of jute is
   a. Corchorus capsularis Linn.
   b. Corchorus capsularious Linn
   c. Corchorus olitorious Linn.
   d. Both a and c

6. How much amount of cellulose is present in jute?
   a. 53%
   b. 54%
   c. 55%
   d. 56%

7. The jute plants grows successfully in areas having ……….soil with pH values …………..
   a. Coarse sand, 4-5
   b. Clay, 7-8
   c. Loamy alluvial soil, 6-8
   d. Black soil, 6-7

8. Gunny bags are prepared from
   a. Cotton
   b. Silk
   c. Jute
   d. wool

9. Biological source of hemp is
   a. Dried flowering tops of female plants of *Cannabis sativa*
   b. Dried seeds of female plant *Cannabis sativa*
   c. Dried flowering tops of male plants of *Cannabis sativa*
   d. Dried seeds of male plant *Cannabis sativa*

10. Only female plants of Cannabis are used in preparation of narcotics because
    a. Resinous material is formed only in femele fertilized plants
    b. Resinous material is formed only in femele unfertilized plants
    c. Both a and b
    d. None of the above

11. In Indian hemp, resin is present in
    a. Seeds
    b. Leaves
    c. Glandular trichomes
    d. flowers

12. Cannabis posses psychotropic properties due to
    a. Cannabinol
    b. Cannabinolic acid
    c. Cannabidiol
    d. Tetrahydrocannbinol

13. Which one of the following is resinous exudation of leaves of the hemp plants?
    a. Bhang
    b. Ganja
    c. Chars
    d. Heroin

14. Substances which causes physical or functional defects in the human embryo or fetus after the pregnant woman is exposed to the substance is called as
    a. Keratogenes
    b. Teratogenes
    c. Heterogenes
    d. None of the above

15. Which one of the following glycoside shows teratogenic activity?
    a. Cardiac glycosides
    b. Anthraquinones glycosides
    c. Flavonoids
    d. Both a and b

16. Which one of the following medicinal plant exerts teratogenic activity?
    a. Ginger
    b. Castor oil
    c. Senna
    d. All of the above

17. Substances of natural origin which causes hypersensitivity in human being are known as
    a. Natural teratogens
    b. Natural allergens
    c. Both a and b
    d. None o the above

18. Which one of the following serves as natural allergens?
    a. Pollen grains
    b. Moulds
    c. Dust particles
    d. All of the above

19. What is pet dander which may cause allergy to person?
    a. Animal hair that has been shed
    b. Microscopic particles of animal skin
    c. Invisible mites that live on animals
    d. Dust that has settled on animal skin

20. Allergenic extracts are prepared by using
    a. 100% glycerine as a diluents
    b. 50% glycerine as a diluents
    c. 60% glycerine as a diluents
    d. 70% glycerine as a diluents

21. Compounds that on hydrolysis produce either polyhydroxy aldehydes or polyhydroxy ketones are called as
    a. Carbohydrates
    b. Proteins
    c. Fats
    d. All of the above

22. Which one of the following is example of low molecular weight sugar with properties like crystalline, soluble in water and sweet in taste?
    a. Fructose
    b. Cellulose
    c. Starch
    d. Pectin

23. Gentianose present in Gentin root on hydroyis yields,
    a. Glucose+Fructose+Sucrose
    b. Glucose+Glucose+Fructose
    c. Glucose+Lactose+Sucrose
    d. Glucose+Glucose+Maltose

24. Rhamniose present in Rhubarb on hydrolysis yields
    a. Rham+rhamnose+Glucose
    b. Rham+rhamnose+ Fructose
    c. Rham+rhamnose+Gelactose
    d. Rham+rhamnose+ Galactose

25. Gums or mucilage as pathological products consisting of calcium, potassium and magnesium salts of complex substances are also known as
    a. Monouronoids
    b. Polyuronoids
    c. Diuronoids
    d. Triuronoids

26. Molisch's test is positive with
    a. Soluble carbohydrate
    b. Insoluble carbohydrate
    c. Both a and b
    d. None

27. Biological source of acacia is
    a. Dried gummy exudates
    b. Dried leaves
    c. Dried latex
    d. Dried milky exudates

28. Arabin is principle constituent of
    a. Tragacanth
    b. Agar
    c. Acacia
    d. Both a and b

29. Which one of the following is given intravenously in hemolysis?
    a. Tragacanth
    b. Guar gum
    c. Starch
    d. Gum acacia

30. *Astragalus gummifer L.* Family, Leguminosae is biological name of
    a. Gum acacia
    b. Tragacanth
    c. Guar gum
    d. None

31. In India, Agar is produced commercially in
    a. Costal regions of Bay of Bengal
    b. Costal regions of Maharashtra
    c. Costal regions of Tamilnadu
    d. None

32. Standard value of acid insoluble ash for agar is
    a. Not more than 0.5per cent
    b. Not more than 1.0 per cent
    c. Not more than 2.0 per cent
    d. Not more than 1.5 per cent

33. Granulated honey contains
    a. Crystalline sucrose
    b. Crystalline fructose
    c. Crystalline dextrose
    d. Crystalline glucose

34. Which one of the following enzyme is used for proteoysis of blood clots and necrotic tissue?
    a. Pepsin
    b. Trypsin
    c. Papain
    d. Pacreatin

35. Papain is obtained from latex of unripe fruit of
    a.   *Cannabis sativa*
    b.   *Carica papaya*
    c.   *Clostridium histoyticum*
    d.   *Bacillus subtilis*

36. Bloom strength is used to measure the quality of
    a.   Gum
    b.   Mucilage
    c.   Agar
    d.   Gelatin

37. What is diameter of plunger used to measure bloom strength of gelatin ?
    a.   12.7 mm
    b.   11.7 mm
    c.   12.7 cm
    d.   11.7 cm

38. Standard gel strength for gelatin is
    a.   150 – 250
    b.   250 – 300
    c.   100 - 150
    d.   150 – 200

39. Casein contains about ………….per cent phosphorus and ………………per cent sulphur.
    a.   0.85 and 0.70
    b.   0.80 and 0.75
    c.   0.85 and 0.75
    d.   None

40. Specific gravity of casein is
    a.   1.25 – 1.31
    b.   1.30 – 1.4
    c.   1.15 – 1.20
    d.   1.20 – 1.30

41. Biological source of bromelain is
    a.   *Carica papaya*
    b.   *Ananas comosus*
    c.   *Aspergillus*
    d.   *Clostridium histolyticum*

42. Which one of the following enzyme has property of activating human plasminogen to plasmin?
    a.   Papain
    b.   Casein
    c.   Pepsin
    d.   Streptokinase

43. Which one of the following enzyme is obtained from human urine and kidney cultures?
    a.   Streptokinase
    b.   Pepsin
    c.   Trypsin
    d.   Urokinase

21. Pepsin degrades proteins in to
    a.   Peptones
    b.   Proteases
    c.   Both a and b
    d.   None

44. The substances which remains liquid at temperature 15.5 – 16.5°C are called as
    a.   Fats
    b.   Fixed oils
    c.   Waxes
    d.   None

45. Caproic acid is obtained from
    a.   Palm kernel oil
    b.   Palm oil
    c.   coconut oil
    d.   Peanut oil

46. Fixed oils and fats can be confirmed by chemical tests using
    a.   Sodium hydroxide
    b.   Sodium hydrogen sulphate
    c.   Sulphuric acid
    d.   Hydrochloric acid

47. Halphen's test is used for detection of
    a.   Seasom oil as an adulterant
    b.   Karanja oil as an adulterant
    c.   Castor oil as an adulterant
    d.   Cotton seed oil as an adulterant

48. Castor oil is derived from
    a. *Arachis hypogaea L.*
    b. *Hydnocarpus heterophylla*
    c. *Ricinus communis*
    d. None

49. Which one of the following oil exerts strong bactericidal effect against *Mycobacterium leprae* and *Mycobacterium tuberculosis*?
    a. Castor oil
    b. Chaulmoogra oil
    c. Lineed oil
    d. Both a and b

50. Choose correct option from following regarding principle active constituents of Chaulmoogra oil
    a. Chaulmoogric acid 27% + Hydnocarpic acid 48% +Gorlic acid
    b. Chaulmoogric acid 48% +Hydnocarpic acid 27% + Gorlic acid
    c. Gorlic acid 48% + Chaulmoogric acid 27% + Gorlic acid
    d. None

51. Chaulmoogra oil is administered in the form of
    a. Oral formulation
    b. Subcutneous injection
    c. Intramuscular injection
    d. Both b and c

52. Wool of the sheep *Ovis aries* Linn family Bovidae, is biological source of
    a. Lanolin
    b. Wool fat
    c. Lard
    d. Bees wax

53. Lanolin is
    a. Hydrous wool fat
    b. Anhydrous wool fat
    c. Both a and b
    d. None

54. Peroxide value of wool fat should be
    a. More than 20
    b. Not more than 20
    c. Less than 20
    d. Both b and c

55. Which one of the following is widely used as water absorbable ointment base in pharmaceuticals?
    a.   Spermaceti
    b.   Bees wax
    c.   Lanoin
    d.   Suet.

56. Cera flava is synonym of
    a.   Carnauba wax
    b.   Yellow bees wax
    c.   Spermaceti
    d.   None

57. The chief constituent of bees wax is
    a.   Palmitin
    b.   Myricin
    c.   stearin
    d.   Both a and b

58. Bees wax is commonly adultrated with
    a.   Colophony
    b.   Spermaceti
    c.   hard paraffin
    d.   all of the above

59. European bees wax differentiated from Indian bees wax by
    a.   High acid value of 17-22
    b.   Low acid value than 17-22
    c.   High ester value 17-22
    d.   Low ester value 17-22

60. Which one of the following marine drug exerted 35 times more potent cardio tonic activity than digoxin during preclinical study?
    a.   Anthopleurin
    b.   Eptatetrin
    c.   Laminine
    d.   Saxitoxin

61. Spongosine occurring in marine Caribbean sponge is naturally a
    a.   Ethoxy derivative of adenoine
    b.   Methoxy derivative of adenosine
    c.   Ethoxy derivative of guanine
    d.   Methoxy derivative of guanine

62. Which one of the following is non steroidal anti-inflammatory compound of marine origin?

    a. Manoalide

    b. Dendalone 3 hydroxy butyrate

    c. Both a and b

    d. Only a

63. Which one of the following compound of marine origin exerts strong antispasmodic activity?

    a. Tetradotoxin

    b. Saxitoxin

    c. Simularin

    d. None

Answer Key

1. a	2. a	3. a	4. c	5. a	6. a	7. c	8. c	9. a	10. B
11. c	12. d	13. c	14. b	15. b	16. d	17. b	18. d	19. a	20. b
21. d	22. a	23. b	24. d	25. b	26. c	27. a	28. c	29. d	30. b
31. a	32. b	33. b	34. c	35. a	36. d	37. b	38. a	39. c	40. a
41. b	42. d	43. d	44. c	45. b	46. a	47. b	48. d	49. c	50. b
51. a	52. d	55. b	54. c	55. d	56. c	57. b	58. b	59. d	60. a
61. a	62. b	63. c	64. a						

Further Readings

1. A.N.M. Alamgir. Therapeutic Use of Medicinal Plants and Their Extracts: Volume 1. [Pharmacognosy- Volume 1]. Springer International Publishing. 2017

2. Alice Kurian, M. Asha Sankar Medicinal Plants. New India Publishing Agency. 2007

3. Amritesh C. Shukla, Jayanta Kumar Patra, Gitishree Das. Advances in Pharmaceutical Biotechnology-Recent Progress and Future Applications. 2020

4. Ashutosh Kar. Pharmacognosy And Pharmacobiotechnology. New Age International (P) Limited. 2003

5. Ayurvedic pharmacopoeia of India Part-I vol.I, 2001.

6. Azhar Ali Farooqi, B. S. Sreeramu. Cultivation of Medicinal and Aromatic Crops. Universities Press (India) Pvt. Limited. 2004

7. Biren Shah, Avinash Seth. Textbook of Pharmacognosy and Phytochemistry. Elsevier Health Sciences. 2014

8. C. S. Shah, J. S. Qadry. A Textbook of Pharmacognosy. Messrs B.S. Shah 1971

9. C.K. Kokate, Purohit, Gokhlae. Text book of Pharmacognosy, 37th Edition, Nirali Prakashan, Pune. 2007

10. Chen, SL., Yu, H., Luo, HM. et al. Conservation and sustainable use of medicinal plants: problems, progress, and prospects. Chin Med 11, 37 (2016).

11. Chi-Tang Ho, Fereidoon Shahidi. Phytochemicals and Phytopharmaceuticals. AOCS Press.2000

12. Cultivation and Utilization of Medicinal Plants. Regional Research Laboratory, Council of Scientific & Industrial Research. 1982

13. Debra K.W. Topham, Mark S. Meskin, Stanley T. Omaye, Wayne R. Bidlack. Phytochemicals as Bioactive Agents. Taylor & Francis.2000

14. Deore SL, Khadabadi SS, Baviskar BA. Pharmacognosy and Phytochemistry-A Comprehensive Approach. PharmMed Press, Hyderabad. 2nd Edition, 2018.

15. Deore SL. Pharmacognosy and Phytochemistry: A Companion Handbook. PharmMed Press, Hyderabad. . 2nd Edition, 2017.

16. Derek J. Chadwick, Joan Marsh. Bioactive Compounds from Plants. Wiley. 2008

17. GS Kumar. KN Jayaveera. A Textbook of Pharmacognosy and Phytochemistry. S Chand & Company Limited. India. 2014.

18. Gunnar Samuelsson. Drugs of Natural Origin-A Textbook of Pharmacognosy. Apotekarsocieteten. 1999

19. H. Ansari. Essentials of Pharmacognosy. Second edition, Birla publications, New Delhi, 2007

20. H. Panda Medicinal Plants Cultivation & Their Uses. Asia Pacific Business Press. 2002

21. Hany El-Shemy. Aromatic and Medicinal Plants-Back to Nature. IntechOpen.2017

22. Indian Pharmacopeia 2018, Ghaziabad: Indian Pharmacopeia Commission; 2018.

23. J.C. Tarafdar, K.P. Tripathi, M. Kumar. Organic Agriculture. Scientific Publishers. 2012

24. James Bobbers, Marilyn KS, VE Tylor. Pharmacognosy & Pharmacobiotechnology. Williams & Wilkins. 1996.

25. Jean Bruneton. Pharmacognosy, Phytochemistry, Medicinal Plants. Technique & Documentation. 1999

26. John T. Arnason, John T. Romeo, Rachel Mata. Phytochemistry of Medicinal Plants. Springer US. 2013

27. K. Chopra. Medicinal Plants-Conservation, Cultivation and Utilization. Daya Publishing House. 2007

28. K. Mangathayaru. Pharmacognosy: An Indian perspective. Pearson Education India. 2013

29. Kaliya A. Text Book of Industrial Pharmacognosy. CBS Publishers & Distributors, Delhi. 2009

30. Kendall Jefferson. Pharmacognosy and Phytotherapy. Foster Academics.2019

31. Khadabadi SS, Deore SL, Baviskar BA. Experimental Phytopharmacognosy. Nirali prakashan, Pune. 1st Edition, 2019.

32. Luqi Huang. Molecular Pharmacognosy. Springer Netherlands. 2012

33. Mallappa Kumara Swamy. Plant-derived Bioactives-Production, Properties and Therapeutic Applications. Springer Singapore. 2020

34. Michael Heinrich, Elizabeth M. Williamson, Joanne Barnes, Simon Gibbons, Jose Prieto-Garcia Fundamentals of Pharmacognosy and Phytotherapy E-Book. Elsevier Health Sciences. 2017

35. Michael Heinrich, Joanne Barnes, Simon Gibbons. Fundamentals of Pharmacognosy and Phytotherapy. Churchill Livingstone/Elsevier. 2012

36. Mohammad Ali. Text book of Pharmacognosy. CBS Publishers & Distribution, New Delhi.2019

37. N P S Sengar, Ashwini Singh, Ritesh Agrawal. A Textbook of Pharmacognosy. PharmaMed Press. 2018

38. Nirmal Joshee, Prahlad Parajuli, Sadanand A. DhekneyMedicinal Plants-From Farm to Pharmacy. Springer International Publishing. 2019

39. R Endress, Plant cell Biotechnology, Springer-Verlag, Berlin, 1994.

40. Rainer Fischer, Stefan Schillberg. Molecular Farming-Plant-made Pharmaceuticals and Technical Proteins. Wiley. 2006

41. Rajesh Arora. Medicinal Plant Biotechnology. CABI. 2010.

42. Rangari VD. Pharmacognosy& Phytochemistry. Career Publication, Nashik. 2008

43. Ravindra Sharma. Agro-Techniques of Medicinal Plants. Daya Publishing House. 2004.

44. S. P. Vyas, V. Dixit. Pharmaceutical Biotechnology. CBS Publishers & Distributors. 2018.

45. S. S. Agarwal, M. Paridhavi. Herbal Drug Technology. Universities Press. 2012

46. S. S. Handa. Pharmacognosy. Vallabh Prakashan, New Delhi. 1989

47. S. S. Purohit, S. P. Vyas.A Scientific Approach: Including Processing and Financial Guidelines. Agrobios (India). 2004

48. Saikat Sen, Raja Chakraborty Herbal Medicine in India-Indigenous Knowledge, Practice, Innovation and Its Value. Springer Singapore. 2019

49. Saurabh Bhatia, Kiran Sharma, Randhir Dahiya, Tanmoy Bera. Modern Applications of Plant Biotechnology in Pharmaceutical Sciences. Elsevier Science. 2015

50. Serdar Oztekin, Milan Martinov. Medicinal and Aromatic Crops-Harvesting, Drying, and Processing. CRC Press. 2014

51. Simone Badal Mccreath. Rupika Delgoda. Pharmacognosy-Fundamentals, Applications and Strategies. Elsevier Science. 2017

52. T. C. Denston. A Textbook of Pharmacognosy. Read Books. 2012

53. The British Pharmacopeia. London: Medicines and Healthcare Products Regulatory Agency; 1993.

54. United States Pharmacopoeia and National Formulary, USP 25 NF 19/National Formulary 20, Rockville, MD, U. S. Pharmacopoeial Convention, Inc. 2002.

55. V. Prakash, N. Tripathi. Basic Concepts of Plant Biotechnology (With MCQ's). Scientific Publishers - Competition Tutor. 2018

56. W.C.Evans, Trease and Evans Pharmacognosy, 16th edition, W.B. Sounders & Co., London, 2009.

57. Website-pps.who.int/iris/handle/10665/42783

58. WHO Guidelines on Good Agricultural and Collection Practices (GACP) for Medicinal Plants By World Health Organization, WHO · 2003

Part – II
Practical Manual

Know Subject: Pharmacognosy

The term 'pharmacognosy' (combination of two Greek words i.e. *pharmakon* means drug and *gnosis* means knowledge) means acquiring knowledge of drugs was coined in 1815 by C. A. Seydler, German medical student in his thesis title *"Analyetica Pharmacognostica"*. Pharmacognosy is defined as scientific and systematic study of structural, physical, chemical and biological characters of crude drugs along with history, method of cultivation, collection and preparation for the market. The American Society of Pharmacognosy defines pharmacognosy as "the study of the physical, chemical, biochemical and biological properties of drugs, drug substances or potential drugs or drug substances of natural origin as well as the search for new drugs from natural sources. It is also called as study of crude drugs.

Thus pharmacognostical studies of plant drugs involves study of synonyms, vernacular names, Biological sources, distribution, morphology, histology, chemistry, qualitative test, various physicochemical tests, pharmacological actions along with commercial varieties, substitutes, adulterants and any other quality control parameters of the drugs.

However, this subject is as old as pharmacy and mankind evolution; recently it is evolved as a multidisciplinary subject focusing many modern disciplines like ethanobotany, ethanopharmcology, phytotherapy, phytochemistry, chemo-taxanomy, biotechnology, clinical trials, herbal drug interaction and even novel drug delivery systems like phytosomes rather only botanical and taxanomical descriptions. Recent advances in extraction methods, analytical hyphenated techniques, screening methods continues to hasten major changes in this subject. Modernization of conventional and/or traditional dosage forms is opening doors to industrial Pharmacognosy.

Due to most recent technologies and innovative chemical concepts, many new drugs or drug candidates still originated from natural products or derivatives thereof. Even in this era of nanotechnology, natural drugs are important part of primary health care which is giving pharmacognosy professionals new possibilities to exploit the huge diversity designed and generated by nature.

There is a shortage of established scientists engaged in pharmacognosy research, which tends to involve subject matter beyond the conventional scientist's knowledge base. Hence, actual secret of opportunities in pharmacognosy research is that only the tip of the iceberg seems to have been discovered yet.

Following materials are required for Pharmacognosy laboratory work.

- Napkin
- Needle
- Filter paper
- Camel hair brushes
- Stains
- slip
- Watch glass
- A sharp razor blades
- Forceps
- Micro-slide
- Cover

Instructions for Students

Students shall read the points given below for understanding theoretical concepts and practical applications.

1. Students should wear white Apron, Cap, Mask, Gloves and Slipper before entering in to laboratory.

2. Students should keep their belongings in locker which are not required during practical like bag, Extra files etc.

3. Students should always carry Laboratory Manual, rough notebook, and practical requirements without fail.

4. Listen carefully to the lecture given by teacher about importance of subject, curriculum philosophy, graphical structure, skills to be developed, information about equipment, instruments, procedure, method of continuous assessment, tentative plan of working laboratory and total amount of work to be done in a year.

5. Students should perform the practical only at the place which allocated to him/her. (No change can be done without permission of subject teacher)

6. Students shall undergo study visit of laboratory for types of equipment, instruments, material to be used, before performing experiment

7. Read write up of each experiment to be performed, a day in advance.

8. Organize the work in the group and make a record of all observations.

9. Understand the purpose of experiment and its practical applications.

10. Write the answer of the questions allotted by teacher during practical hours if possible or afterwards, but immediately.

11. Students should not hesitate to ask any difficulty faced during conduct of practical.

12. The students shall study all the questions given in the laboratory manual and practice to write the answers to these questions

13. Students shall develop maintenance skill as expected by the industries.

14. Students should develop the habits of pocket discussion, group discussion related to the experiments so that exchanges of knowledge, skills could take place.

15. Students shall attempt to develop related hands on skills and gain confidence.

16. Students shall visit nearby workshops, workstation, industries, technical exhibitions, trade fair etc. even not included in the lab manual. In short, students should have exposure to the area of work right in the student's hood.

17. Students shall insist for the completion of recommended laboratory work, industrial visits, answers to the given questions, etc

18. Students shall develop habits of evolving more ideas, innovations skills etc. than included in the scope of manual

19. Students shall develop technical magazines, proceedings of seminars, refers websites related to the scope of the subjects and update their knowledge and skills.

20. Students should develop the habit of not to depend totally on the teachers but to develop self learning techniques

21. Students should develop the habit to react with the teacher without hesitation with respect to the academic involved.

22. Students should develop the habit to submit the practical exercise continuously and progressively on the scheduled dated and should get the assessment done

23. Student should be well prepared while submitting the write up of the experiments. This will develop the continuity of the studies and he will be over laded at the end of the term.

24. Students should clean platform before leaving the laboratory.

Index

Sr. No	Aim	Date	Page	Marks	Sign
1	To perform analysis of crude drugs by chemical tests				
2	To determine stomatal number and stomatal index of given leaf crude drug				
3	To determine vein-islet number of given leaf crude drug- Indian senna (Cassia angustifolia				
4	To determine vein-termination number of given leaf crude drug- Indian senna (*Cassia angustifolia*)				
5	To determine palisade ratio of given leaf crude drug- Indian senna (*Cassia angustifolia*				
6	To determine percentage purity by *Lycopodium* spore method				
7	To measure size of starch grain by eye piece micrometer in a given crude drug powder				
8	To measure size of calcium crystals by eye piece micrometer in a given crude drug powder				
9	To measure length of phloem fibers in given crude drug powder				
10	To determine different ash values as per IP				
11	To determine different extractive values as per IP				
12	To determine moisture content by Loss on Drying (LOD) method				
13	To Determine Swelling Index of a given Crude Drug-Isapgol				
14	To Determine Foaming Index of Saponin containing Crude Drug-Licorice				
15	To Determine Foaming Index of Saponin containing Crude Drug- Safed musali				
	Further Reading				

Aim 01: To perform analysis of crude drugs by chemical tests: (i) Acacia (ii) Agar (iii) Castor oil (iv) Gelatin (v) Honey (vi) Starch (vii) Tragacanth

Requirements: All pharmacognosy chemical tests reagents, test tubes, Gas burners, water bath

Theory: The unorganized drugs possess no specific cellular structure but consist of extracts, exudation, secretions, latex and other products of the plants. These may be solid, semi-solid or liquid. Physical and chemical parameters are most important in identification of unorganized drugs.

Excipient	Morphology and Chemical analysis tests		Observation
Acacia/ Indian Gum/ Acasia, Babul or kikar gond(Hindi) ***Biological Source:*** Dried gummy exudation obtained from the stem and branches of *Acacia arabica* belonging to family Leguminoseae *Use:* Pharmaceutical aid, binding, emulsifying agent, suspending agent, demulcent	Colour: Tears are cream brown to red in colour, powder is light brown in colour Odour: Odourless Taste: Bland and mucilaginous Size and shape: Irregular brown tears of varying size Extra features: Tears with minute fissures, brittle in nature, glossy and occasionally iridescent		
	Take 5 ml of 2% w/v solution and add 1 ml of strong lead subacetate solution.	Flocculent white precipitate	
	Take 5% aqueous solution; add 0.5 ml hydrogen peroxide solution and 0.5 ml of 1% alcoholic benzidine. Shake well and allow to stand for 5 minutes.	Deep blue color	
	Treat powder with ruthenium red solution and examine microscopically.	No red color indicates that it is different from agar	
	Take 10 ml of 2% w/v solution and add 0.2 ml of 20% w/v lead acetate solution.	No precipitation indicates it is different from agar and tragacanth	
	Take 0.1 g of powder and add 1 ml of N/50 iodine to it.	No crimson color indicates that it is different from agar and tragacanth	
	Take 1 ml of solution, add 4 ml of water, and dilute hydrochloric acid; boil for few min. Add Fehling's solution and heat.	Red precipitate of cuprous oxide	

Contd...

Agar/ Agar – agar/ Japanese Isinglass ***Biological Source:*** Dried gelatinous substance, obtained from *Gelidium amansii, G. Cartilagineum, G. Pristodes, Gracilaria confervoides, pteocladialucida, P. Capollacea* and other closely allied members of Family. Rhodophyceae ***Uses:*** Bulk laxative, Pharmaceutical aid , in the preparation of culture media	**Morphology:** Strips: Colourless, slender, translucent, 4 mm wide Bands: Yellowish, 4 cm wide Sheets: 45-60 cm long and 10-15 cm wide Flakes or Course Powder: Greyish white, odourless Taste : Mucilaginous Solubility: Practically insoluble in cold water, but swells to gelatinous mass. Soluble in boiling water.	
	Take aqueous solution and add ruthenium red.	Red color
	Take aqueous solution and add N/50 iodine.	Deep crimson to brown color
	Take 5% aqueous solution; and add 5 ml of dilute hydrochloric acid and heat on water bath for 30 min. Add to the first part, 3 ml of 10% caustic soda solution and 2 ml of Fehling solution. Heat on water bath.	Reduction takes place due to galactose
	Take 5% aqueous solution and add 5 ml of dilute hydrochloric acid, and heat on water bath for 30 min. Add barium chloride solution (10%) to second part.	White precipitate of barium sulphate
	Prepare ash of Agar, add dilute hydrochloric acid, and observe under microscope.	Skeleton and sponge spicules of diatoms will be observed.
	Take 5% aqueous solution and add tannic acid to it.	No precipitate
Castor oil /Ricinus oil ***Biological Source:*** The fixed oil obtained by cold expression from kernels of seeds of *Ricinus communis* Linn Family : Euphorbiaceae	**Morphology** Colour: Pale yellow or almost colourless liquid Odour : Nauseating Taste: First bland, then slightly acrid and usually nauseating Extra features : A viscous and transparent liquid	
	Completely miscible with half of its volume of light petroleum ether	
	Oil + equal volume of alcohol = Clear liquid. Cool at 0°C	Clear liquid for three hours.
	Acidified petroleum ether + oil; shake, add a drop of ammonium molybdate	white turbidity

Contd...

Gelatin ***Biological Source:*** A protein extracted by partial hydrolysis of animal collagenous tissue like skin, tendons, ligaments and bones with boiling water ***Uses:*** Pharmaceutical aid, capsule shell preparation; in pessaries, plasters etc	**Morphology** Colour: Colourless or pale yellow Odour: Very slight Taste: Characteristic and bouillon like. Shape: Translucent sheets, flakes, shred or a course to fine powder. Solubility: Insoluble in cold water but swells and softens, absorbs water but soluble in hot water forms jelly on cooling.	
	Heat a small quantity of gelatin with soda lime.	Ammonia is evolved
	Take 0.5% aqueous solution and add a few drops of 10% tannic acid.	White precipitate
	Take 0.5% aqueous solution and add Millon's Reagent.	White precipitate which becomes red on heating
	Take 0.5% aqueous solution and add 10% picric acid solution to it.	Yellow precipitate
Honey Madhu (Hindi) Honey purified, Mel. ***Biological Source:*** A sugar secretion deposited in honey comb by the bee, *Apis dorsata*, and other species of *Apis* e.g. A Indica, A florea etc Family: Apidae ***Uses:*** Sweetening agent	**Morphology** Colour: Pale yellow or yellowish brown. Odour: Characteristic , Pleasant Taste: sweet and faintly acrid Extra features: Syrup thick liquid translucent when fresh, then opaque and granular due to the crystallization of glucose	
	Fehling solution test	Red ppt
	Fiehe's test: It is used to detect adulteration of honey with invert sugar (Acid hydrolyzed sugar). It actually detects the presence of HMF (Hydroxymethyl furfural) content in honey. Invert sugar has high HMF content whereas, honey has lesser HMF content (around 10 mg/kg). Fiehe's reagent (seliwanoff reagent) which contains Resorcinol and HCL gives Cherry Red colour on reacting with Furfural.	Cherry Red colour

Contd...

Starch It comprises polysac-charide obtained from fully grown grains of Corn [*Zea mays* Linn.]; Rice [*Oryza sativa* Linn.]; and Wheat [*Triticum aestivum* Linn.] belonging to the family *Gramineae* and also from the tubers of Potato [*Solanum tuberosum* Linn.] family *Solanaceae*. **Uses:** It is used as absorbent, demulcent and employed as a disintegrating agent, diluent (or filler) and lubricant.	**Morphology** **Color: White** **Odor: Odorless** **Taste: Characteristic called as starchy** **Shape and Size** • Corn [*Zea mays* Gramineae] : Round poly-hedral of 5-35 um, distinct centric hilum, stria-tions absent • Wheat [*Triticum aestivum* Gramineae] : Lenti-cular or oval in shape of 5-50 um, concentric hilum, faint striations • Potato [*Solanum tuberosum* Solanaceae] : • Irregularly ovoid and sub spherical, 20-100um, eccentric hilum, distinct striations • Rice [*Oryza sativa*, Gramineae] : • Polyhedral, of 2-12 um, minute centric hilum, striations absent	
	Boil 1 g of starch with 15 ml of water and cool.	The translucent viscous jelly is produced.	
	Add solution of iodine to starch powder.	The blue colour disappears on warming and reappears on cooling.	
Tragacanth/ Gum ***Biological Source:*** Tragacanth Dried gummy exudation obtained by incision from stems and branches of *Astrogalus gummifer* Labill and other species of Astragalus Family : Leguminosae ***Uses:*** Pharmaceutical aid; Demulcent, emollient, laxative.	Morphology Colour : White or pale yellowish - white flakes. Odour : Odourless Taste: Tasteless Shape: Thin flattered ribbon like flakes Size: Flakes are 25 × 12 × 2 mm. Solubility : Partly soluble in water, swells, insoluble in alcohol	
	Take 4 ml of 0.5% w/v solution; add 0.5 ml of hydrochloric acid and heat it for 30 min on a water bath; add 1.5 ml of sodium hydroxide solution and Fehling's solution, Heat solution using water bath.	Red precipitate	
	Take 4 ml of 0.5% w/v solution; add 0.5 ml of hydrochloric acid and heat for 30 min on a water bath; add 10% barium chloride solution.	No precipitate indicates it is different from agar	

Contd...

Take 0.5% w/v solution of the gum and add 20% w/v solution of lead acetate.	Flocculent precipitate is obtained which indicates it is different from acacia	
Treat powder with ruthenium red solution and examine microscopically.	No pink color (distinction from Indian tragacanth)	
Treat powder with N/50 iodine solution.	Olive green color (distinction from acacia and agar)	
Warm powder with 5% aqueous caustic potash (KOH).	Canary yellow color	

Results: All given crude drugs are analysed by chemical tests.

Questions:

1. How to differentiate between Agar and Acacia based on chemical testing?
2. What is Fiehe's test?
3. How to detect adulteration in Honey?
4. How to differentiate Indian tragacanth from Gum Tragacanth?

Aim 02: To determine stomatal number and stomatal index of given leaf crude drug.- Datura [*Datura stramonium*]

Requirements: Microscope, slides, brush, glycerin, water, camera lucida, black drawing sheet, white colored pencil, scale.

Theory: Stomatal number is average number of stomata per square mm of epidermis of the leaf. Stomatal index is percentage of the number of stomata forms to the total number of epidermal cells; each stoma also being counted as one epidermal cell.

Procedure: Clear the piece of the leaf (middle part) by boiling with chloral hydrate solution or alternatively with chlorinated soda. Peel out upper and lower epidermis separately by means of forceps. Keep it on slide and mount in glycerin water. Arrange a camera lucida and drawing board (black paper) for making drawings to scale. Draw a square of 1 mm by means of stage micrometer on black colored drawing paper using white pencil. Place the slide with cleared leaf (epidermis) on the stage. Trace the epidermis cell and stomata. Count the number of stomata present in the area of 1 sq. mm. Include the cell if at least half of its area lies within the square. Record the result for each of the ten fields and calculate the average number of stomata per sq. mm. To calculate stomatal index, count the number of stomata, as well as the number of epidermal cells in each field. Calculate the stomatal index using the above formula. Determine the values for upper and lower surface (epidermis) separately.

$$\text{Stomatal index} = \frac{\text{Stomatal number}}{\text{Total number of stomata + Total number of epidemal cells}} \times 100$$

Observation/Calculations:

No. of Field	Readings Upper Epidermis		Readings Lower Epidermis	
	Stomatal number	Stomatal index	Stomatal number	Stomatal index
1				
2				
3				
4				
5				
6				
7				
8				
9				
10				
Average				
Range				

Results: Stomatal number and Stomatal index determined for given sample of crude drug
..........................and found as follows:

Parameter	Details	Calculated Value	Standard value mentioned Pharmacopoeia or published research paper	Remark (Authentic or adulterated sample of crude drug)
Stomatal number	Upper epidermis		59-140	
	Lower Epidermis		145-255	
Stomatal index	Upper epidermis		20.3-26.2	
	Lower Epidermis		19.7-27.7	

Questions

1. What is stomata?
2. What are different types of stomata?
3. What are key steps in determination of stomatal number and index?
4. Define stomatal number.
5. Define stomatal index.
6. Why do need to determine stomatal number and index of both upper and lower epidermis?

Aim 03: To determine vein-islet number of given leaf crude drug- Indian senna (Cassia angustifolia)

Requirements: Microscope, slides, brush, glycerin, water, camera lucida, black drawing sheet, white colored pencil, scale.

Theory: This is number of vein-islets per square mm of the leaf surface midway between midrib and margin.

Procedure: Clear a piece of the leaf by boiling in alkali solution for about 30 minutes. Arrange camera lucida and drawing board for making drawings to scale. Place stage micrometer on the microscope and using 16 mm objectives, draw a line equivalent to 1mm as seen through the microscope. Construct a square on this line. Move the paper so that the square is seen in the eye piece, in the centre of the field. Place the slide with the cleared leaf (epidermis on the stage). Trace off the veins which are included within the square, completing the outlines of those islets which overlap two adjacent sides of the square. Count the number of vein islets in the square millimeter. Where the islets are intersected by the sides of the square, include those on two adjacent sides and exclude those islets on the other sides. (To obtain a critical result for a leaf, 4 sq. mm. should be used, preferably in one large area of 4 sq. mm.). Find the range as well as average number of vein islets from the four adjoining squares, to get the values for one sq. mm.

Observation/Calculations:

No. of Field	Readings
	Vein-Islets
1	
2	
3	
4	
5	
6	
7	
8	
9	
10	
Average	
Range	

Results: Vein islet number determined for given sample of crude drug ....and found as follows:

Name of leaf crude drug	
Calculated Vein islet number	
Standard value mentioned Pharmacopoeia or published research paper for **Cassia angustifolia**	**19.5-22.5** **(Average 21)**
Remark (Authentic or adulterated sample of crude drug)	

Questions

1. What is vein-islet?
2. What are key steps in determination of veinlet number and vein-termination number?
3. What is significance of vein-islet number determination?

Aim 04: To determine vein-termination number of given leaf crude drug- Indian senna (*Cassia angustifolia*)

Requirements: Microscope, slides, brush, glycerin, water, alkali solution, camera lucida, black drawing sheet, white colored pencil, scale.

Theory: This is number of vein- termination per square mm of the leaf surface midway between midrib and margin.

Procedure: Clear a piece of the leaf by boiling in alkali solution for about 30 minutes. Arrange camera lucida and drawing board for making drawings to scale. Place stage micrometer on the microscope and using 16 mm objectives, draw a line equivalent to 1mm as seen through the microscope. Construct a square on this line. Move the paper so that the square is seen in the eye piece, in the centre of the field. Place the slide with the cleared leaf (epidermis on the stage). Trace off the veins which are included within the square, completing the outlines of those islets which overlap two adjacent sides of the square. Count the number of veinlet terminations present within the square. Calculate average number of veinlet termination number from the four adjoining squares, to get the values per square mm.

Observation/Calculations:

No. of Field	Readings
	Vein- termination
1	
2	
3	
4	
5	
6	
7	
8	
9	
10	
Average	
Range	

Results: Veinlet- termination number determined for given sample of crude drug ....and found as follows:

Name of leaf crude drug	
Calculated Vein- termination number	
Standard value mentioned Pharmacopoeia or published research paper for **Cassia angustifolia**	25.9-32.8 (Average-31.5)
Remark (Authentic or adulterated sample of crude drug)	

Questions

1. What is vein-termination?
2. What are key steps in determination of vein-termination number?
3. What is significance of vein-islet number determination?

Aim 05: To determine palisade ratio of given leaf crude drug- Indian senna (*Cassia angustifolia*)

Requirements: Microscope, slides, brush, glycerin, water, alkali solution, camera lucida, black drawing sheet, white colored pencil, scale.

Theory: This is an average number of palisade cells beneath each epidermal cell. It can be also determined with powdered drugs.

Procedure: Clear a piece of the leaf by boiling in alkali solution for about 30 minutes. Arrange camera lucida and drawing board for making drawings to scale. Place stage micrometer on the microscope and using 16 mm objectives, draw a line equivalent to 1mm as seen through the microscope. Construct a square on this line. Move the paper so that the square is seen in the eye piece, in the centre of the field. Place the slide with the cleared leaf (epidermis on the stage). Trace off at least four epidermal cells using 4 mm objective. Then focus down and draw palisade cells beneath each epidermal cell. Count palisade cells under four epidermal cells including half of palisade cell within walls of epidermal cell. Calculate range as well as average number of palisade cells beneath each epidermal cell.

Observation/Calculations:

No. of Field	Readings
	Veinlet- termination
1	
2	
3	
4	
5	
6	
7	
8	
9	
10	
Average	
Range	

Results: Palisade ratio determined for given sample of crude drug ....and found as follows:

Name of leaf crude drug	
Calculated Palisade ratio	
Standard value mentioned Pharmacopoeia or published research paper for **Indian senna (Cassia angustifolia)**	**Upper epidermis: 7.5-9.5** **Lower epidermis- 5.1-7.0**
Remark (Authentic or adulterated sample of crude drug)	

Questions

1. What is Palisade ratio?
2. What are key steps in determination of Palisade ratio?
3. What is significance of Palisade ratio determination?

Aim 06: To determine percentage purity by *Lycopodium* spore method.

Requirements: Microscope, slides, brush, glycerin, water, weighing balance, Lycopodium spores, crude drug sample containing starch grains like ginger

Theory: *Lycopodium* is composed of the spores of *Lycopodium clavatum* L. Lycopodium is a genus of club mosses, also known as ground pines or creeping cedar, in the family Lycopodiaceae. Each spore of *Lycopodium* is tetrahedral in shape, the base is rounded and the three flat sides meet to form three well-marked covering ridges, which join one another at the apex. The whole surface of the spore is covered with minute reticulations and the interior is filled with fixed oil. The spores are exceptionally uniform in size (25μm) and 1 mg always contains an average of 94000 spores. If any crude drug powder contains characteristic particles of uniform size and shape like starch grains, pollen grains, trichomes, calcium crystals, fibers, cells then the number of characteristic particles per unit weight is often constant and is useful in assessing the quality of a sample.

$$\text{Percentage Purity} = \frac{N \times W \times 940000}{S \times M \times P} \times 100$$

where,

N   =   Number of characteristic particles of sample in 25 fields

W   =   Weight of Lycopodium spores taken in mg

S   =   Number of Lycopodium spores in 25 fields

M   =   Weight of sample in mg

P   =   Standard value of number of characteristic samples per mg in taken sample material (e.g. 1 mg ginger powder contains 2,86,000 starch grains)

Note: Lycopodium spore method is useful for any type of crude drug while leaf constants determination is restricted only to leaf crude drugs.

Procedure: Take accurately weighed powder of sample drug as well as Lycopodium separately and mix it. Prepare smooth paste in any oil or glycerin: water mixture. Apply as a thin layer on glass slide. Observe and calculate characteristic particles from sample powder and spores from Lycopodium sample in 25 different fields. Add values in formula and calculate the percentage purity by mentioned formula.

Observation and Calculations:

S.No.	N = Number of characteristic particles of sample in 25 fields	S = Number of Lycopodium spores in 25 fields
1		
2		
3		
4		
5		
6		
7		

Contd...

S.No.	N = Number of characteristic particles of sample in 25 fields	S = Number of Lycopodium spores in 25 fields
8		
9		
10		
11		
12		
13		
14		
15		
16		
17		
18		
19		
20		
21		
22		
23		
24		
25		

Calculations: Percentage Purity $= \dfrac{N \times W \times 940000}{S \times M \times P} \times 100$

Results: Percentage purity of crude drugs………………………… **determined by** *Lycopodium* **spore method and found** ……………………………

It complies with standard value……………………………….. mentioned in Pharmacopoeia or published research paper.

Questions

1. What is Lycopodium spore method?
2. Why lycopodium spores are selected for development of this method?
3. What is significance of Lycopodium spore method in crude drug evaluation?
4. What are advantages of Lycopodium spore method over leaf constants?

Aim 07: To measure size of starch grain by eye piece micrometer in a given crude drug powder.

Requirement: Micrometers (Eyepiece and stage), Starch powder (preferable potato due to relatively big size starch grains), microscope, slides, brush, iodine solution

Theory: Starch is chemically polysacharide containing amylopectin and beta-amylose. Size, shape and dimensions of starch grains are useful as diagnostic features to identify adulteration and confirm purity. Most popular starch grains useful in study are:

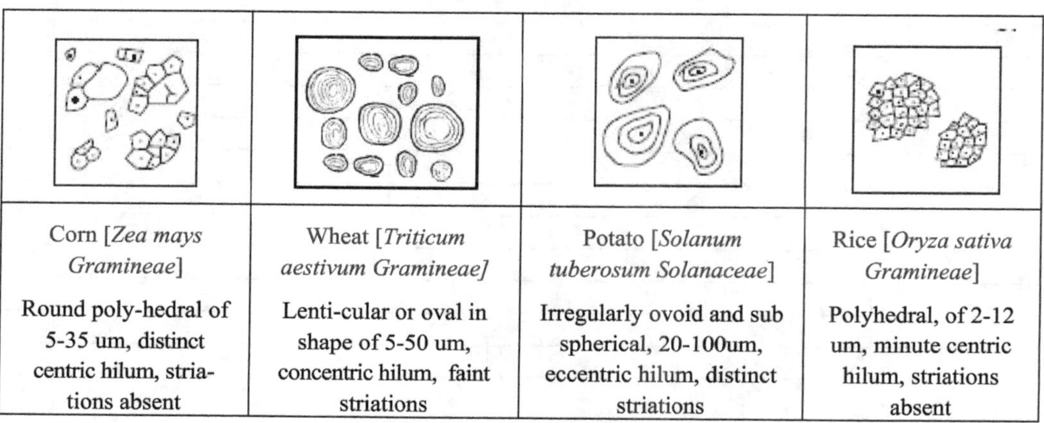

Corn [*Zea mays Gramineae*]	Wheat [*Triticum aestivum Gramineae]*	Potato [*Solanum tuberosum Solanaceae*]	Rice [*Oryza sativa Gramineae*]
Round poly-hedral of 5-35 um, distinct centric hilum, striations absent	Lenti-cular or oval in shape of 5-50 um, concentric hilum, faint striations	Irregularly ovoid and sub spherical, 20-100um, eccentric hilum, distinct striations	Polyhedral, of 2-12 um, minute centric hilum, striations absent

Micrometer is a device having a scale to measure dimensions of magnified microscopic characters. Micrometers are of two types: eyepiece micrometer and stage micrometer. Both micrometers have 1 mm scale etched on surface which is divided into 100 divisions and hence 1 division is equal to 10 microns. But as value of divisions of eyepiece micrometer varies with combination of eyepiece lenses due to different manufacturing brands of microscopes, hence it is a must to calibrate eyepiece micrometer by stage micrometer.

Step-1: Calibrate eyepiece micrometer by stage micrometer.

Procedure: Replace ocular lenses with eyepiece micrometer. Put stage micrometer on stage of microscope. Co-incide first line of '0' of stage micrometers with eyepiece mirometer. Then observe the next superimposed line. Now count divisions of eyepiece and stage micrometer between these two superimposed lines. Then convert divisions of stage micrometer in microns. Further calculate calibration factor of one division of eyepiece micrometer.

For example:

If 3 divisions of stage micrometer = 25 divisions of eyepiece micrometer

But 1 division of stage micrometer = 10 microns

And hence 3 divisions of stage micrometer = 30 microns

So 30 microns = 25 divisions of eyepiece micrometer

1 division of eyepiece micrometer = 25/30 = 0. 83 microns

Step-2: Measure dimensions of starch grain

Procedure: Calibrate eyepiece micrometer and calculate calibration factor. Take 2 mg powder and stain with iodine solution to differentiate starch grains. Spread the slurry as a thin layer over slide. Observe under microscope. Rotate the eyepiece micrometer and count divisions occupied by each starch grain. Repeat it for at least 25 grains. Multiply each value with the calibration factor. Now express the results in the form of range and average dimension of starch grains.

Observation and Calculations:

S.No.	Diameter of Starch grains	Calibration factor	Diameter after multiplication with Calibration factor
1			
2			
3			
4			
5			
6			
7			
8			
9			
10			
11			
12			
13			
14			
15			
16			
17			
18			
19			
20			
21			
22			
23			
24			
25			
Average value: Mean of 25 readings/25			

Results: The average value of starch grains of ……………is found ……………… and in range…………to…………..It complies with standard value…………………………….. mentioned in Pharmacopoeia or published research paper.

Questions

1. What is micrometer?
2. What are types of micrometer?
3. Why to calibrate eyepiece micrometer ?
4. What are uses of micrometry in Pharmacognosy ?
5. How to determine dimensions by micrometery?

Aim 08: To measure size of calcium crystals by eye piece micrometer in a given crude drug powder.

Requirement: Micrometers (Eyepiece and stage), Crude drug powder (preferable squill due to relatively big size crystals), microscope, slides, brush

Theory:

Micrometer is a device having a scale to measure dimensions of magnified microscopic characters. Micrometers are of two types: eyepiece micrometer and stage micrometer. Both micrometers have 1 mm scale etched on surface which is divided into 100 divisions and hence 1 division is equal to 10 microns. But as value of divisions of eyepiece micrometer varies with combination of eyepiece lenses due to different manufacturing brands of microscopes, hence it is a must to calibrate eyepiece micrometer by stage micrometer.

Calcium Crystals

Calcium crystals have great diagnostic value. Presence and absence of crystals, and their dimensions are useful in correct identification of crude drugs. This helps in detection of adulterants.

Calcium carbonate	These are rare and generally associated with cell wall. They are also called as "cystoliths" as they appear in the form of grapes in the tissues. Cystoliths have been seen in the leaves of the plants of Cucurbitaceae, Acanthaceae, Urticaceae, Cannabinaceae, Ulmaceae. Example: Cannabis leaf, Indian rubber plant leaf
Calcium oxalate	These crystals are very common and present in almost each part of plant. They are either tetragonal (using three water molecules and very rare in plants) or monoclinic (using one water molecules and common in plants).
	Prisms/single crystals: They are large, single or small groups and well developed. Cluster crystals/ spheraphides: They are group of numerous prisms/pyramids. The crystal are projecting, pointed, acute angled, and more or less spherical. Rosette crystals: They are large number of crystals in spherical mass (in the centre of which is an organic substance). Components of crystals radiate from the centre to the periphery and form a toothed circumference. Acicular crystals/ raphids: They are needle like, slender, long pointed at the ends. They may be single or in bundles. Microcrystal/ crystal sand / micro sphenoid: They occur like an amorphous mass in cell. They are very minute and are present in large number in a single cell which is usually enlarged than other cells and is called idioblast. (a) Prismatic crystal; (b) Rosette crystal; (c) Acicular crystal

Table 8.1 Presence of Calcium crystals in crude drugs

Crude drug	Type of calcium crystals
Asparagus, aloe, Centella, Clove flower bud, Digitallis, Digitallis lanata, Ephedra, Ginger, Isapgol, Nuxvomica, Quassia	Absent
Azadircata, Senna, Rhubarb, Clove stalk, Wild cherry bark, Tinosperma	Prism and cluster
Bacopa, Rauwolfia, Vasaka, Liquorice	Prism

Contd...

Crude drug	Type of calcium crystals
Caraway	Rosette
Cassia, cinnamon, gentian	Acicular
Cinchona	Microprism
Cinnamon	Tubular
Coriander, Dill, Fennel	Microrosette
Datura	Spherophide crystals
Eucalyptus, Podophyllum	Clusters
Gentian	Needle shaped
Ipecac, Squill	Raphides
Kurchi	Rhomboidal
Vinca	Microtubular, tactoid or needle shaped
Withania, Cinchona, Belladonna	Microsphenoid

Crude Drug	Calcium crystal length	Starch grain
Licorice	25-35 µ	10-20 µ
Squill	20 – 150 to 900 µ	2-4 µ

Step-1: Calibrate eyepiece micrometer by stage micrometer.

Procedure: Replace ocular lenses with eyepiece micrometer. Put stage micrometer on stage of microscope. Co-incide first line of '0' of stage micrometers with eyepiece mirometer. Then observe the next superimposed line. Now count divisions of eyepiece and stage micrometer between these two superimposed lines. Then convert divisions of stage micrometer in microns. Further calculate calibration factor of one division of eyepiece micrometer.

For example:

If 3 divisions of stage micrometer = 25 divisions of eyepiece micrometer

But 1 division of stage micrometer = 10 microns

And hence 3 divisions of stage micrometer = 30 microns

So 30 microns = 25 divisions of eyepiece micrometer

1 division of eyepiece micrometer = 25/30 = 0. 83 microns

Step-2: Measure dimensions of starch grain in a given crude drug powder

Procedure: Calibrate eyepiece micrometer and calculate calibration factor. Take 2 mg powder and observe under dark to differentiate calcium crystals. Spread the slurry as a thin layer over slide. Observe under microscope. Rotate the eyepiece micrometer and count divisions occupied by each calcium crystals. Repeat it for at least 25 grains. Multiply each value with the calibration factor. Now express the results in the form of range and average length of calcium crystals.

Observation and Calculations:

S.No.	Diameter of calcium crystals	Calibration factor	Length after multiplication with Calibration factor
1			
2			
3			
4			
5			
6			
7			
8			
9			
10			
11			
12			
13			
14			
15			
16			
17			
18			
19			
20			
21			
22			
23			
24			
25			
Average value: Mean of 25 readings/25			

Results: The average value of calcium crystals of ……………is found ……………… and in range…………to…………..

It complies with standard value…………………………….. mentioned in Pharmacopoeia or published research paper.

Questions

1. What is micrometer?

2. What are types of micrometer?

3. Why to calibrate eyepiece micrometer ?

4. What are types of calcium crystals?

5. How calcium crystals plays important role in evaluation of crude drugs?

Aim 09: To measure length of phloem fibers in given crude drug powder.

Requirement: Micrometers (Eyepiece and stage), microscope, slides, brush, crude drug sample containing abundant phloem fibers like licorice, cinchona

Theory: Presence, absence, size and shape of phloem fibers is important diagnostic tool in quality control of crude drugs especially roots, rhizomes and bark.

Procedure: Calibrate eyepiece micrometer and calculate calibration factor. Take 2 mg powder and stain with Phloroglucinol-HCl. Spread the slurry as a thin layer over slide. Observe under microscope. Rotate the eyepiece micrometer and count divisions occupied by each fiber. Repeat it for at least 25 fibers. Multiply each value with the calibration factor. Now express results in the form of range and average length of fiber. Similarly width can be calculated.

Observation and Calculations:

S.No.	Length of phloem fibers	Calibration factor	Length of phloem fibers after multiplication with Calibration factor
1			
2			
3			
4			
5			
6			
7			
8			
9			
10			
11			
12			
13			
14			
15			
16			
17			
18			
19			
20			
21			
22			
23			
24			
25			
Average value: Mean of 25 readings/25			

Results: The average value of starch grains of ……………is found ……………… and in range…………to………….. It complies with standard value………………………………….. mentioned in Pharmacopoeia or published research paper.

Questions

1. What is micrometer?

2. What are types of micrometer?

3. Why to calibrate eyepiece micrometer ?

4. How phloem fiber plays important role in evaluation of crude drugs?

Aim 10: To determine different ash values as per IP

Requirement: Incinerator (Muffle furnace), Silica crucible, weighing balance, ashless filter paper, funnel, filtration assembly, hydrochloric acid (HCl), water

Theory: An ash value indicates total inorganic matter present in crude drug which always remains constant and hence considered as important diagnostic parameter in determination of purity and correct identity of crude drugs. Many times additional inorganic foreign matter content is naturally adhering or added unintentionally either in collection and or preparation of drug for market or during storage. But sometimes it is added deliberately as a practice of adulteration. While preparing ash, it is necessary to remove all traces of black organic material inferring in an analysis of total inorganic elements.

Ash value is defined as the residue remains after incineration which can be sand, silica, soil, calcium crystals, and or elements. There are following types of ash values need to be determined as per guidelines given in many pharmacopoeias:

1. Total Ash value

This method is designed to measure the total amount of material remaining after ignition. It includes both physiological ash and non-physiological ash. The physiological ash is derived from plant tissue itself and non - physiological ash is residue of extraneous matter (ex. Sand and Soil) adhering to plant surface. Total ash usually consists of carbonates, phosphates, silicates and silica.

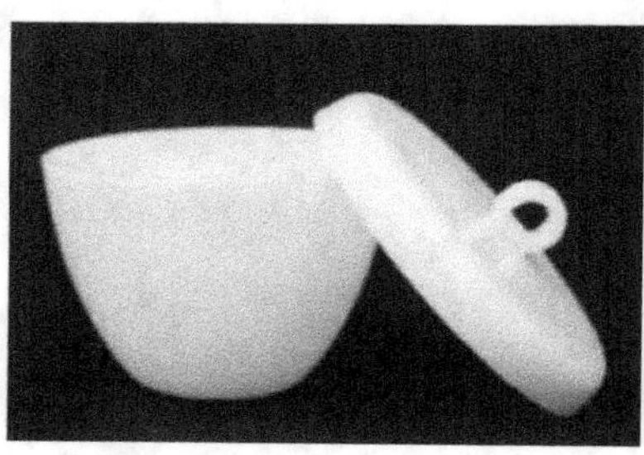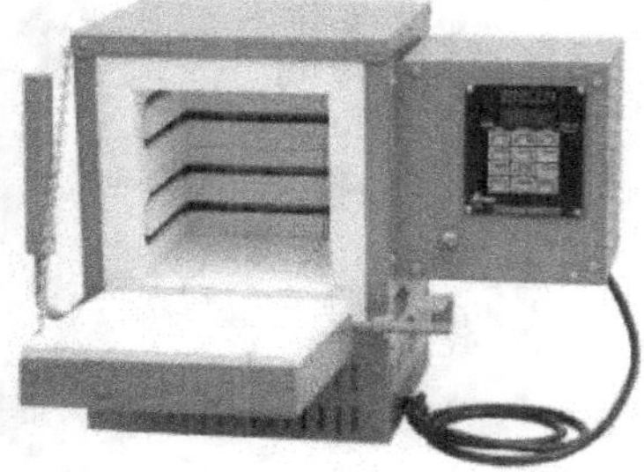

Procedure: Weigh accurately 2gm of air-dried powdered drug and take in tarred platinum crucible. Spread the drug material in affine even layer at bottom of the platinum crucible. Keep this platinum crucible with a drug material in muffle furnace for ignition at high temperature up to 450^0C only for 6 hours.

Continue ignition till to obtain complete white ash. Weigh intermittently till constant weight of crucible. Now take out crucible from furnace; cool and weigh.

Calculate the total ash by subtracting the weight of crucible with ash of drug after ignition from weight of crucible with a drug powder before ignition. Percentage of total ash is calculated with reference to air-dried drug.

2. Acid insoluble ash value

Acid insoluble ash is actually part of total ash insoluble in dilute hydrochloric acid. Acid insoluble ash indicates adhering dirt, sand as well as variation caused by calcium oxalate.

Procedure: Take weighed total ash and boil with 25 ml 2N HCl solution for 5 minute. Cool and filter insoluble matter on ash less filter paper and wash with hot water. Ignite residue and weigh. Calculate percentage of acid insoluble ash with reference to air-dried material.

3. Water soluble ash value

The water extract of crude drugs possesses various biological activities and hence it is possible that water extracted means exhausted powder may be used as adulterant for original drug. Therefore water-soluble ash value can be quite reliable parameter which should be investigated to judge such type of adulteration

Procedure: Take weighed total ash and boil with 25 ml water for 5 minute. Collect insoluble matter on ash less filter paper and wash with hot water and further ignite for 15 minute at the temperature not exceeding 450^0C.

Calculate the percentage of water soluble ash by subtracting weight of insoluble matter from weight of total ash.

This difference between weights represents water soluble ash. Percentage of water soluble ash is calculated with reference to air dried drug.

Calculations:

Total Ash value	➤ Weight of sample crude drug powder : 2 gm ➤ Weight of Total Ash: ➤ Percentage of total Ash value: Weight of total ash*100/Weight of sample
Acid insoluble ash	➤ Weight of Insoluble matter : ➤ Percentage of Acid insoluble ash: Weight of Insoluble matter*100/Weight of sample
Water soluble ash value	➤ Weight of sample total Ash: ➤ Weight of Insoluble matter: ➤ Weight of Acid insoluble ash = Weight of sample total Ash- Weight of Insoluble matter ➤ Percentage of Acid insoluble ash: Weight of Acid insoluble ash *100/Weight of sample

Results: Ash value are determined for given sample of crude drug ....and found as follows:

Type of Ash value	Percentage found	Percentage reported in Pharmacopoeia or Research papers	Complies (Yes/No)
Total Ash value			
Acid insoluble ash			
Water soluble ash value			

Questions

1. What is Ash value?

2. What are types of Ash value?

3. What is significance of Ash value determination?

4. Why to determine ash value of crude drugs?

5. What are possible contents of water soluble ash?

6. What are possible components of Acid insoluble ash?

Aim 11: To determine different extractive values as per IP

Requirement: Glass stoppered conical flask, Water bath, weighing balance, filter paper, funnel, filtration assembly, water, alcohol, Solvent ether

Theory:: Extractive values are measure total soluble chemical constituents in specific solvents from crude drug which always remain constant and hence can be used standard for correct identity, evaluation, quality control and in determination of purity.

Procedure:

According to many pharmacopoeias, generally three extractive values need to be determined i.e. ether, alcohol and water which actually refers to soluble non-polar, semi-polar and polar constitutes respectively. Following are different types of extractive values:

1. **Water soluble extractive value**

   Water soluble extractive value represents number of polar active constituent of crude drug, such as sugars, tannins, glycosides, specific alkaloids and or flavonoids etc.

   Procedure: Take 5 gm of powdered crude drug in the glass stopered conical flask and macerate with 25 ml of distilled water (containing 5% chloroform to avoid microbial growth) for 6 hours with frequent shaking, and then allow standing for 18 hours. After completion of 18 hours, filter the contents of flask and transfer the filtrate in the tarred flat bottom porcelain dish. Then evaporate the filtrate to dryness on water bath at 105°C for 6 hours. Cool in dessicator for 30 min and weigh. Calculate percentage content of extractable matter by water in milligrams per gram of air-dried material.

2. **Alcohol soluble extractive value**

   Alcohol is very preferred solvent to extract various natural chemicals constituents like sugars, tannins, oils, glycosides, resins, phenolics and few alkaloids etc. Therefore this extractive value is frequently employed to determine semi-polar content of crude drug.

   Procedure: Take 5 gm of powdered crude drug in the glass stopered conical flask and macerate with 25 ml of 95 % alcohol for 6 hours with frequent shaking, and then allow standing for 18 hours. After completion of 18 hours, filter the contents of flask and transfer the filtrate in the tarred flat bottom porcelain dish. Then evaporate the filtrate to dryness on water bath at 105°C for 6 hours. Cool in dessicator for 30 min and weigh. Calculate percentage content of extractable matter by alcohol in milligrams per gram of air-dried material.

3. **Ether soluble extractive value**

   This ether soluble extractive value represents both non-polar volatile and non volatile ether soluble constituents like steroids, resins, lipids, pigments, aglycone moieties and few alkaloids and phenolic constituents.

   Procedure: Take 5 gm of powdered crude drug in the glass stopered conical flask and macerate with 25 ml of ether for 6 hours with frequent shaking, and then allow standing for 18 hours. After completion of 18 hours, filter the contents of flask and transfer the filtrate in the tarred flat bottom porcelain dish. Then evaporate the filtrate to dryness on water bath at

105°C for 6 hours. Cool in dessicator for 30 min and weigh. Calculate percentage content of extractable matter by ether in milligrams per gram of air-dried material.

Observations/Calculations:

Extractive values	Calculations
Water soluble	Weight of sample crude drug powder : Weight of dried extract: Percentage of Water soluble extractive value : Weight of dried extract × 100/Weight of sample
Alcohol soluble	Weight of sample crude drug powder : Weight of dried extract: Percentage of Alcohol soluble extractive value: Weight of dried extract × 100/Weight of sample
Ether soluble	Weight of sample crude drug powder : Weight of dried extract: Percentage of Ether soluble extractive value: Weight of dried extract × 100/Weight of sample

Results: Extractive values are determined for given sample of crude drug (Common name/ Biological source)..and found as follows:

Type of Extractive values	Percentage found	Percentage reported in Pharmacopoeia or Research papers	Complies (Yes/No)
Water soluble			
Alcohol soluble			
Ether soluble			

Questions

1.   What is Extractive value?

2.   What are types of Extractive value?

3.   What is significance of Extractive value determination?

4.   Why to determine Extractive value of crude drugs?

5.   Which phytochemical can be present in Water Extractive value?

6.   Which phytochemical can be present in Alcohol Extractive value?

7.   Which phytochemical can be present in ether extractive value?

Aim 12: To determine moisture content by Loss on Drying (LOD) method

Requirement: Hot air oven, desiccator, weighing bottle, weighing balance, weighing paper, crude drug sample powder

Theory: Loss on drying (LOD) means the weight loss due to hygroscopic moisture and volatile substances determined in a substance after it is dried to a constant weight or for the period of time specified in the Pharmacopoeia. It is the loss of mass on drying expressed as percent w/w. The moisture content was considered essential to determine because the presence of moisture affects the proportion of active compounds from formulation. Also excess moisture present in the formulation may facilitate the growth of microbes.

Procedure:

Method 1 (For thermostable substance)

Take 2g quantity of the sample and place in the previously dried weighing bottle. Dry the sample in an oven at a temperature 105°C until the constant mass of the substance is obtained.

Method 2 (For thermolabile substance)

Take 2g quantity of the sample and place in the previously dried weighing bottle. Dry the sample in an desiccator over phosphorus (V) oxide at atmospheric pressure and room temperature (or in a vacuum, at room temperature or the temperature specified in the Pharmacopoeia) until the constant weight of the substance is obtained.

Observations/Calculations:

➢ Weight of sample crude drug powder:

➢ Weight after drying to constant weight:

➢ Loss on drying (LOD): Weight of sample crude drug powder - Weight after drying to constant weight

➢ Percentage of moisture : Loss on drying (LOD) × 100/Weight of sample

Results: Moisture content determined for given sample of crude drug (Common name/Biological source)...and found as follows:

Parameter	Percentage found	Percentage reported in Pharmacopoeia or Research papers	Complies (Yes/No)
Percentage of moisture content			

Questions

1. What are different methods of determination of moisture content?
2. What is significance of moisture content determination?
3. Why to determine moisture content of crude drugs?
4. Which is most sensitive method of moisture content determination?

Aim 13: To Determine Swelling Index of a given Crude Drug-Isapgol

Requirement: 25 ml glass stoppered measuring cylinder (length-125mm, internal diameter about 16 mm subdivided in 0.2 ml and marked from 0 to 25 ml), mucilage containing crude drug sample

Theory: This test is very useful for materials with swelling properties, especially gums and mucilage, pectin and hemicelluloses. The swelling index is the volume in ml taken up by the swelling of 1g of plant material under specified conditions.

Isapgol consists of dried seed and dried seed coats of plant known as *Plantago ovata*. Family: Plantaginaceae. Swelling index of ispaghula seeds is 10–13.

Procedure

1. Introduce the quantity of the individual plant material, previously reduced to the required fitness and accurately weighed into a 25 ml glass stoppered measuring cylinder. The length of the graduated portion of cylinder should be 125mm and internal diameter about 16 mm subdivided in 0.2 ml and marked from 0 to 25 ml in an upward direction.

2. Take 1 gm of plant material. Add 25 ml of water unless otherwise indicated in the test procedure and shake the mixture thoroughly at intervals of every 10 min for 1 hour. Allow to stand for 3 hours at room temperature or as otherwise given. Measure the volume in ml occupied by the plant material, including any sticky mucilage. Calculate the mean value of the individual determinations related to 1g of plant material.

Observations/Calculations:

➤ Weight of sample crude drug powder (gram): One gram

➤ Volume in occupied by the plant material (ml):

➤ Swelling Index: Average of three readings of Volume in occupied by the plant material (ml)

Results: Swelling index determined for given sample of crude drug (Common name/Biological source)..and found as follows:

Parameter	Value obtained	Value reported in Pharmacopoeia or Research papers	Complies (Yes/No)
Swelling index			

Questions

1. What is swelling index?

2. What is significance of swelling index determination?

3. Why to determine swelling index of crude drugs?

4. Which type of crude drugs should be evaluated for swelling index?

5. Is swelling index need to determined for every crude drug?

Aim 14: To Determine Foaming Index of Saponin containing Crude Drug-Licorice

Requirement: Saponin containing crude drug powder, 100 ml volumetric flask, water bath, stoppered test tubes, scale

Theory: This test is to measure the foaming ability of an aqueous decoction of saponin containing medicinal plant materials which possesses property to form persistent foam when an aqueous decoction is shaken.

Procedure

1. Prepare aqueous decoction of about 1g of coarse powder plant material in 100 ml water by boiling for 30 min.

2. Cool and filter into a 100 ml volumetric flask and add sufficient water to make up the volume to 100 ml.

3. Now prepare 10 stoppered test tubes (height-16cm and diameter-16 mm) in a series containing successive portions of above decoction 1, 2, 3, up to 10 ml and adjust the volume of the liquid in each tube with water to 10 ml.

4. Stopper the tubes and shake them in a lengthwise motion for 15 sec, 2 frequencies per second. Allow to stand for 15 min and measure the height of the foam.

5. If the height of the foam in every tube is less than 1 cm, the foaming index is less than 100.

6. If height of foam is more than 1cm in every test tube, the foaming index is over 1000. In this case, the determination needs to be made on a new series of dilutions of the decoction in order to obtain results.

7. If in any tube a height of foam of 1cm is observed, the dilution of the plant material in this tube is the index sought.

8. If this tube is the first or second tube in a series, it is necessary to have an intermediate dilution prepared in a similar manner to obtain more precise results.

Formula for foaming index: 1000/A where A= volume of decoction having exact 1 cm height

Observations/Calculations:

➢ A= volume of decoction having exact 1 cm height : -------------

➢ Foaming index: 1000/A

Results: Foaming index determined for given sample of crude drug (Common name/Biological source)...and found as follows:

Parameter	Percentage found	Percentage reported in Pharmacopoeia or Research papers	Complies (Yes/No)
Foaming index			

Questions

1. What is foaming index?
2. What is significance of foaming index determination?
3. Why to determine foaming index of crude drugs?
4. Which type of crude drugs should be evaluated for foaming index?
5. Is foaming index need to determine for every crude drug?

Aim 15: To Determine Foaming Index of Saponin containing Crude Drug- Safed musali

Requirement: Saponin containing crude drug powder, 100 ml volumetric flask, water bath, stoppered test tubes, scale

Theory: This test is to measure the foaming ability of an aqueous decoction of saponin containing medicinal plant materials which possesses property to form persistent foam when an aqueous decoction is shaken.

Procedure

1. Prepare aqueous decoction of about 1g of coarse powder plant material in 100 ml water by boiling for 30 min.

2. Cool and filter into a 100 ml volumetric flask and add sufficient water to make up the volume to 100 ml.

3. Now prepare 10 stoppered test tubes (height-16cm and diameter-16 mm) in a series containing successive portions of above decoction 1, 2, 3, up to 10 ml and adjust the volume of the liquid in each tube with water to 10 ml.

4. Stopper the tubes and shake them in a lengthwise motion for 15 sec, 2 frequencies per second. Allow to stand for 15 min and measure the height of the foam.

5. If the height of the foam in every tube is less than 1 cm, the foaming index is less than 100.

6. If height of foam is more than 1cm in every test tube, the foaming index is over 1000. In this case, the determination needs to be made on a new series of dilutions of the decoction in order to obtain results.

7. If in any tube a height of foam of 1cm is observed, the dilution of the plant material in this tube is the index sought.

8. If this tube is the first or second tube in a series, it is necessary to have an intermediate dilution prepared in a similar manner to obtain more precise results.

Formula for foaming index: 1000/A where A= volume of decoction having exact 1 cm height

Observations/Calculations:

➢ A= volume of decoction having exact 1 cm height : -------------
➢ Foaming index: 1000/A

Results: Foaming index determined for given sample of crude drug (Common name/Biological source)...and found as follows:

Parameter	Percentage found	Percentage reported in Pharmacopoeia or Research papers	Complies (Yes/No)
Foaming index			

Questions

1. What is foaming index?
2. What is significance of foaming index determination?
3. Why to determine foaming index of crude drugs?
4. Which type of crude drugs should be evaluated for foaming index?
5. Is foaming index need to determine for every crude drug?

Further Reading

1. A.N.M. Alamgir. Therapeutic Use of Medicinal Plants and Their Extracts: Volume 1

2. Alice Kurian, M. Asha Sankar Medicinal Plants. New India Publishing Agency. 2007

3. Anjoo Kamboj, Moronkola Dorcas Olufunke Practical Pharmacognosy. Scitus Academics LLC. Thomas Edward Wallis. Practical Pharmacognosy. Churchill. 2018

4. Ashutosh Kar. Pharmacognosy And Pharmacobiotechnology. New Age International (P) Limited. 2003

5. Biren Shah, Avinash Seth. Textbook of Pharmacognosy and Phytochemistry. Elsevier Health Sciences. 2014

6. C. S. Shah, J. S. Qadry. A Textbook of Pharmacognosy. Messrs B.S. Shah 1971

7. C.K. Kokate, Purohit, Gokhlae. Text book of Pharmacognosy, 37th Edition, Nirali Prakashan, Pune. 2007

8. Christophe Wiart, Ashok Kumar. Practical Handbook of Pharmacognosy-Preliminary Techniques of Identification of Crude Drugs of Plant Origin. 2000

9. Deore SL. Pharmacognosy and Phytochemistry: A Companion Handbook. PharmMed Press, Hyderabad. . 2nd Edition, 2017.

10. Deore SL, Khadabadi SS, Baviskar BA. Pharmacognosy and Phytochemistry-A Comprehensive Approach. PharmMed Press, Hyderabad. 2nd Edition, 2018.

11. GS Kumar. KN Jayaveera. A Textbook of Pharmacognosy and Phytochemistry. S CHAND & Company Limited. India. 2014.

12. Gunnar Samuelsson. Drugs of Natural Origin-A Textbook of Pharmacognosy. Apotekarsocieteten. 1999

13. H. Ansari. Essentials of Pharmacognosy. Second edition, Birla publications, New Delhi, 2007

14. James Bobbers, Marilyn KS, VE Tylor. Pharmacognosy & Pharmacobiotechnology. Williams & Wilkins. 1996.

15. Jean Bruneton. Pharmacognosy, Phytochemistry, Medicinal Plants. Technique & Documentation. 1999

16. Joshi Saroja, Vidhu Aeri. Practical Pharmacognosy. Frank Brothers. 2009.

17. Khadabadi SS, Deore SL, Baviskar BA. Experimental Phytopharmacognosy. Nirali prakashan, Pune. 1st Edition, 2019.

18. K. Mangathayaru. Pharmacognosy: An Indian perspective. Pearson Education India. 2013

19. K. R. Khandelwal. Practical Pharmacognosy. Nirali Prakashan, Pune. 2008

20. Kaliya.A. Text Book of Industrial Pharmacognosy. CBS Publishers & Distributors, Delhi. 2009

21. Kendall Jefferson. Pharmacognosy and Phytotherapy. Foster Academics.2019

22. Kokate CK. Practical Pharmacognosy. Vallabh Prakashan, Delhi. 2005

23. Luqi Huang. Molecular Pharmacognosy. Springer Netherlands. 2012

24. M A Iyengar, S G K Nayak. Pharmacognosy Lab Manual. PharmaMed Press. 2019

25. M A Iyengar. Pharmacognosy of Powdered Crude Drugs. PharmaMed Press. 2017

26. M A Iyengar. Study of Crude Drugs. PharmaMed Press. 2016

27. Michael Heinrich, Elizabeth M. Williamson, Joanne Barnes, Simon Gibbons, Jose Prieto-Garcia Fundamentals of Pharmacognosy and Phytotherapy E-Book. Elsevier Health Sciences. 2017

28. Michael Heinrich, Joanne Barnes, Simon Gibbons. Fundamentals of Pharmacognosy and Phytotherapy. Churchill Livingstone/Elsevier. 2012

29. Mohammad Ali. Pharmacognosy and Phytochemistry, CBS Publishers & Distribution, New Delhi.

30. N P S Sengar, Ashwini Singh, Ritesh Agrawal. A Textbook of Pharmacognosy. PharmaMed Press. 2018

31. Nilambari S. Gurav, Shailendra S. Gurav Indian Herbal Drug Microscopy. Springer New York. 2013

32. Rangari VD. Pharmacognosy& Phytochemistry. Career Publication, Nashik. 2008

33. S. S. Agarwal, M. Paridhavi. Herbal Drug Technology. Universities Press. 2012

34. S. S. Handa. Pharmacognosy. Vallabh Prakashan, New Delhi. 1989

35. Saikat Sen, Raja Chakraborty Herbal Medicine in India-Indigenous Knowledge, Practice, Innovation and Its Value. Springer Singapore. 2019

36. Simone Badal Mccreath. Rupika Delgoda. Pharmacognosy-Fundamentals, Applications and Strategies. Elsevier Science. 2017

37. Steven E. Ruzin. Plant Microtechnique and Microscopy.1999

38. T. C. Denston. A Textbook of Pharmacognosy. Read Books. 2012

39. Vidhu Aeri, D.B. Anantha Narayana, Dharya Singh. Powdered Crude Drug Microscopy of Leaves and Barks. Elsevier Science. 2019

40. W.C.Evans, Trease and Evans Pharmacognosy, 16th edition, W.B. Sounders & Co., London, 2009.

41. The British Pharmacopeia. London: Medicines and Healthcare Products Regulatory Agency; 1993.

42. Indian Pharmacopeia 2018, Ghaziabad: Indian Pharmacopeia Commission; 2018.

43. United States Pharmacopoeia and National Formulary, USP 25 NF 19/National Formulary 20, Rockville, MD, U. S. Pharmacopoeial Convention, Inc. 2002.

44. Ayurvedic pharmacopoeia of India Part-I vol.I, 2001.